Veal Picatta, Curried Beef, Lemon Chicken, Broiled Stuffed Mushrooms, Pesto, Fresh Vegetable Souffle, Dessert Crepes with Fruit, Chili Con Carne, Zucchini Muffins, Citrus Salad . . .

You'll find recipes for these and many other palate-pleasing meals in this indispensable cookbook. For culinary variety, medical reliability, and practicality, THE ALL-IN-ONE DIABETIC COOKBOOK is a bonanza for anyone concerned with the well-being and dining pleasure of a diabetic. Each recipe has been carefully tested at home by out-patients of the famous Mayo Clinic. The whole family will enjoy these wonderful, nutritionally sound dishes.

"Skillfully explores the latest innovations in diabetes treatment."—*Publishers Weekly*

"Finally, a cookbook for those with diabetes . . . meets a long-standing need."—*Asbury Park Press*

P.J. PALUMBO, M.D., F.A.C.P., is Consultant in Internal Medicine, Division of Endocrinology and Metabolism, at the Mayo Clinic and Mayo Foundation in Rochester, Minnesota, as well as Professor of Medicine and Vice-Chairman for Education, Department of Internal Medicine, Mayo Medical School. JOYCE DALY MARGIE, M.S., is former Research Nutritionist at the Mayo Cinic.

THE ALL-IN-ONE DIABETIC COOKBOOK

P. J. PALUMBO, M.D., F.A.C.P.
AND
JOYCE DALY MARGIE, M.S.

With Recipes for Young Cooks by Paul Margie

A PLUME BOOK

PLUME
Published by the Penguin Group
Penguin Books USA Inc., 375 Hudson Street, New York, New York 10014, U.S.A.
Penguin Books Ltd, 27 Wrights Lane, London W8 5TZ, England
Penguin Books Australia Ltd, Ringwood, Victoria, Australia
Penguin Books Canada Ltd, 10 Alcorn Avenue, Toronto, Ontario, Canada, M4V 3B2
Penguin Books (N.Z.) Ltd, 182–190 Wairau Road, Auckland 10, New Zealand

Penguin Books Ltd, Registered Offices: Harmondsworth, Middlesex, England

Published by Plume, an imprint of Dutton Signet, a division of Penguin Books USA Inc. This book was formerly titled *The Complete Diabetic Cookbook* and published in a hardcover edition by New American Library and simultaneously in Canada by The New American Library of Canada Limited (now Penguin Books Canada Limited).

First Plume Printing, March 1989
30 29 28 27 26 25 24 23 22 21 20

LIBRARY OF CONGRESS CATALOGING IN PUBLICATION DATA:

Palumbo, P. J.
The all-in-one diabetic cookbook.

1. Diabetes—Diet therapy—Recipes. I. Margie, Joyce Daly. II. Title.
RC622.P35 1987 641.5'6314 86-23457
ISBN 0-452-26467-7

Printed in the United States of America
Original hardcover design by Marilyn Ackerman

Note to the Reader
The ideas, procedures, and suggestions contained in this book are not intended as a substitute for consulting with your physician. All matters regarding your health require medical supervision.

ACKNOWLEDGMENTS

All nutrient analysis was done at the Ohio State University. Information on their continually updated data base is available from:

Dianne Clapp, M.S., R.D.
Department of Dietetics
Ohio State University Hospital
410 West 10th Avenue
Columbus, Ohio 43210

Jill Metcalfe, who has had extensive experience with diabetics and who now is working for the British Diabetes Association, reviewed the manuscript.

Peggy Thielen Schreck, M.S., R.D., Consultant Nutritionist, Summit, New Jersey, was responsible for coding the recipes for nutritional analysis and for determining the appropriate food group exchanges for each recipe.

The dietitians at the Mayo Clinic, Saint Marys Hospital, and Rochester Methodist Hospital in Rochester, Minnesota, contributed suggestions, guidance, and recipes. Virginia Anderson, B.S., R.D., was particularly helpful.

Margaret Powers, M.S., R.D., and Harold Haller, R.D., of the Diabetes Care and Education Practice Group of the American Dietetic Association contributed guidance and suggestions, particularly concerning the revised food exchange lists.

All recipes were home-tested. The recipes in the children's section of the book were also tested by Andrew Margie and Barbara Fleissner.

FOREWORD

The All-in-One Diabetic Cookbook meets a long-standing need. It incorporates all points of today's dietary strategies for the treatment of both non-insulin-dependent diabetes mellitus and insulin-dependent diabetes mellitus.

The book contains over 400 tested recipes with nutrient analyses in terms of caloric value, food exchanges, and protein, carbohydrate, fat, sodium, and cholesterol contents. Recipe categories include appetizers, soups, salads, first courses, main courses, meats, breads, combination dishes, and desserts. Ideas for breakfast, lunch, supper, and snacks are given.

Paul Margie, a teenager himself, wrote the section "Recipes for Young Cooks," including an explanation of terms, kitchen safety rules, how to measure ingredients, and meal preparation techniques. Encouraging young diabetics to prepare food for themselves and for the family should be a very effective method of teaching principles of nutrition.

The book emphasizes the desirability of following a diet low in fat and cholesterol, high in complex carbohydrates and fiber (up to 25 grams per 1,000 calories), with a caloric content that produces weight loss in those with non-insulin-dependent diabetes mellitus, yet is sufficient to permit adequate weight gain and growth in children and in pregnant women. Techniques for helping the patient make a personal commitment to adhere to an appropriate diet and ways of reinforcing that commitment are highlighted.

Methods of measuring food at home, the content of foods served in fast-food restaurants, and advice for planning food intake during travel, on sick days, and in the presence of diabetic ketoacidosis and long-term complications are thoroughly described.

Dr. P. J. Palumbo and Joyce Daly Margie have integrated the material in the book in an extremely effective way, giving excellent descriptions of both types of diabetes, of symptoms and signs that the patient may note before diagnosis, and of how to establish the diagnosis of each type. Goals of treatment by a team (physician, dietitian, nurse, and patient) and how to coordinate their efforts to individualize education and therapy for the patient (*the most important team member*) are emphasized. Thus, the book contains essentially all of the information that a person would need to live successfully with diabetes.

Readers will also find a glossary of frequently used terms and lists of addresses of Diabetes Associations in the United States and Canada and the International Diabetes Federation.

—John K. Davidson, M.D., Ph.D.
Professor of Medicine (Endocrinology)
Department of Medicine
Emory University School of Medicine
and Director of the Diabetes Unit
Grady Memorial Hospital
Atlanta, Georgia

CONTENTS

(continued)

PART III
RECIPES FOR YOUNG COOKS 213

by Paul Margie

PART IV
UNDERSTANDING DIABETES 291

by P. J. Palumbo, M.D., F.A.C.P.

PART I

Good Nutrition for Diabetics

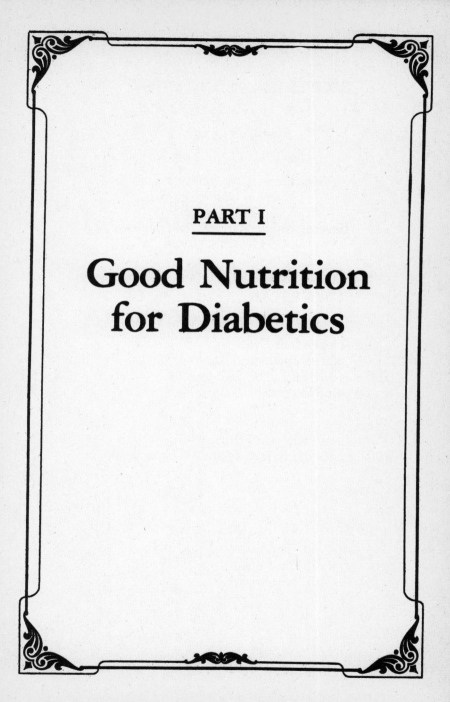

1

THE NEW DIABETIC DIET

In recent years there has been a major shift in the diet that doctors recommend for their diabetic patients. New scientific findings have led to new diet guidelines.

Today, the diabetic patient is instructed to follow a diet that is *low* in fat and cholesterol and *high* in fiber and complex carbohydrates. In addition, the diabetic is now permitted limited amounts of sugar and is discouraged from using artificial sweeteners.

These new guidelines are reflected in our recipes. Some are simple and some more sophisticated. All have been chosen so the *whole family* can enjoy the *same* meals. You should never again have to cook special, separate, uninteresting dishes for the diabetic member of the family.

For children, diabetes can be a special problem if following the diet means not eating the same foods that other children enjoy. Therefore, we have included a section specifically addressed to the medical and nutritional needs of diabetic children. This section was written by Paul Margie, a teenager himself. It contains easy-to-follow recipes for dishes favored by children.

Diabetes is not a short-term illness. It requires a lifetime of careful control if serious complications are to be avoided. Regardless of whether he or she is taking a drug, every diabetic must constantly control his or her diet. This book explains how to translate the diet treatment plan that your doctor has recommended into delicious recipes and easy cookery.

There are two ways your doctor and dietitian may work with you to implement your diet prescription. First, you may be taught how to use the ADA Exchange Lists to plan your daily meals. Second, you may be given instructions on how to use more specific carbohydrate, fat, and protein analyses. Both the exchanges and the key nutrient analyses have been provided with each recipe to assist you with whichever plan you are using.

We hope that you enjoy using our book and that it is helpful to you or the diabetic in your family.

THE DIET PRESCRIPTION

Diet control is the fundamental component of all programs of treatment for diabetes. For the majority of non-insulin-dependent diabetics, and particularly those who are obese, dietary management may be the only treatment necessary to control blood sugar levels. For insulin-dependent diabetics, eating and insulin dosages are closely related.

The physician actually writes a diet prescription for a diabetic patient. This prescription specifies the number of calories per day, the amounts of carbohydrate, protein, and fat to be eaten, and the distribution of these nutrients throughout the day. If you invest some time initially in learning about the diet prescription, you will be able to adapt it to almost any circumstance without disrupting the treatment program.

The physician considers numerous goals in developing a diet prescription. The main ones are:

- To provide an adequate calorie intake to promote growth in children.
- To maintain ideal body weight in lean adults or to decrease body weight in obese patients.
- To decrease breakdown of body fat (ketoacidosis) and body protein.
- To avoid hyperglycemia (high blood sugar level) and hypoglycemia (low blood sugar level).
- To control blood levels of cholesterol and triglycerides.

We discuss each of those goals in detail in a complete section called Understanding Diabetes (pages 291–315). There are two basic principles, however, that we want to emphasize as you begin to use our book. First, a diabetic patient's diet must be nutritious. It should be balanced with the right amounts of nutrients necessary to promote and to maintain good health. Calorie intake must be divided throughout the day in a way that will best avoid fluctuations in blood sugar levels. This division of calories and the number of calories consumed need tc be consistent from day to day. Second, the diet must be personal. It should be flexible and palatable so that it can be followed willingly. It also must be adaptable to changing situations—for example, among family and guests, when traveling, eating out or at a party, or during illness.

You are probably wondering how the basic recommended diet has changed in recent years. The changes can be summed up fairly easily. Previously, calories were made up by restricting carbohydrates and increasing the fat and protein contents. Sugar was strictly forbidden, and use of artificial sweeteners was encouraged. No attention was paid to the amounts of cholesterol and fiber in the diet. This chapter explains what the recommendations are and how they can help you or the diabetic in your family.

DISTRIBUTING THE CALORIES

The total number of calories consumed daily is the most fundamental element of the diabetic's diet prescription. For patients who are within 10 to 15 percent of their ideal weight, an allowance of 12 to 15 Calories per pound is usually adequate.

The calorie intake should be spread as evenly as possible throughout the day. Generally, three to six meals are recommended, depending on the specific treatment program. Diabetics who are being treated by diet alone usually need only three meals a day, unless a bedtime snack is a personal preference. Those taking an oral medication usually only need three meals a day, but a bedtime snack may be added to avoid a low blood sugar level during the night.

Most diabetics taking insulin require four to six meals a day, depending on the type and scheduling of the insulin doses. The timing of meals for the insulin-dependent diabetic is very important because carbohydrate intake needs to be timed to correspond to the circulating insulin level. If a meal is skipped or insufficient food is consumed, there will not be enough circulating sugar available and hypoglycemia can occur.

Each meal should be a mixture of carbohydrate, protein, and fat. Because of the way the timing of meals, the distribution of calories, and the type of food consumed affect the blood sugar and insulin levels, it is extremely important that an individualized meal plan be developed to meet each patient's particular needs. Once the meal plan is set up, it should be followed in as regular and consistent a manner as possible. Our recipes will make it easier for you to prepare tempting, irresistible meals and to monitor their calorie content.

BALANCING THE ESSENTIAL NUTRIENTS

The three basic nutrients—protein, fat, and carbohydrate—all supply calories. About 50 to 60 percent of the daily calorie intake should be in the form of carbohydrate. Of this amount of carbohydrate, 70 percent should be complex carbohydrate—whole grains, beans, pasta, rice, vegetables, and fruits. The remaining 40 to 50 percent of calories are divided between protein and fat. Usually, fat intake should contribute no more than 25 to 30 percent of the total calorie intake. For a patient with cardiovascular disease, the prescribed fat intake may be even lower. Protein content should be 12 to 20 percent of calories.

CARBOHYDRATES

Carbohydrates are the first nutrients considered in planning the diabetic's diet. There are two types of carbohydrates. Simple carbohydrates, such as sugar, are quickly absorbed into the body. Complex carbohydrates, such as starch, have a more complicated chemical structure and must be broken down (digested) before they can be absorbed. Therefore, they produce a later and a slower increase in the blood sugar level.

Concentrated simple carbohydrates are more readily absorbed when they are the only food eaten. Their absorption is slower when they are eaten as part of a mixed meal—one containing a mixture of carbohydrate, protein, and fat. This blunts the peaks in blood sugar levels after a meal. Fat and protein also tend to decrease the speed at which the stomach empties, which also decreases blood sugar peaks after meals. This effect of protein and fat makes it possible to include some concentrated simple carbohydrates in the diet, but *only* when they are consumed as part of a mixed meal. This action also makes it possible to include small amounts of concentrated carbohydrates, such as sugar, in recipes that also include protein and fat.

Recently, a way has been developed to measure how effective various carbohydrate foods are in raising the blood sugar level—this is called the glycemic index. Previously, it was believed that carbohydrates that had the same chemical structure had the same effect on the blood sugar level. Now it is known that carbohydrate consumed in liquid form (for example, as orange juice) is absorbed more rapidly than the same carbohydrate in solid form (for example, a whole fresh orange). The absorption of carbohydrate is also affected by the manner in which a food is processed and cooked. It was found that foods containing complex carbohydrates (starches) do not affect the blood sugar level in the same way. For example, bread, potato, and rice increase the blood sugar level more than bran, oatmeal, legumes, pasta, soybeans, peanuts, and ice cream do.

Because most people do not eat a meal consisting of only potatoes or rice, it is difficult to predict exactly what will happen as the result of a given meal. When a meal contains a mixture of nutrients, each nutrient influences the absorption of other nutrients contained in the meal.

SUGAR

Small amounts of concentrated carbohydrate, in the form of sugar, sweets, and desserts, can be part of the daily intake. This is not to say that diabetics can now eat anything and everything they want. Preferably, this refers to small amounts of sugar used in the preparation of foods that also incorporate protein and fat. This would include such things as breads, muffins, pancakes, waffles, and some low-calorie desserts.

Most artificial sweeteners, dietetic gelatin, and sugar-free beverages contain almost no calories and may be used in small amounts if the doctor approves. However, the controversy concerning the safety of the various artificial sweeteners continues, and we have chosen not to use them in this book. If you choose to use them, they should be used judiciously and only if your doctor agrees. Artificial sweeteners allow flexibility in meal planning and may be very helpful for the obese diabetic who must reduce calories. Be cautious in the selection of an artificial sweetener and discuss its proper use with the dietitian and the physician.

Likewise, "dietetic" foods designed for various modified diets—diabetic, low-salt, weight-reduction, low-lactose, etc.—should only be used cautiously. Many foods labeled "diet" or "dietetic" or "sugar-free" contain some form of sugar (sucrose, fructose, lactose, dextrose, sorbitol, or mannitol). Therefore, dietetic candy, cookies, chocolate, ice cream, jelly, jam, and syrup may still contain a significant number of calories and should not be used unless approved by a doctor or dietitian.

FOODS TO AVOID

Any food that contains a large amount of added sugar should be avoided, except in special circumstances or when it is incorporated into an approved recipe. This is because this kind of food causes a relatively rapid increase in the blood sugar level. The following foods should be avoided (an asterisk indicates that you will find acceptable recipes in our book):

Cake*
Candy
Chewing gum
Cookies*
Honey
Jam
Jelly
Marmalade
Molasses
Pastries*
Pies*
Pudding*
Sugar
Sweet rolls
Sweetened condensed milk
Sweetened soft drinks
Syrup

FIBER

Dietary fiber is defined as that part of plant foods that contains nondigestible and nonabsorbable carbohydrate. There are several general types of fibers. Each type has different physical properties and therefore produces a different effect when consumed. Some increase gastric bulk and decrease the time it takes the food to pass through the gastrointestinal tract. Others bind cholesterol and thereby lower the blood cholesterol level. High-fiber diets decrease calorie intake because they contribute to a feeling of fullness or satisfaction. A diet high in fiber content can decrease the insulin needs in some diabetics. The bulk provided by fiber slows down absorption of sugar without increasing calorie intake.

A food that is high in fiber usually is in its whole, natural state as opposed to being processed: for example, whole-grain products such as bran or oat cereal or whole wheat bread instead of refined products such as white bread; fresh, whole fruits with their skins instead of juices and canned fruits; vegetables, especially raw ones, instead of canned vegetables. Legumes, lentils, dried beans, barley, brown rice, kasha, cornmeal, and nuts and seeds also are excellent sources of fiber.

Products such as methyl cellulose, pectin, and guar can be incorporated into the diet to increase fiber content. Bran provides a good source of cellulose, and fruits provide a good source of pectin. Guar is a powder that can be used to thicken soups or to make gelatin desserts, bread, or cookies. (Guar tends to impart a thick and heavy texture to bread and cookies and therefore has to be used judiciously. Do not use guar or other such products without first obtaining the advice of a physician.)

The average intake of dietary fiber in North America is about 15 to 20 grams per day. A high-fiber diet contains approximately 25 grams of fiber (from natural foods or purified fiber) per 1,000 Calories daily.

Dietary fiber contributes to good bowel motility. However, too much may produce abdominal cramps and diarrhea. It is best to build up the amount of fiber in the diet gradually over a period of time. High-fiber diets may be inappropriate for those with gastric problems and in some elderly persons. Before greatly increasing the amount of fiber in your diet, check with your physician.

PROTEIN AND FAT

Protein is used by the body to build and to maintain the tissues. It also contributes calories to meet energy requirements. Good sources are meat, milk, fowl, fish, cheese, eggs, and legumes. It is now clear, however, that there is no benefit in having extra protein in the diet. Furthermore, many of the protein-containing foods contain saturated fat.

Saturated fats increase the blood cholesterol level. They are found primarily in foods of animal origin—meat and dairy products. Most physicians now recommend cutting down on saturated fat. The way to do that is to eat red meat no more than once a day, select lean cuts of meat, and trim away all visible fat. Skim and discard the fat from stews and soups; do not make gravy from meat drippings. Substitute poultry, fish, and game hens for red meat.

Legumes are also an excellent alternate source of protein. Their protein is "incomplete" in that it does not contain all the protein components needed by the body. Therefore, other foods that contain these missing components must be added, such as whole-grain products, nuts, seeds, and low-fat dairy products. Because legumes can cause intestinal bloating and gas in persons not accustomed to eating them in large amounts, you should increase your consumption of them slowly.

EVEN LESS CHOLESTEROL

It is a good idea to cut down drastically on foods that contain large amounts of cholesterol. Limit yourself to two or three egg yolks per week. Substitute whites of two eggs or a commercial egg substitute for one whole egg. Organ meat (liver, kidneys, sweetbreads, heart, tongue, chitlings, and brains) should be eaten only once or twice a month. Use polyunsaturated margarine instead of butter, and only use cream on special occasions.

Switch from whole-milk products to skim-milk products. Cheese is a highly concentrated form of whole milk. Swiss cheese has the lowest fat content. Look for the new skim-milk cheese products.

Most common vegetable oils are polyunsaturated. However, some have been saturated during processing. Hydrogenated or partially hydrogenated vegetable oils contain saturated fat. Coconut, palm, and macadamia nut oil are saturated. Read labels carefully when selecting a vegetable oil or purchasing a prepared food product.

GENERAL RECOMMENDATIONS

The fundamental dietary principles for the non-insulin-dependent diabetic are the same as those for the insulin-dependent diabetic. To sum up:

- For an adult at or near ideal weight, the ideal weight is used to calculate calorie needs. Generally, 12 to 15 Calories per pound of ideal weight represents an adequate caloric intake for the diabetic. For the overweight patient an appropriate calorie-restricted diet, 1,000 to 1,400 Calories, may be prescribed.
- Calorie intake needs to be distributed throughout the day (in amounts that match the times of the insulin effect for insulin-dependent patients).
- At least 50 percent of the calorie intake should be from carbohydrates, 12 to 20 percent from protein, and 25 to 30 percent from fat.
- Most of the carbohydrates should be in the form of complex carbohydrates and fiber in order to avoid too rapid absorption and quick upswings in the blood sugar level.
- Meals must be mixed (i.e., include carbohydrate, fat, and protein to provide for slower absorption of carbohydrate and therefore lead to smoother control of the blood sugar level).
- Unsaturated fats should be limited for a lower cholesterol level.
- Refined sugar can be eaten in mixed meals, in limited quantities.

2

MEAL PLANNING

MEAL PLANNING WITH FOOD EXCHANGES

Unless you have been instructed to use specific nutrient analyses in planning your meals, you will be using the diabetic food exchange list system. It was worked out to simplify meal planning according to the diet prescribed by the physician for the vast majority of patients. The original lists of basic food groups were redefined by The American Diabetes Association (ADA) and the American Dietetic Association to create the ADA Exchange Lists for Meal Planning included in this chapter. The exchange lists divide foods into six different categories: starch/bread, meat, vegetable, fruit, milk, and fat. These food groups form the basis of the nutritional program. The foods within each group contain approximately the same number of calories and the same amount of protein, fat, and carbohydrate when served in the specified portions. The portion of food is just as important as the kind of food. At first, using these lists does not appear to be simple. Learning to think about food in a totally new way is not easy. But once one gets the hang of it, the exchange list system becomes second nature.

For all practical purposes, all of the foods included in any one list are interchangeable. For example, if you eat one slice of whole wheat bread *or* ½ cup of cooked pasta, your body receives the same number of calories and the same amounts of protein, fat, and carbohydrate. In other words, as long as the correct portions are used, the foods in any one group can be substituted or traded for each other. Therefore, if you are permitted two servings from the starch/bread group, you could select one slice of whole wheat toast and ½ cup of bran flakes *or* you could select two slices of whole wheat toast. However, you cannot exchange one slice of bread for one egg or for a glass of juice. Foods in one group usually cannot be traded for foods in another group.

The meat and milk lists are divided into subgroups based on the amount of fat and calories. If it is necessary to control the amount of cholesterol and saturated fat in the diet, only foods from the low-fat groups should be selected.

BALANCED DIET

No one food supplies all the nutrients needed for a well-balanced diet. A balanced diet contains poultry, fish, and meat, vegetables and fruits, breads and cereals, and dairy products. It is a good idea to vary the foods selected from each group each day. For example, do not always choose the same fruit or the same vegetable. A varied diet is more appetizing as well as healthier.

MEASURING FOODS

Unless you have been instructed by your physician or dietitian to use a special scale, standard kitchen scales and measuring cups and spoons are all that are needed for measuring food portions. It is a good idea to measure all the foods at first until you develop the knack of estimating correct portion sizes. However, it is very easy to become more generous, so it is a good idea to measure the portion sizes periodically to make sure that you are still estimating them correctly.

FOOD EXCHANGE LISTS

The food exchange lists given on the next few pages were developed by the American Diabetes Association and the American Dietetic Association. They are from *Exchange Lists for Meal Planning*, American Diabetes Association and American Dietetic Association, 1986, and are reprinted by permission.

Starch/Bread Exchanges

Nutrient analysis of one exchange:
Protein, 3 grams
Carbohydrate, 15 grams
Fat, trace
Calories, 80

Cereals/grains/pasta	
Bran cereals, concentrated*	1/3 cup
Bran cereals, flaked (such as Bran Buds, All Bran)*	1/2 cup
Bulgur (cooked)	1/2 cup
Cooked cereals	1/2 cup
Cornmeal (dry)	2 1/2 tablespoons
Grape-Nuts	3 tablespoons
Grits (cooked)	1/2 cup
Other ready-to-eat unsweetened cereals	3/4 cup
Pasta (cooked)	1/2 cup
Puffed cereal	1 1/2 cups
Rice, white or brown (cooked)	1/3 cup
Shredded wheat	1/2 cup
Wheat germ*	3 tablespoons
Dried beans/peas/lentils	
Beans and peas (cooked) (such as kidney, white, split, blackeye)*	1/3 cup
Lentils (cooked)*	1/3 cup
Baked beans*	1/4 cup
Starchy vegetables	
Corn*	1/2 cup
Corn on cob, 6 inches long*	1
Lima beans*	1/2 cup
Peas, green (canned or frozen)*	1/2 cup
Plantain*	1/2 cup
Potato, baked	1 small (3 ounces)
Potato, mashed	1/2 cup
Squash, winter (acorn, butternut)	3/4 cup
Yam, sweet potato, plain	1/3 cup
Bread	
Bagel	1/2 (1 ounce)
Bread sticks, crisp, 4 inches long x 1/2 inch	2 (2/3 ounce)

* 3 grams or more of fiber per serving.

Croutons, low fat	1 cup
English muffin	½
Frankfurter or hamburger bun	½ (1 ounce)
Pita, 6 inches across	½
Plain roll, small	1 (1 ounce)
Raisin, unfrosted	1 slice (1 ounce)
Rye, pumpernickel*	1 slice (1 ounce)
Tortilla, 6 inches across	1
White (including French, Italian)	1 slice (1 ounce)
Whole wheat	1 slice (1 ounce)
Crackers/snacks	
Animal crackers	8
Graham crackers, 2½ inches square	3
Matzo	¾ ounce
Melba toast	5 slices
Oyster crackers	24
Popcorn (popped, no fat added)	3 cups
Pretzels	¾ ounce
Rye crisp, 2 inches x 3½ inches	4
Saltine-type crackers	6
Whole wheat crackers, no fat added (crisp breads, such as Finn, Kavli, Wasa)	2-4 slices (¾ ounce)
Starch foods prepared with fat†	
Biscuit, 2½ inches across	1
Chow mein noodles	½ cup
Corn bread, 2-inch cube	1 (2 ounces)
Cracker, round butter type	6
French fried potatoes, 2 inches to 3½ inches long	10 (1½ ounces)
Muffin, plain, small	1
Pancake, 4 inches across	2
Stuffing, bread (prepared)	¼ cup
Taco shell, 6 inches across	2
Waffle, 4½-inch square	1
Whole wheat crackers, fat added (such as Triscuits)	4-6 (1 ounce)

* 3 grams or more of fiber per serving.
† Count as 1 starch/bread serving, plus 1 fat serving.

Meat Exchanges: Lean Meat

Nutrient analysis of one exchange:
Protein, 7 grams
Fat, 3 grams
Calories, 55

Beef	
USDA Good or Choice grades of lean beef, such as round, sirloin, and flank steak; tenderloin; and chipped beef*	1 ounce
Pork	
Lean pork, such as fresh ham; canned, cured or boiled ham*; Canadian bacon*; tenderloin	1 ounce
Veal	
All cuts are lean except for veal cutlets (ground or cubed). Examples of lean veal are chops and roasts	1 ounce
Poultry	
Chicken, turkey, Cornish hen (without skin)	1 ounce
Fish	
All fresh and frozen fish	1 ounce
Crab, lobster, scallops, shrimp, clams (fresh or canned in water*)	2 ounces
Oysters	6 medium
Tuna* (canned in water)	¼ cup
Herring (uncreamed or smoked)	1 ounce
Sardines (canned)	2 medium
Wild Game	
Venison, rabbit, squirrel	1 ounce
Pheasant, duck, goose (without skin)	1 ounce
Cheese	
Any cottage cheese	¼ cup
Grated parmesan	2 tablespoons
Diet cheeses* (with less than 55 calories per ounce)	1 ounce
Other	
95% fat-free luncheon meat	1 ounce
Egg whites	3 whites
Egg substitutes with less than 55 calories per ¼ cup	¼ cup

* 400 mg or more of sodium per exchange.

Meat Exchanges: Medium-Fat Meat

Nutrient analysis of one exchange:
Protein, 7 grams
Fat, 5 grams
Calories, 75

Beef	
Most beef products fall into this category Examples are: all ground beef, roast (rib, chuck, rump), cubed, Porterhouse, T-bone), and meatloaf	1 ounce
Pork	
Most pork products fall into this category Examples are: chops, loin roast, Boston butt, cutlets	1 ounce
Lamb	
Most lamb products fall into this category Examples are: chops, leg, and roast	1 ounce
Veal	
Cutlet (ground or cubed, unbreaded)	1 ounce
Poultry	
Chicken (with skin), domestic duck or goose (well drained of fat), ground turkey	1 ounce
Fish	
Tuna* (canned in oil and drained)	¼ cup
Salmon* (canned)	¼ cup
Cheese	
Skim or part-skim milk cheeses, such as:	
Ricotta	¼ cup
Mozzarella	1 ounce
Diet cheeses* (with 56-80 calories per ounce)	1 ounce
Other	
86% fat-free luncheon meat*	1 ounce
Egg (high in cholesterol, limit to 3 per week)	1
Egg substitutes with 56-80 calories per ¼ cup	¼ cup
Tofu (2½ inches x 2¾ inches x 1 inch)	4 ounces
Liver, heart, kidney, sweetbreads (high in cholesterol)	1 ounce

* 400 mg or more of sodium per exchange.

Meat Exchanges: High-Fat Meat

Nutrient analysis of one exchange:
Protein, 7 grams
Fat, 8 grams
Calories, 100

Remember, these items are high in saturated fat, cholesterol, and calories, and should be used only three (3) times per week.
(One exchange is equal to any one of the following items.)

Beef	
Most USDA Prime cuts of beef, such as ribs, corned beef*	1 ounce
Pork	
Spareribs, ground pork, pork sausage* (patty or link)	1 ounce
Lamb	
Patties (ground lamb)	1 ounce
Fish	
Any fried fish product	1 ounce
Cheese	
All regular cheeses*, such as American, Blue, Cheddar, Monterey, Swiss	1 ounce
Other	
Luncheon meat,* such as bologna, salami, pimiento loaf	1 ounce
Sausage,* such as Polish, Italian	1 ounce
Knockwurst, smoked	1 ounce
Bratwurst*	1 ounce
Frankfurter* (turkey or chicken)	1 frank (10/pound)
Peanut butter (contains unsaturated fat)	1 tablespoon

Count as one high-fat meat plus one fat exchange:

Frankfurter* (beef, pork, or combination)	1 frank (10/pound)

Guidelines

Meat should be weighed after cooking and after bone, skin, and excess fat have been removed. A 3-ounce portion of cooked meat is equal to approximately 4 ounces of raw meat.

Meat and meat substitutes may be prepared by baking, boiling, broiling, roasting, steaming, or microwave cooking. Use a rack while meat is cooking so fat can drain off.

* 400 mg or more of sodium per exchange.

Use a nonstick-coated pan or nonstick vegetable spray for pan-fried foods.

If fats are used in cooking, count them as part of the total fat allowance.

If starches (such as flour, batter, crackers, bread crumbs, or cereal) are used in meat dishes, count them as part of the starch allowance.

Vegetable Exchanges

Nutrient analysis of one exchange:
Protein, 2 grams
Carbohydrate, 5 grams
Calories, 25

Artichoke (½ medium)	Greens	Rutabaga
Asparagus	Collard	Sauerkraut*
Beans (green, wax, Italian)	Mustard	Spinach, cooked
	Turnip	Summer squash (crookneck)
Bean sprouts	Kohlrabi	
Beets	Leeks	Tomato (one large)
Broccoli	Mushrooms, cooked	Tomato/vegetable juice
Brussels sprouts	Okra	Turnips
Carrots	Onions	Water chestnuts
Cauliflower	Pea pods	Zucchini, cooked
Eggplant	Peppers (green)	

For all items, one exchange portion is ½ cup of cooked vegetables or juice or 1 cup of raw vegetables.

Guidelines

If fat (butter, margarine, cream sauce, bacon, nuts, cheese sauce, oil, salad dressing, or sour cream dip) is used to season vegetables, count this as part of the fat allowance.

Season vegetables with herbs, spices, lemon, or vinegar to avoid additional calories from fat.

*Salt content, 400 milligrams or more per serving.

Fruit Exchanges

Nutrient analysis of one exchange:
Carbohydrate, 15 grams
Calories, 60

Fresh, frozen, and unsweetened canned fruit	
Apple (raw, 2 inches across)	1 apple
Applesauce (unsweetened)	½ cup
Apricots (medium, raw) or	4 apricots
Apricots (canned)	½ cup, or 4 halves
Banana (9 inches long)	½ banana
Blackberries (raw)*	¾ cup
Blueberries (raw)*	¾ cup
Cantaloupe (5 inches across)	⅓ melon
(cubes)	1 cup
Cherries (large, raw)	12 cherries
Cherries (canned)	½ cup
Figs (raw, 2 inches across)	2 figs
Fruit cocktail (canned)	½ cup
Grapefruit (medium)	½ grapefruit
Grapefruit (segments)	¾ cup
Grapes (small)	15 grapes
Honeydew melon (medium)	⅛ melon
(cubes)	1 cup
Kiwi (large)	1 kiwi
Mandarin oranges	¾ cup
Mango (small)	½ mango
Nectarine (1½ inches across)*	1 nectarine
Orange (2½ inches across)	1 orange
Papaya	1 cup
Peach (2¾ inches across)	1 peach, or ¾ cup
Peaches (canned)	½ cup, or 2 halves
Pear	½ large, or 1 small
Pears (canned)	½ cup, or 2 halves
Persimmon (medium, native)	2 persimmons
Pineapple (raw)	¾ cup
Pineapple (canned)	⅓ cup
Plum (raw, 2 inches across)	2 plums
Pomegranate*	½ pomegranate
Raspberries (raw)	1 cup
Strawberries (raw, whole)*	1¼ cup
Tangerine (2½ inches across)	2 tangerines
Watermelon (cubes)	1¼ cup

(continued)

* 3 grams or more of fiber per serving.

FRUIT EXCHANGES ***(continued)***

Dried fruit	
Apples*	4 rings
Apricots*	7 halves
Dates	2½ medium
Figs*	1½
Prunes*	3 medium
Raisins	2 tablespoons
Fruit juice	
Apple juice/cider	½ cup
Cranberry juice cocktail	⅓ cup
Grapefruit juice	½ cup
Grape juice	⅓ cup
Orange juice	½ cup
Pineapple juice	½ cup
Prune juice	⅓ cup

Guidelines

Fruit may be fresh, canned, cooked, dried, or frozen.

All fruit should be used without added sugar.

The label on canned or frozen fruits and juices should state "no sugar added" or "unsweetened."

Juice-packed fruits should be drained. Count the drained juice as a separate fruit portion.

Fruits that are canned or frozen in syrup should not be used, even if the syrup is rinsed off.

---

* 3 grams or more of fiber per serving.

Milk Exchanges

Nutrient analysis of one exchange:
Protein, 8 grams
Carbohydrate, 12 grams
Fat, trace (skim), 5 (low-fat), 8 (whole)
Calories, 90 (skim), 120 (low-fat), 150 (whole)

Skim and very lowfat milk	
Skim milk	1 cup
½% milk	1 cup
1% milk	1 cup
Lowfat buttermilk	1 cup
Evaporated skim milk	½ cup
Dry nonfat milk	⅓ cup
Plain nonfat yogurt	8 ounces
Lowfat milk	
2% milk	1 cup fluid
Plain lowfat yogurt (with added nonfat milk solids)	8 ounces
Whole milk	

The whole milk group has much more fat per serving than the skim and lowfat groups. Whole milk has more than 3¼% butterfat. Try to limit your choices from the whole milk group as much as possible.

Whole milk	1 cup
Evaporated whole milk	½ cup
Whole plain yogurt	8 ounces

Guidelines

If milk is used in cooking, count it as part of the milk allowance.

Fat Exchanges

Nutrient analysis of one fat exchange:
Fat, 5 grams
Calories, 45

Unsaturated fats	
Avocado	1/8 medium
Margarine	1 teaspoon
Margarine, diet*	1 tablespoon
Mayonnaise	1 teaspoon
Mayonnaise, reduced-calorie*	1 tablespoon
Nuts and seeds:	
Almonds, dry roasted	6 whole
Cashews, dry roasted	1 tablespoon
Pecans	2 whole
Peanuts	20 small or 10 large
Walnuts	2 whole
Other nuts	1 tablespoon
Seeds, pine nuts, sunflower (without shells)	1 tablespoon
Pumpkin seeds	2 teaspoons
Oil (corn, cottonseed, safflower, soybean, sunflower, olive, peanut)	1 teaspoon
Olives*	10 small or 5 large
Salad dressing, mayonnaise-type	2 teaspoons
Salad dressing, mayonnaise-type, reduced-calorie	1 tablespoon
Salad dressing (all varieties)*	1 tablespoon
Salad dressing, reduced-calorie†	2 tablespoons

(Two tablespoons of low-calorie salad dressing is a free food.)

Saturated fats	
Butter	1 teaspoon
Bacon*	1 slice
Chitterlings	1/2 ounce
Coconut, shredded	2 tablespoons
Coffee whitener, liquid	2 tablespoons
Coffee whitener, powder	4 teaspoons
Cream (light, coffee, table)	2 tablespoons
Cream, sour	2 tablespoons
Cream (heavy, whipping)	1 tablespoon
Cream cheese	1 tablespoon
Salt pork*	1/4 ounce

Guidelines

Polyunsaturated fats should be used more than saturated fats. The preferred kinds of oil are safflower, corn, sunflower, soy, and cotton-

* If more than one or two servings are eaten, these foods have 400 mg or more of sodium.

† 400 mg or more of sodium per serving.

seed. Products such as margarine, salad dressing, and nondairy creamers that are made with oil should list one of these oils as the first ingredient.

If fats are used in cooking, count them as part of the total fat allowance.

HOW TO CALCULATE NUTRITIVE VALUES OF OTHER RECIPES AND FOODS

If you want to eat a favorite food or make a favorite recipe, but the nutrient value has not been given in this book, you can consult one of the following sources:

Adams, C. F.: *Nutritive Value of American Foods in Common Units* (Agriculture Handbook 456). Washington, D.C., Superintendent of Documents, U.S. Government Printing Office, 1975.

Bowes, A. de P., and Church, C. F.: *Bowes and Church's Food Values of Portions Commonly Used,* thirteenth edition. (Revision by J. A. T. Pennington and H. N. Church.) New York, Harper & Row, Publishers, 1980.

Kraus, B.: *The Dictionary of Sodium, Fats, and Cholesterol.* New York, Grosset and Dunlap, 1977.

These sources give the exact numbers for the ingredients you need for the recipe. The nutrient values are often given in milligrams (mg) or grams (g). To calculate the nutrient value for one serving from a given recipe, add the nutrient values for each food item and divide the total by the number of servings in the recipe. If the data are given for a 100-gram portion, keep in mind that 1 ounce equals approximately 30 grams and calculate the nutrient content as shown below. Follow the same procedure for each ingredient in the recipe. Then add up the nutrient values for each item for the overall value of the recipe. Divide this number by the number of servings or cups the recipe yields to arrive at the exact nutrient value of one serving.

A		B		C		D		E
Nutrient value for a specific item per 100 g	÷	100 g	=	Nutrient value for 1 g	×	Weight of serving in g	=	Nutrient value of serving

For example, to calculate the caloric value of crackers weighing 15 grams (½ ounce), calculate:

A		B		C		D		E
475	÷	100	=	4.75	×	15	=	71 calories

3

GUIDELINES FOR LOW-SALT MEALS

LOW-SALT MEALS

Under normal circumstances, most people can consume as much sodium as they want. However, in some people, sodium is not handled in the normal fashion. Your doctor will prescribe a low-salt diet for you if you must be careful about sodium intake.

Sodium is a necessary component of the blood and an essential nutrient in our diet. It is found in varying amounts in almost everything we eat. The main source of sodium in the diet is table salt (sodium chloride), which is about 40 percent sodium. One teaspoon of salt contains about 2 grams of sodium. The average person in the United States consumes 4 to 10 grams of sodium per day. Of this amount, about 1 gram occurs naturally in the food itself. The rest comes from salt that is added. Cured foods (such as ham, luncheon meat, and bacon), condiments (steak sauce, mustard, catsup, and soy sauce), and many of the preservatives used in processing foods are major sources of dietary sodium. Most fresh foods, and particularly fruits and vegetables, contain lesser amounts of sodium. Antacids, some diet soft drinks, laxatives, cough medicines, and some artificial sweeteners also contain significant amounts of sodium. It is important to read all labels carefully or to ask your dietitian about the sodium content of these products.

A person's taste for salt depends on how much that person is exposed to it. Even those who salt their food heavily before they taste it will gradually lose the desire for salt over a period of a few months, once they stop using it. The sodium content for all the recipes in this book appears, along with other nutrient information, at the end of each recipe. If sodium is a problem for you, keep track of your daily intake and avoid recipes that have a high sodium content.

SOME PRACTICAL SUGGESTIONS

Start by taking the salt shaker off the table and eliminating obviously salty foods—ham, bacon, steak sauce, potato chips, bologna, regular canned or dried soups, and salted salad dressings and condiments—from the diet. Then, gradually cut down the amount of salt used in cooking. In most instances, you will not have to use special low-sodium food products. If you do have to use them, there are many available. But, before you spend extra money to buy them, see if you find the same food in the regular food sections of your market. Although most fresh fruits, vegetables, meats, poultry, and fish are fine to use, many of the same items, when canned or frozen, contain salt or a sodium preservative. A list of low-sodium diabetic exchanges appears at the end of this chapter.

Check the ingredient list on all processed foods for the words "salt," "sodium," "sodium chloride," "soda," "sodium compounds," or "Na" (the chemical symbol for sodium). If one of these words appears among the first three ingredients listed, you probably should avoid that product. Most cheeses are quite high in sodium; however, several low-sodium, low-fat cheeses are now available. Be sure that the product is truly *low* in sodium and not just slightly lower than the regular product.

USING HERBS AND SPICES

Learning to cook with less salt is a challenge that is easier to meet if you learn to substitute the exciting tastes of herbs and spices for salt. If you have not cooked with herbs and spices before, the following guidelines should be helpful.

1. Use herbs and spices sparingly. They should accentuate, not overpower, the flavor of the food.
2. When you start cooking with herbs, use no more than ¼ teaspoon of dried herbs or ¾ teaspoon of fresh herbs for a dish that serves four people. If you like the taste, you can always increase it the next time.
3. If you are preparing a recipe that is to be cooked for a long time—for example, a soup or a stew—add the herbs during the last hour of cooking.
4. Add herbs to hamburgers, meat loaf, and stuffing before cooking.
5. Sprinkle roasts, steaks, and chops with herbs before cooking, or add an herb-flavored margarine after cooking. Herb-flavored margarine is also tasty on vegetables. Meats can be brushed with oil and then sprinkled with herbs 1 hour before cooking.
6. Add herbs to vegetables, sauces, and gravies while you are cooking them.
7. Add herbs to cold foods (tomato juice, salad dressings, and cottage cheese) several hours before serving. Storing these foods in the refrigerator for several hours or overnight will bring out the flavor of the herbs.
8. Heat and moisture bring out the fragrance and flavor of herbs. To add a subtle herb taste to food, place the dried herbs in a tea strainer, dip the strainer into piping hot water for 20 seconds, drain the water, and add the moistened herbs to the food.

9. To avoid having bits of the herb itself in the food, tie the herbs in a small piece of cheesecloth and remove the bag before serving.

10. Marinating meat in a wine and herb mixture before cooking will greatly enhance its flavor.

11. To hasten flavor release, crush herbs in the palm of the hand before adding them to food.

12. When substituting fresh herbs for dried herbs, use 3 or 4 times as much of the fresh herbs.

13. Do not combine too many different herbs and spices in one dish or at one meal.

COOKING WITH WINE

Most of the alcohol used in cooking evaporates during the cooking process, leaving behind a wonderful taste and very few calories. Because only 1 or 2 tablespoons of alcohol per serving are used in most recipes, these calories do not have to be calculated into the diet. When the right amount of wine is used, it will enhance the flavor of the foods. However, the whole is only as good as its parts, so be sure to use a good wine for cooking.

SEASONINGS AND FREE FOODS

The following foods and seasonings contain negligible amounts of protein, fat, or carbohydrate. They may be used as desired without substitution in the meal plan.

- Beverages
  - Coffee
  - Tea
  - Decaffeinated coffee
- Seasonings
  - Salt (use only as allowed)
  - Pepper
  - Herbs
  - Spices
- Condiments
  - Salt-free catsup (limit, 1 tablespoon)
  - Fresh horseradish
  - Salt-free prepared mustard
  - Dry mustard
- Garlic and onion powder
- Bouillon or broth (fat-free, salt-free)
- Flavoring extracts
- Gelatin (½ cup sugar-free)
- Cranberries (½ cup unsweetened)
- Rhubarb (½ cup unsweetened)
- Lemon juice
- Lime juice
- Vinegar
- Salt-free low-calorie salad dressing (limit, 1 tablespoon)

FOODS TO AVOID

The following foods contain large amounts of sodium. You should avoid these foods.

Bottled meat sauce and barbecue sauce
Bouillon
Celery flakes
Celery salt
Club soda
Garlic salt
Meat tenderizers
Monosodium glutamate
Onion salt
Pickles and pickled vegetables
Prepared catsup
Prepared horseradish
Prepared mustard
Regular low-calorie salad dressing
Seasoning salts and mixes
Soy sauce
Worcestershire sauce

SEASONING SUGGESTIONS

Meats and Eggs

Beef: dry mustard, marjoram, nutmeg, onion, sage, thyme, pepper, mushrooms,* bay leaf
Chicken: paprika, mushrooms,* thyme, sage, parsley, dill
Eggs: pepper, green pepper, mushrooms,* dry mustard, paprika, curry powder, oregano, tarragon
Fish: dry mustard, paprika, curry powder, bay leaf, lemon juice, mushrooms*
Lamb: mint, garlic, rosemary, curry powder, broiled pineapple rings†
Pork: onion, garlic, sage, applesauce,† spiced apples†
Veal: bay leaf, ginger, marjoram, curry powder

Vegetables

Asparagus: lemon juice, toasted sesame seeds
Beans, green: marjoram, lemon juice, nutmeg, unsalted French dressing, dill
Broccoli: lemon juice, oregano
Cabbage: dill, savory, caraway seeds
Carrots: parsley, mint, nutmeg
Cauliflower: nutmeg, tarragon
Corn: green pepper, tomatoes,* chives
Lima beans: minced chives, onion, parsley, marjoram
Peas: mint, mushrooms,* parsley, onion
Potatoes: parsley, mace, chopped green pepper, onion
Squash: ginger, mace
Sweet potatoes: cinnamon, nutmeg, ginger
Tomatoes: basil, sage, green pepper, onion, oregano

*If salted vegetables are allowed, tomatoes and mushrooms used as seasoning may be salted. If only unsalted vegetables are allowed, tomatoes and mushrooms used for seasoning should be fresh, frozen, or unsalted canned.
†Fruits used as seasoning should be counted as 1 fruit exchange in the meal plan.

The Exchange Lists are the basis of a meal-planning system designed by a committee of the American Diabetes Association and the American Dietetic Association. While designed primarily for people with diabetes and others who must follow special diets, the Exchange Lists are based on principles of good nutrition that apply to everyone.

LOW-SODIUM DIABETIC EXCHANGES

Starch/Bread Exchanges

One exchange of starch contains:
- 3 grams of protein
- 15 grams of carbohydrate
- 80 Calories
- 20–25 milligrams of sodium

Bread: Unsalted breads are those that do not have salt added in preparation or processing and are labeled "salt-free"; regular bakery bread is salted.

White (including French and Italian)	1 slice (1 ounce)
Whole wheat	1 slice (1 ounce)
Rye or pumpernickel*	1 slice (1 ounce)
Raisin, unfrosted	1 slice (1 ounce)
Pita bread, 6 inches across	½
Bagel	½ (1 ounce)
English muffin	½ small
Plain roll	1 (1 ounce)
Hamburger or frankfurter bun	½ (1 ounce)
Dried bread crumbs	3 tablespoons
Tortilla, 6-inch diameter	1
Bread sticks, unsalted, 4 inches long by ½ inch	2 (⅔ ounce)

Cereals: Unsalted cereals are those that do not have salt added in preparation or processing; shredded wheat, puffed wheat, puffed rice, and cornflakes are available "salt-free" (check label); other ready-to-eat cereals contain added salt; all other cereal products such as rice and noodles are unsalted, unless salt is used in cooking.

Bran flakes*	½ cup
Bran cereal, concentrated*	⅓ cup

Adapted from: *Your Diet for Diabetes with Sodium Control,* Department of Internal Medicine, Mayo Clinic, Rochester, Minnesota, Mayo Foundation, 1980. By permission.

* Contains 3 grams or more of fiber per serving.

Puffed cereal (unfrosted)	1½ cups
Grape-Nuts	3 tablespoons
Other ready-to-eat unsweetened cereal	¾ cup
Cooked cereal	½ cup
Grits (cooked)	½ cup
Rice or barley (cooked)	⅓ cup
Pasta (cooked, including spaghetti, noodles, macaroni)	½ cup
Popcorn, large kernel (popped, without added fat or salt)	3 cups
Popcorn, small kernel (popped, without added fat or salt)	1½ cups
Cornmeal (dry)	2½ tablespoons
Flour	2½ tablespoons
Tapioca	2 tablespoons
Wheat germ*	3 tablespoons

Crackers: Unsalted crackers are those that do not contain any salt in preparation or processing; they should be labeled "salt-free" or "low-sodium"; if salted starches are allowed, crackers that do not have salted tops may be used.

Graham, 2½-inch square	3
Matzo	¾ ounce
Melba toast	5
Soda, unsalted, 2½-inch square	6
Rye crisp, unsalted, 2 by 3½ inches	4

Dried beans, peas, lentils, and starchy vegetables: Unsalted beans and other starchy vegetables are those that do not have salt added in preparation or processing, including fresh, frozen (no salt added), canned (low-sodium), or dried beans and other vegetables; regular canned vegetables or frozen vegetables with salt added are salted vegetables; additional salt should not be added in cooking.

Beans, peas, lentils (cooked)*	⅓ cup
Corn*	½ cup
Corn on the cob*	1 small (6 inches)
Lima beans*	½ cup
Parsnips	⅔ cup
Peas, green (fresh)*	½ cup
Plantain*	½ cup
Potato, baked	1 small (3 ounces)

(continued)

* Contains 3 grams or more of fiber per serving.

STARCH/BREAD EXCHANGES *(continued)*

Potato (mashed)	½ cup
Pumpkin	¾ cup
Winter squash, acorn or butternut	¾ cup
Yam or sweet potato, plain	⅓ cup

Other bread products and starch exchanges: Other bread and cereal products are unsalted only if they are homemade without any salt and contain low-sodium baking powder rather than regular baking powder; if salted starches are allowed, they may be made from a home recipe that includes salt and regular baking powder or baking soda; commercial mixes and commercially prepared refrigerator doughs should not be used (add 1 fat exchange).

Animal crackers	8
Biscuit, 2½-inch diameter	1
Cornbread, 2 by 2 by 1 inch	1 (2 ounces)
Corn muffin, 2-inch diameter	1 (2 ounces)
Muffin, plain, small	1
Pancake, 4 inches across	2
Waffle, 4½ inches square	1

Additional starch exchanges: Many of the following foods contain some added sugar; they should be used only occasionally and as part of a planned meal or snack.

		Exchanges
Sherbet	¼ cup	1 starch
Angel food cake	1/12 of 10-inch cake or 1½-inch slice	2 starch
Gingersnaps, 1 inch	3	1 starch
Vanilla wafers, 1 inch	6 small	1 starch, 1 fat
Ice cream (any flavor)	½ cup	1 starch, 2 fat
Ice milk (any flavor)	½ cup	1 starch, 1 fat

Avoid: Salted snack foods; salted crackers; potato chips; pretzels; salted popcorn; corn chips; commercial mixes; commercially frozen convenience foods; canned soups; dried soup mixes; broth or bouillon.

Meat Exchanges

One exchange of meat contains:
- 7 grams of protein
- 3–8 grams of fat
- 55–100 Calories
- 23 milligrams of sodium if unsalted
- 70 milligrams of sodium if salted (¼ teaspoon of salt per pound of meat)

Meat should be weighed after cooking and after bone, skin, and excess fat have been removed. A 3-ounce portion of cooked meat is equal to approximately 4 ounces of raw meat.

Lean Meat (these meat and meat substitutes are lowest in fat and calories; use meat from the lean and medium-fat categories most often)

Beef: baby beef, tenderloin, chuck, flank steak, plate ribs, plate skirt steak, round (bottom, top) rump, spare ribs, tripe, ground (above meats trimmed of fat and then ground)	1 ounce
Pork: leg (whole rump, center shank)	1 ounce
Veal: leg, loin, rib, shank, shoulder cutlets	1 ounce
Poultry (meat without skin): chicken, turkey, Cornish hen, guinea hen, pheasant	1 ounce
Fish:	
Any fresh or frozen	1 ounce
Unsalted canned tuna, salmon, or crab	¼ cup
Lobster or mackerel	1 ounce
Clams, scallops, shrimp	1 ounce (about 5)
Oysters	3 ounces (5 to 7 medium)
Cottage cheese	¼ cup
Parmesan cheese	3 tablespoons
Egg substitute	¼ cup
Dried beans and peas (add 1 starch/bread exchange)	1 cup

Medium-Fat Meat (these meats and meat substitutes contain a moderate amount of fat and calories; use meats from the lean and medium-fat categories most often)

Beef (not prime)	1 ounce

(continued)

MEAT EXCHANGES ***(continued)***

Lamb: chops, leg, or roast	1 ounce
Pork: loin (all cuts of tenderloin), shoulder, arm (picnic), shoulder blade, Boston butt	1 ounce
Poultry: capon, duck (domestic), goose	1 ounce
Veal, cutlet	1 ounce
Egg (limit to 3 per week)	1
Tofu (2½ inches by 2¾ inch by 1 inch)	4 ounces

High-Fat Meat (these meats and meat substitutes are high in fat and calories; use these meats only occasionally, especially if you are following a low-calorie diet for weight reduction)

Beef: prime cuts	1 ounce
Lamb, ground	1 ounce
Liver, heart, kidney, sweetbreads	1 ounce
Pork: spare ribs, loin (back ribs), ground pork	1 ounce
Peanut butter, unsalted (contains no saturated fat)	1 tablespoon
Roasted soybeans	1 ounce

Avoid: Salt-cured meats; salted canned or processed meats, fish, or fowl; bacon; ham; dried beef; frankfurters; processed cold cuts; sausages; sardines; salted cheese and cheese foods; salted peanuts; salted peanut butter; commercial casserole mixes; frozen dinners.

The following meats and meat substitutes are higher in sodium. Limit to 2 servings per week from this group: organ meats (such as liver, heart, kidney, sweetbreads, and tripe); duck and goose; shellfish (such as lobster, crab, clams, oysters, scallops, and shrimp).

Meat and meat substitutes may be prepared by baking, broiling, boiling, or roasting. If you use fats in cooking, reduce the number of fat exchanges allowed at that meal. If you use starches (such as flour, batter, crackers, bread crumbs, or cereal) to prepare meat dishes, reduce the number of starch exchanges allowed at that meal.

Vegetable Exchanges

One exchange of vegetable contains:

2 grams of protein
5 grams of carbohydrate
25 Calories
23 milligrams of sodium if unsalted
275 milligrams of sodium if salted (1/8 teaspoon salt per serving)

Unsalted vegetables are those that do not have salt added in preparation or processing, including fresh, frozen (no-salt-added), and canned (low-sodium) vegetables. Regular canned vegetables or frozen vegetables with salt added in processing are salted vegetables; additional salt should not be used in cooking.

One exchange of the following vegetables is ½ cup (or 100 grams).

Artichoke (½ medium)
Asparagus
Bean sprouts
Beets
Broccoli
Brussels sprouts
Cabbage, cooked
Carrots
Cauliflower
Eggplant
Greens, cooked:
 Chard
 Collards
 Dandelion
 Kale
 Mustard
 Spinach
 Turnip greens
Kohlraki
Leeks
Mushrooms, cooked
Okra
Onion
Rutabaga
String beans, green or yellow
Tomatoes (1 large)
Tomato juice, unsalted
Tomato paste, unsalted
Turnips
Vegetable juice cocktail, unsalted
Water chestnuts
Zucchini

The following vegetables have little protein, fat, carbohydrate, or calories (1 cup raw).

Cabbage
Celery
Chicory
Chinese cabbage*
Cucumber
Endive
Escarole
Greens
Green pepper
Lettuce
Mushroom
Parsley
Radishes
Romaine
Spinach
Summer squash
Watercress

Avoid: Sauerkraut; pickled vegetables; salted tomato juice; salted vegetable juice cocktail; seasoned tomato sauce; commercially frozen vegetable mixes with sauce.

---

* Contains 3 grams or more of fiber per serving.

Fruit Exchanges

One exchange of fruit contains:
15 grams of carbohydrate
60 Calories
Trace of sodium

Fruit may be fresh, canned, cooked, dried, or frozen. All fruit should be used without added sugar. If fruit is canned or frozen, the label should state one of the following: "no sugar added," "juice-packed," "water-packed," or "unsweetened." Fruits that are canned or frozen in syrup should not be used, even if the syrup is rinsed off. Unless otherwise noted, the serving size for fruits is: ½ cup fresh fruit or juice; ¼ cup dried fruit.

Apple	
Fresh	1 small
Juice	½ cup
Applesauce	½ cup
Apricots	
Fresh	4 medium
Canned	½ cup
Dried*	7
Banana (9 inches long)	½
Berries	
Blackberries*	¾ cup
Blueberries*	¾ cup
Raspberries (raw)	1 cup
Strawberries (raw, whole)	1¼ cups
Cherries	
Fresh	10 large
Canned	½ cup
Cider	½ cup
Cranberry, juice cocktail	⅓ cup
Dates	2½ medium
Figs (2 inches across)	
Fresh	2
Canned	½ cup
Dried*	1½
Fruit cocktail	½ cup
Grapefruit	
Fresh	½ medium
Juice	½ cup
Sections	¾ cup

* Contains 3 grams or more of fiber per serving.

Grapes	15
Juice	⅓ cup
Kiwi (large)	1
Mandarin oranges	¾ cup
Mango	½ small
Melon	
Cantaloupe (5 inches across)	⅓ melon
Honeydew	⅛ medium
Watermelon (cubes)	1¼ cups
Nectarine* (1½ inches across)	1
Orange	
Fresh (2½ inches across)	1 small
Juice	½ cup
Sections	½ cup
Papaya	1 cup
Peach (2¾ inches across)	
Fresh	1
Canned	½ cup
Dried	¼ cup
Pear	
Fresh	1 small
Canned	½ cup
Dried	¼ cup
Persimmon, native	2 medium
Pineapple	
Raw	¾ cup
Canned	⅓ cup
Plums	
Fresh (2½ inches across)	2
Pomegranate*	½
Prunes	
Whole*	3 medium
Juice	⅓ cup
Raisins	2 tablespoons
Tangerine* (2½ inches across)	2

Avoid: Fruits that have been crystallized or dried with a sodium compound. Check the label on dried foods closely.

* Contains 3 grams or more of fiber per serving.

Milk Exchanges

One exchange of milk contains:
- 8 grams of protein
- 12 grams of carbohydrate
- Trace of fat to 8 grams
- 90–150 Calories
- 115 milligrams of sodium

Nonfat and 1% fat-fortified milk	
Skim, nonfat, or 1% fat milk	1 cup
Powdered (nonfat dry, before adding liquid)	⅓ cup
Canned, evaporated skim	½ cup
Yogurt made from skim milk (plain, unflavored)	1 cup
2% fat-fortified milk (omit 1 fat exchange)	
2% milk	1 cup
Yogurt made from 2% milk (plain, unflavored)	1 cup
Whole milk (omit 2 fat exchanges)	
Whole milk	1 cup
Canned, evaporated whole milk	½ cup
Yogurt made from whole milk (plain, unflavored)	1 cup

Avoid: Cultured buttermilk, instant beverage mixes.

Fat Exchanges

One exchange of fat contains:
- 5 grams of fat
- 45 Calories
- 20 milligrams of sodium if unsalted
- 46 milligrams of sodium if salted

These fats are predominantly polyunsaturated or monounsaturated. They should be used in preference to saturated fats. The preferred kinds of oil are safflower, corn, sunflower, soy, and cottonseed oil. Products made with oil, such as margarine, salad dressing, and nondairy creamers, should list one of these oils as the first ingredient.

Margarine	1 teaspoon
Margarine, diet	1 tablespoon
Oil	1 teaspoon
Salad dressings	
Salt-free French- or Italian-style	1 tablespoon
Mayonnaise	1 teaspoon
Mayonnaise, reduced calorie	1 tablespoon
Nondairy cream substitutes	2 tablespoons
Avocado	1/8 medium
Almonds, unsalted	6 whole
Pecans, unsalted	2 large
Peanuts, unsalted	20 small or 10 large
Walnuts, unsalted	2 whole
Other nuts, unsalted	1 tablespoon

These fats are predominantly saturated fats. They should be used only occasionally.

Butter	1 teaspoon
Cream, light or sour	2 tablespoons
Cream, heavy	1 tablespoon
Other nondairy cream substitutes	2 tablespoons
Gravy, unsalted	2 tablespoons
Cream cheese	1 tablespoon
Lard	1 teaspoon

Avoid: Salted nuts; commercially prepared salted salad dressings; bacon; salt pork; olives; commercial gravy or gravy mixes.

Salt Substitutes

Salt substitutes are permitted unless your physician or dietitian indicates otherwise.

4

GUIDELINES FOR SPECIAL SITUATIONS

LOSING WEIGHT

For obese or overweight persons, the calorie content of the diet prescription is set at a level designed to produce loss of weight without causing a loss of lean body mass (muscle). The ideal weight reduction diet results in a slow, progressive weight loss of 1 to 2 pounds each week and allows new eating patterns to develop that will enable the individual to keep the weight off.

Losing weight and keeping it off is not easy to do alone. Joining a weight control group can lend support to a person's efforts.

One useful approach to losing weight and keeping it off is behavior modification. This approach is based on the belief that, in order to lose weight and keep it off, one needs to change those habits that encourage eating, and the easiest way to do this is to replace them with new habits that permit weight control. Here are specific steps that can help:

1. Chew food slowly.
2. Never shop for food when hungry.
3. Always make out a shopping list in advance. Do not add to it during shopping.
4. Do not leave open bowls of food on the table.
5. Always sit down to eat.
6. Restrict eating to one or two places, such as the kitchen and dining room.
7. Never eat while engaging in another activity, such as watching television.
8. Become aware of your own individual eating pattern so that you can identify problems and make appropriate changes. It helps to keep a diary of when and where you eat and under what circumstances—for example, in response to frustration, anger, boredom, hunger, or at certain times of day.
9. Do not keep high-calorie foods or snacks around. Keep a supply of low-calorie foods readily available as snacks.
10. Enlist your family to assist you in changing your eating habits.
11. Do not skip meals.
12. Develop a reward system for weight loss.
13. Develop a plan, and continually evaluate and update it.
14. Make only one change at a time.

15. Make a personal commitment to weight loss.
16. Whenever possible, institute a regular exercise program.
17. Never drive when you can walk.
18. Use stairs instead of elevators.
19. Plan to take a walk or to exercise at the times when you usually snack.
20. Do not be afraid to make more than one trip up the stairs each day.

FOODS TO AVOID

The following foods contain large amounts of sugar. You should avoid these foods.

Cake
Candy
Chewing gum
Cookies
Honey
Jam
Jelly
Marmalade
Molasses
Pastries
Pie
Pudding
Sugar
Sweet rolls
Sweetened condensed milk
Sweetened soft drinks
Syrup

SPECIAL SITUATIONS

The regular diet is planned for the diabetic's regular pattern of activities, but special situations arise—meals away from home, travel across time zones, and occasional illness. Circumstances such as these require adjustments in the regular routine. The information in this chapter is designed to help in making the appropriate adjustment to a situation. However, this information does not replace the advice and instructions of your physician. It is always a good practice to check with your physician when you encounter a new situation that has not been discussed before. It is particularly important for the diabetic to stay in close contact with his or her physician during an illness.

EATING AWAY FROM HOME

Being a diabetic is in no way a hindrance to eating out. In fact, the diabetic diet is probably one of the easiest to follow in almost any type of restaurant. Once you know your meal plan and feel comfortable about estimating portion sizes, you will be able to select your diet from any menu.

Try to select a meal that resembles, as closely as possible, your regular meal plan. It helps to carry a copy of your meal plan in your purse or wallet.

If the serving size is too generous, ask for a doggy bag. Occasionally, when eating out in the evening, you may wish to save one or two meat exchanges from your earlier meals to add to your dinner meat exchanges.

Because the medication doses are taken at times related to food intake, it is important to eat at approximately the same times each day. If you plan to eat later than usual, eat the fruit or milk exchange from your dinner meal plan at the regular time to tide you over. If dinner will be very late, eat your evening snack at your normal dinner time to prevent the blood sugar level from getting too low.

Until you feel secure about your diet and about estimating portion sizes, avoid ordering dishes that contain a mixture of ingredients. If you ask, most restaurants will prepare simple foods such as broiled chicken or broiled fresh fish. Ask that sauces, gravies, mayonnaise, and salad dressings be served on the side so you can measure them accurately. Order fresh vegetables and specify that they be cooked without additional fat. Select clear instead of creamed soups, and avoid fried foods and mixed casserole dishes.

Try fresh melon, fresh fruit cup, juice, or broth as an appetizer and fresh fruit for dessert. If you cannot live without a sweet dessert, you can occasionally order plain vanilla ice cream (½ cup is equal to 1 starch/bread plus 2 fat exchanges).

To control fat and cholesterol intake, order margarine instead of butter or skim milk instead of regular milk and trim the fat and skin from poultry and meat.

Here are some ideas to assist in selecting a meal from a restaurant menu. Remember, the portion sizes are important and should conform as closely as possible to the regular meal plan. On a low-salt diet, avoid items marked * and request that your food be cooked without added salt.

Breakfast

Fruit Exchanges:

Fresh melon
Freshly squeezed orange juice
Grapefruit half
Banana
Fresh fruit cup
Any other fruit or juice, fresh or canned unsweetened

Fat Exchanges:

Margarine
Cream
Nondairy cream substitutes
*Bacon

Starch/Bread Exchanges:

Unsweetened hot or cold cereal (puffed wheat or rice are unsalted)
Plain roll
Unbuttered toast, preferably whole-grain
English muffin
Waffle
Pancake
Bagel
Muffin
Biscuit
Grits

Milk Exchanges:

Milk, preferably skim
Low-fat yogurt

Meat Exchanges:

Eggs (ask that the eggs be cooked in vegetable oil if fried or scrambled; eat no more than two or three fresh eggs per week if your cholesterol intake is being controlled)
Egg substitutes
Cottage cheese
*Cheese
*Canadian bacon
*Ham
*Lean sausage

Lunch or Supper

Fruit Exchanges:

Canned fruit or juice, fresh or unsweetened
Applesauce, unsweetened
Pineapple, fresh or unsweetened
Grapefruit half
Fresh melon
Fruit cocktail, fresh or unsweetened canned

Meat Exchanges:

Lean roast beef, lamb, pork, or veal; trim away all visible fat
*Lean cold cuts, sliced chicken, turkey
Small steak; trim away visible fat
Lean hamburger, broiled
Fish
Cottage cheese
*Cheese
Egg
*Peanut butter (omit 2 fat exchanges)
Dried peas or beans

Vegetable Exchanges:
- Artichoke
- Lettuce and tomato
- Tossed greens
- Sliced tomato
- Hearts of lettuce
- Fresh or canned cooked vegetables (make sure that vegetables are cooked without extra fat, and have salad dressing served on the side so you can measure it yourself)

Starch/Bread Exchanges:
- Bread, preferably whole-grain
- Plain roll
- Frankfurter or hamburger bun
- Pita bread
- Bread sticks
- Melba toast
- *Saltines
- Rice or barley
- Pasta
- Lentils, peas, or beans
- Corn
- Potato
- Biscuit
- Muffin
- *Chips

Milk Exchanges:
- Milk, preferably skim
- Low-fat yogurt

Fat Exchanges:
- Margarine
- Oil
- Cream
- *Salad dressing (use oil and vinegar if you are on a low-salt diet)
- Mayonnaise
- Nondairy cream substitutes
- *Olives
- Gravy
- *Nuts
- Avocado
- *Bacon

FAST FOOD FACTS

There is no reason why the diabetic cannot eat in fast-food restaurants, provided selections are made carefully. Follow the regular meal plan and avoid high-sugar items such as milkshakes and desserts unless these foods are eaten just before intense exercise.

Those who are following a weight-loss diet should pay special attention to the calorie values of foods served in the fast-food restaurant. If you are on a low-salt diet, ask that your food be prepared without salt.

	Serving Size	Calories (1 serving)	Carbo. (gm)	Protein (gm)	Fat (gm)	Sodium (mg)
Arby's						
Roast Beef Sandwich	1 (5 oz)	350	32	22	15	880
Junior Roast Beef Sandwich	1 (3 oz)	220	21	12	9	530
Ham and Swiss Croissant Sandwich	1 (4 oz)	330	33	15	15	995
French Dip Sandwich	1 (5.5 oz)	386	47	29	21	1745
Potato Cakes	2 (3.5 oz)	190	24	2	9	476
Kentucky Fried Chicken						
Original Dinner (2 pieces chicken, mashed potatoes, gravy, cole slaw, roll)	11.2 oz	604	48	30	32	1528
Extra Crispy Dinner	12 oz	755	60	33	43	1544
Long John Silver's						
Fish in Fish/Fries Meal	3 Fish	606	33	39	36	2019
Fish Fillet w/Sauce in Baked Fish Meal	5.5 oz	151	0	33	2	361
Shrimp in Chilled Shrimp Dinner	20	120	–	20	–	380
Cole Slaw (as part of meal)	4 oz	182	11	1	15	367

(continued)

FAST FOOD FACTS ***(continued)***

	Serving Size	Calories (1 serving)	Carbo. (gm)	Protein (gm)	Fat (gm)	Sodium (mg)
McDonald's						
Hamburger	1 (3.5 oz)	263	28	12	11	506
Quarter Pounder with Cheese	1 (6.6 oz)	525	31	30	32	1220
Filet-O-Fish	1 (5.0 oz)	435	36	15	26	799
Chicken McNuggets	6 pieces (3.8 oz)	323	14	19	21	512
French Fries (Regular order)	1 order (2.4 oz)	220	26	3	12	109
Egg McMuffin	1 (4.9 oz)	340	31	19	16	885
Pizza Hut						
Thin 'N Crispy Pizza, 10-inch pie	½ pie (3 slices)	490	51	29	19	N/A
Thick 'N Chewy, 10-inch pie	½ pie (3 slices)	620	73	38	20	N/A
Taco Bell						
Burrito	1 (5.8 oz)	343	48	11	12	272
Taco	1 (3 oz)	186	14	15	8	79
Tostada	1 (5 oz)	179	25	9	6	101

N/A=Not available

This chart was excerpted from a more extensive version in Fast Food Facts, *© 1985 by the International Diabetes Center, 5000 W. 39th St., Minneapolis, MN 55416. The booklet is available for $2.50 (plus 75¢ postage and handling) from the Center.*

EATING AND EXERCISE

For the insulin-dependent diabetic, the timing and level of intensity of exercise can affect the blood sugar level and in turn your food intake. So, before starting a new exercise program, be sure to check with your doctor to work out any adjustments that may be necessary in your treatment program. A good time to exercise is 1 or 2 hours before meals. Don't exercise immediately after an insulin dose or when insulin is at its peak level of effectiveness. Check the blood sugar level before starting any *extra* exercise and eat a snack. If your doctor has not instructed you concerning your blood sugar level, exercise, and food intake, refer to the table on pages 314–15 for some recommendations.

No matter what exercise you choose, be sure to select the proper equipment. Also be sure to drink plenty of water to replace fluids lost by perspiring. Allow for warm-up and cool-down periods for short-term activities and be well prepared for all-day activities like skiing or backpacking by carrying extra food with you. Read pages 309 to 315 in Part IV for a more complete discussion of exercise and diabetes.

EATING IN ETHNIC RESTAURANTS

When eating in an ethnic restaurant, you need to be well-versed in your diet so you can recognize the ingredients in various dishes. Estimate as closely as possible the number of bread, meat, fat, vegetable, and fruit exchanges in the particular dish you are interested in. For example, if food is fried, add 2 or 3 fat exchanges. If it is breaded, add 1 starch exchange. Be sure to count mayonnaise, oil, or salad dressing. It is better to err on the side of slightly overestimating the food exchanges involved rather than underestimating them.

EATING ON AIRPLANES

Most airlines offer a variety of meals to meet special religious or other dietary specifications. Just notify the reservations personnel at least 24 hours in advance of your flight so that the proper preparation can be made. Remind the flight attendant or the gate agent when you check in that you ordered a special meal. It is a good idea to always carry some food with you on a trip in case of delays or mixups with your meal. Let the flight attendant know when you have to eat so your meal is not delayed.

If there is a problem, you should be able to select appropriate foods from the regular airline meal.

EATING AT THE HOME OF A FRIEND

Being invited to dinner at the home of a friend need not pose a problem if you tell your hostess in advance that you are a diabetic and must watch your diet. This will save embarrassment for both of you. She can plan her menu accordingly and it will alleviate the problem of being urged to eat "just a little more" or "to have a piece of chocolate cake." Your hostess will understand if you ask for smaller portions or pass up dessert. Planning ahead will avoid any unnecessary problems.

ALCOHOLIC BEVERAGES

Alcoholic beverages supply calories and should not be used if a low-calorie diet for weight reduction has been prescribed. Alcohol may be used in moderation by some persons with diabetes; however, alcohol may be harmful to others. You should ask your physician or dietitian whether you may use alcoholic beverages and, if so, in what amounts. If alcohol is allowed, it should be taken slowly and with food. Do not use sweet wines, liqueurs, or mixes that contain sugar.

Using wine or other alcoholic beverages is an excellent low-calorie, low-sodium way to flavor food. The calories do not have to be calculated into the diet if alcoholic beverages are used in small amounts. Usually, only 1 or 2 tablespoons of alcohol per serving are used in cooking, and the alcohol evaporates during the heating. The calories that remain are from the carbohydrate or protein contained in the beverage.

An *occasional* cocktail or glass of wine usually is not a problem for diabetics. But talk to the doctor about it first and find out exactly how much and how often you may drink alcoholic beverages. If you drink, do so in moderation. Never drink on an empty stomach. Drink slowly, and avoid sugary or sweet drinks. And do not forget to count the calories and make the necessary adjustments in your meal plan to compensate for the alcoholic beverage. Some of the more common alcoholic beverages are listed below along with some ideas for exchanges between alcoholic beverages and foods on your meal plan.

	Exchanges
Spirits:	
1 ounce gin, rum, vodka, whiskey	2 fat
Wine:	
3½ ounces dry wine	½ starch, ½ fat
2 ounces dry sherry	½ starch, 2 fat
Beer:	
12 ounces regular	1 starch, 2 fat
12 ounces Lite	2 fat

TRAVELING ACROSS TIME ZONES

Traveling by air across time zones can pose a problem for the diabetic. You should always check with your doctor for specific individual instructions concerning the timing of your medications. In general, the diabetic may take meals and insulin doses according to the time of day he or she arrives at the destination. An afternoon dose of insulin usually can be taken on arrival at the destination if it is beyond the time the insulin is normally given. The next day's insulin dose can be administered at the usual time (utilizing the time of the new time zone). When traveling across the Atlantic (west to east), the morning and afternoon insulin doses are taken at the usual times on the day of departure, and the morning dose of insulin is taken at arrival at the destination. When returning (east to west), again follow the time on land—morning insulin dose in Europe and afternoon insulin dose on arrival in the United States. When traveling across the Pacific (east to west), the same rule of following the treatment program depending on the time of day at the destination applies. The afternoon insulin dose can be given on arrival at the destination or en route if necessary. The next day's dose is given according to the time at the destination. When returning (west to east), use the same rules for traveling west to east across the Atlantic. Food should be readily available while you are traveling, and you should eat at appropriate intervals, regardless of the time, to avoid long periods without food.

If you are being treated by diet alone, there are no special precautions necessary when traveling long distances other than to follow the prescribed dietary plan. Those on oral hypoglycemic agents should take their medication at meals, depending on the time of day they plan to arrive at their destination. Be sure to eat at appropriate intervals during the trip to avoid hypoglycemia.

SICK DAYS

When an acute illness occurs, such as an upset stomach, sore throat, or bad cold, it is still necessary to maintain your calorie intake and drug doses even though you may have no appetite or are vomiting. If you are not able to take solid food but can tolerate liquids, you can maintain calorie intake with sweetened juices, regular sweetened soft drinks, sherbets, etc. In this way, you will be able to meet your energy requirements and provide an adequate amount of sugar for insulin action. *When you are ill, stay in close contact with your physician for advice regarding diabetes management.* The blood and urine sugar levels should be checked more frequently, usually every 4 to 6 hours, and you should always test for ketoacids in the urine.

If control of fever or cough is necessary, any standard remedy such as aspirin and sugar-free cough syrup can be used. Sugar-free medications are preferred. In the event of hypoglycemic reaction, administration of the hormone glucagon may be necessary.

Insulin should never be stopped during an illness, regardless of decreased appetite or nausea and vomiting. A physician should help you adjust the dosage as necessary. Usually, more, not less, insulin is needed during an acute illness. If persistent vomiting occurs and the blood sugar remains over 400 mg/dl and the urine ketoacid test remains positive despite the best efforts at control, hospitalization probably will be necessary.

Attempt to eat small amounts frequently. Include water, clear broth, tea, and other fluids to replace lost salt and water. Take sips of carbonated beverages or fruit juices hourly. The need for insulin and food may be increased during illness. Consult your physician if you are ill for more than a day and are unable to maintain your normal routine.

MEAL PLANNING DURING ILLNESS

The diet may need to be modified during a period of illness. If the regular diet cannot be eaten, replace the carbohydrate content of the diet by the following steps:

1. Determine the carbohydrate content of a meal by adding the carbohydrate contents of the fruit, milk, and bread exchanges in the meal plan. For example:

   One milk exchange (12 grams each) = 12 grams
   Two starch/bread exchanges (15 grams each) = 30 grams
   One fruit exchange (15 grams each) = 15 grams
   Total: 57 grams

2. Select a combination of foods from the list below that will give approximately the same amount of carbohydrate as the regular meal. For example:

   1 cup carbonated beverage = 20 grams
   5 saltines = 15 grams
   ¾ cup Jell-O = 20 grams
   Total: 55 grams

Group I

One fruit exchange will provide 15 grams of carbohydrate. The following foods may be substituted for one fruit exchange:

½ cup orange or grapefruit juice
¼ cup grape juice
½ cup regular sweetened carbonated beverage
(gingerale, cola drink, or Seven-Up)
½ of double-stick popsicle

5–6 pieces of hard candy
2 teaspoons granulated sugar, corn syrup, or honey

When nausea occurs, let the carbonated beverage stand open at room temperature before it is served.

Group II

One milk exchange will provide 12 grams of carbohydrate. The following are equal to one milk exchange:

1 cup milk
1 cup buttermilk
1 cup plain yogurt
1 cup milkshake (½ cup milk plus ½ cup vanilla ice cream)

Group III

One starch/bread exchange will provide 15 grams of carbohydrate. The following foods may be substituted for one starch/bread exchange:

1 slice dry toast
½ cup cooked cereal
1 cup creamed soup
½ cup vanilla ice cream
¼ cup sherbet
4 to 5 crackers or melba toast
½ cup sweetened gelatin
1 cup eggnog (1 egg, 6 ounces milk, ¼ cup vanilla ice cream)

If the illness makes it impossible to eat or causes vomiting, clear liquids containing sugar and salt should be taken. Be sure to monitor blood glucose every 2 to 3 hours. If this fluid cannot be taken or vomiting continues, call your physician.

PART II

General Recipes

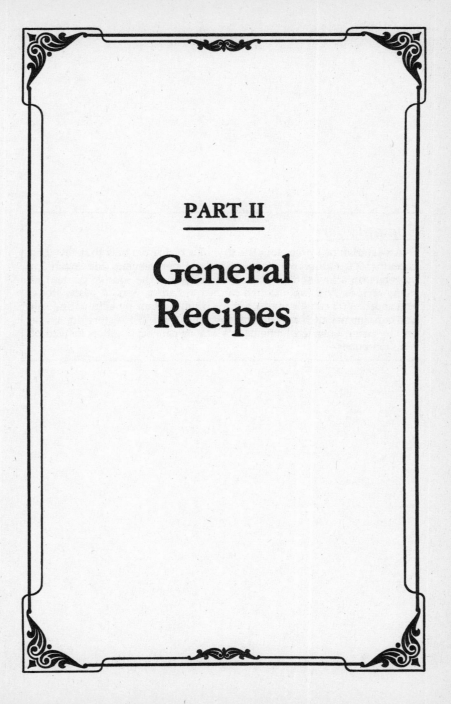

Sodium Alert

An asterisk (*) preceding the title of a recipe denotes that this dish contains 400 milligrams or more sodium per serving, too much for someone on a low-sodium diet. You can lower the sodium content of many recipes by using *unsalted* canned tomatoes, tomato paste, stock, and soups. You can also reduce the sodium content by eliminating salt and condiments such as mustard, soy sauce, and Worcestershire sauce, and by using unsalted homemade stock or canned bouillon instead of bouillon cubes.

NOTES

1. Every effort has been made to be as accurate as possible in the nutrient analysis of the recipes and in the specific yields of each recipe, but variations will occur because of differences in ingredients and in personal cooking techniques. Therefore, the analysis given with each recipe represents the *approximate* nutrient content per serving. These analyses were used to determine the food exchanges for each recipe. Exchanges were calculated to correlate as closely as possible to the nutrient analyses. This is not always absolutely accurate, so you may find some discrepancies.

2. The nutrient content of the recipes will change if ingredients are left out or substituted.

3. In most recipes in this book, 2 egg whites may be substituted for ¼ cup of "egg substitute." One whole egg may be substituted for ¼ cup of "egg substitute," but this greatly increases the cholesterol content of the recipe. The reverse is also true. You can reduce the cholesterol content of many recipes by using egg substitutes or egg whites for whole eggs.

4. If you are using a sugar substitute for sugar in a recipe, follow the specific instructions on the label of the product you select regarding sugar equivalents and specific cooking instructions. These products are different from one another and cannot always be used in the same way. Sugar substitutes *do* contain calories, and these calories can add up when large amounts are used.

5. Follow directions carefully concerning size of portions served because the nutrient content per serving is based on this size. If a larger or a smaller serving is eaten, make the appropriate adjustments in the nutrient content per serving.

6. Unless otherwise specified, medium-sized fruit and vegetables were used for recipes.

7. You can increase your fiber intake by selecting whole-grain products such as whole wheat bread or pasta.

8. The nutrient analysis given for each recipe *does not* include the foods that are suggested as accompaniments to the recipe (i.e., "serve with").

9. Fresh or reconstituted (without added sugar) juices may be used interchangeably unless otherwise specified.

10. Recipes calling for "salt to taste" were calculated to contain ⅛ teaspoon or less of salt per serving.

11. The sodium content of recipes calling for stock, broth, or bouillon can be greatly reduced by using homemade salt-free or low-salt chicken or beef broth. Also, canned chicken and beef broths are lower in sodium content than broths made with cubes or granules.

KITCHEN ARITHMETIC

Sometimes it is difficult to know exactly what size pan or baking dish to use for a recipe. At other times you may not know exactly how much of an ingredient you need to obtain a specific measurement, such as 2 tablespoons of lemon juice or 4 cups of sliced apples. The following information should help you when you are trying to make these decisions.

Baking Dishes	*Equivalents*
4-cup baking dish:	8-inch pie pan
	8 x 1½-inch layer pan
	7⅛ x 3⅝ x 2¼-inch loaf pan
6-cup baking dish:	8- or 9½-inch layer pan
10-inch pie pan:	8½ x 3⅝ x 2⅝-inch loaf pan
8-cup baking dish:	8 x 8 x 2-inch baking pan
	11 x 7 x 1½-inch baking pan
	9 x 5 x 3-inch loaf pan
10-cup baking dish:	8 x 9 x 2-inch baking pan
	11¾ x 7½ x 1¾-inch baking pan
	15½ x 10½ x 1-inch jelly roll pan
12-cup and over baking dish:	13½ x 8¾-inch baking dish equals 12 cups
	15 x 9 x 2-inch baking pan equals 15 cups
	14 x 10½ x 2-inch roasting pan equals 19 cups

Volume of Various Baking Pans

Tubes:	7½ x 3-inch bundt tube pan	6 cups
	9 x 3½-inch fancy tube or bundt pan	9 cups
	9 x 3½-inch angel cake pan	12 cups
	10 x 4-inch angel cake pan	18 cups

Melon mold:	7 x 5½ x 4-inch mold	6 cups
Ring molds:	8½ x 2¼-inch mold	4½ cups
	9¼ x 2¾-inch mold	8 cups

Measurement with Metric Equivalents

Measure	*Equivalent*	*Metric: milliliters (ml), grams (g), or kilograms (kg)*
1 tablespoon	3 teaspoons	14.8 ml
2 tablespoons	1 ounce	29.6 ml
1 jigger	1½ ounces	44.4 ml
¼ cup	4 tablespoons	59.2 ml
⅓ cup	5 tablespoons plus 1 teaspoon	78.9 ml
½ cup	8 tablespoons	118.4 ml
1 cup	16 tablespoons	236.8 ml
1 pint	2 cups	473.6 ml
1 quart	4 cups	947.2 ml
1 liter	4 cups plus 3⅓ tablespoons	1,000 ml
1 ounce (dry)	2 tablespoons	28.35 g
1 pound	16 ounces	453.59 g
2.2 pounds	35.3 ounces	1 kg

Kitchen Substitutions

When the recipe calls for:	*You can use:*
1 tablespoon cornstarch	2 tablespoons flour (for thickening)
1 egg	¼ cup liquid imitation egg substitute
1 cup milk	1 cup skim milk plus 2 tablespoons unsalted margarine; ½ cup evaporated milk plus ½ cup water; 4 tablespoons powdered milk plus 1 cup water; 4 tablespoons nonfat dry milk plus 2 teaspoons oil and 1 cup water
1 cup sour milk	1 cup sweet milk plus 1 tablespoon lemon juice or vinegar
1 cup cake flour	⅞ cup all-purpose flour (⅞ cup is 1 cup less 2 tablespoons)
½ cup margarine	7 tablespoons vegetable shortening
1 cup buttermilk	1 tablespoon white vinegar plus milk to equal 1 cup

1 clove garlic	1 teaspoon garlic salt or 1/8 teaspoon garlic powder
2 teaspoons minced onion	1 teaspoon onion powder
1 tablespoon finely chopped chives	1 teaspoon freeze-dried chives
1 teaspoon dried herbs	1 tablespoon chopped fresh herbs
1 cup sour cream	1 tablespoon lemon juice plus evaporated milk to equal 1 cup
1 tablespoon molasses	1 tablespoon honey

When the recipe calls for:	*You start with:*
1 cup cooked spaghetti or noodles	1½ ounces uncooked noodles
1 cup macaroni	½ cup uncooked macaroni
4 cups sliced potatoes	4 medium potatoes
1 cup cooked rice	6 level tablespoons uncooked rice
2½ cups sliced carrots	1 pound carrots
1 cup canned tomatoes	1½ cups chopped fresh tomatoes, simmered 20 minutes
4 cups shredded cabbage	1 small cabbage (1 pound)
1 teaspoon grated lemon peel	1 medium lemon
2 tablespoons lemon juice	1 medium lemon
1 lemon rind	1 tablespoon grated rind
4 teaspoons grated orange peel	1 medium orange
4 cups sliced apples	4 medium apples
2 cups shredded Swiss or Cheddar cheese	8 ounces Swiss or Cheddar cheese
1 cup cracker crumbs	23 soda crackers
½ cup soft bread crumbs	1 slice fresh bread
2 cups chopped walnuts or pecans	½ pound shelled walnuts or pecans
1 cup cooked dried beans or peas	½ cup plus 1 tablespoon
1 cup cooked dried lentils	6 tablespoons

Meat Roasting Chart

Meat	Weight in pounds	Minutes per pound	Oven temp.	Temp. inside meat
Fresh Pork			°F	°F
Rib and loin	3–7	30–40	325	185
Leg	5	25–30	325	185
Picnic shoulder	5–10	40	325	185
Shoulder, butt	3–10	40–50	325	185
Shoulder, boned and rolled	3–6	60	325	185
Beef				
Standing rib				
Rare	3–7	20	325	135
Medium	3–7	22–25	325	165
Well done	3–7	25–30	325	170
For rolled and boned roasts, increase cooking time 5 to 12 minutes per pound				
Lamb				
Shoulder, well done	4–10	30–40	325	190
Shoulder, boned and rolled	3–6	40	325	182
Leg, medium	5–10	40	325	175
Leg, well done	3–6	40–50	325	182
Crown, well done	3–6	40–50	325	182
Smoked Pork				
Shoulder and picnic hams	5	30–40	325	170
	8	30–40	325	175
Boneless	2	40	325	180
	4	25	325	170
Ham	12–20	16–18	325	170
	Under 10	20	325	175
	Half hams	25	325	170
Veal				
Loin	4–6	35	325	175
Leg	5–10	35	325	175
Boneless shoulder	4–10	45	325	175
Poultry				
Chicken, stuffed	3–5	20–25	325	170
	Over 5	30	325	170
Turkey	8–10	20	325	175
	18–20	14	325	175
Duck	5–10	15	325	175

APPETIZERS AND SOUPS

Feta Cheese Spread with Garlic and Chives

8-ounce package cream cheese, softened
6 ounces feta cheese, soaked in cold water 5 minutes and then drained
4 anchovy fillets, drained
6 tablespoons unsalted margarine (¾ stick), cut into 6 pieces
¼ cup dairy sour cream
2 cloves garlic, minced
2 tablespoons snipped chives
6 drops hot pepper sauce
Freshly ground white pepper

Place cheeses and anchovy fillets in blender container or food processor. Cover and blend, stopping machine and scraping sides of container with rubber scraper. Blend in margarine, 1 tablespoon at a time.

Transfer mixture to bowl and stir in remaining ingredients. Cover and refrigerate at least 5 hours. Remove spread 1 hour before serving (if serving as a dip, keep several hours at room temperature to soften).

Yield: 2 cups

Nutrient analysis of 2 tablespoons: ½ medium-fat meat exchange; 1½ fat exchanges; 97 Calories; 3 g protein; 9 g fat; 1 g carbohydrate; 179 mg sodium; 25 mg cholesterol.

Camembert with Toasted Almonds

4½-ounce can Camembert cheese
1 tablespoon sliced almonds
1½ teaspoons margarine

Preheat oven to 325°F. Remove cheese from can. Unwrap and set aside. Place almonds in can and bake for 5 minutes.

Add margarine to can; place cheese on top of margarine in can. Bake 5 minutes longer. (For spreadable cheese, bake an additional 5 minutes.) Turn cheese onto serving plate.

Yield: ¾ cup

Nutrient analysis of 2 tablespoons: 1 lean meat exchange; 1 fat exchange; 94 Calories; 6 g protein; 8 g fat; 0 g carbohydrate; 190 mg sodium; 16 mg cholesterol.

Oeufs avec Mayonnaise

6 hard-cooked eggs, shelled and chilled
1 cup mayonnaise (see below)
2 tablespoons capers, drained
2 tablespoons snipped parsley

Cut eggs lengthwise into halves. Place halves cut side down on serving platter. Spoon mayonnaise over eggs; garnish with capers and parsley.

Yield: 6 servings

Nutrient analysis of 1 serving: 1 medium-fat meat exchange; 2 fat exchanges; 167 Calories; 7 g protein; 15 g fat; 1 g carbohydrate; 188 mg sodium; 292 mg cholesterol.

Mayonnaise

1 tablespoon plus 1½ teaspoons lemon juice
1 teaspoon prepared Dijon-style mustard
½ teaspoon salt
1 egg
⅓ cup olive oil†
⅔ cup vegetable oil†

Measure lemon juice, mustard, salt, egg, and olive oil into blender container or food processor. Cover and blend for 30 seconds. On high speed, slowly add vegetable oil; continue processing until mixture is consistency of mayonnaise.

Yield: 1½ cups

Nutrient analysis of 2 tablespoons: 4 fat exchanges; 172 Calories; 1 g protein; 19 g fat; 0 g carbohydrate; 92 mg sodium; 22 mg cholesterol.

†1 cup olive or vegetable oil can be substituted for the combined oils.

Crab and Water Chestnut Spread

1 cup flaked cooked crabmeat (6-ounce package frozen cooked crabmeat)
1 cup minced water chestnuts
1 tablespoon soy sauce
2 tablespoons minced scallions
½ cup low-calorie mayonnaise

Mix all ingredients. Serve with whole-grain crackers.

Yield: 2½ cups

Nutrient analysis of 2 tablespoons: 1 lean meat exchange; 51 Calories; 4 g protein; 2 g fat; 3 g carbohydrate; 343 mg sodium; 29 mg cholesterol.

Tuna Amandine

2 ¼-ounce envelopes unflavored gelatin
½ cup cold water
1 cup boiling water
2 8-ounce packages cream cheese, softened
2 tablespoons lemon juice
1 tablespoon curry powder
½ teaspoon salt
¼ teaspoon garlic powder
⅓ cup minced scallions (include tops)
2-ounce jar pimiento, drained and chopped
2 7-ounce cans tuna in water, drained and flaked
1¼ cups sliced almonds, toasted

Sprinkle gelatin on cold water to soften. Stir in boiling water until gelatin is dissolved. Cut cream cheese into pieces; beat into gelatin mixture until smooth. Stir in the lemon juice, curry powder, salt, and garlic powder. Fold in scallions, pimiento, tuna, and ½ cup of the almonds. Pour into 5½-cup mold; chill until firm.

Unmold onto serving platter. Garnish with remaining almonds and, if desired, sliced stuffed olives, parsley, and pimiento strips.

Yield: 5½ cups

Nutrient analysis of 2 tablespoons: ½ lean meat exchange; ½ fat exchange; 48 Calories; 3 g protein; 4 g fat; 1 g carbohydrate; 54 mg sodium; 10 mg cholesterol.

Marinated Mushrooms

2 cups quartered mushrooms
¼ cup Vinaigrette Français (page 91)
1 tablespoon prepared Dijon mustard
1 tablespoon snipped parsley

Place mushrooms in bowl. Mix dressing, mustard, and parsley; pour on mushrooms and toss to coat. Serve immediately or marinate for 2 to 3 hours.

Yield: 4 servings (½ cup each)

Nutrient analysis of 1 serving: ½ vegetable exchange; 1 fat exchange; 58 Calories; 1 g protein; 6 g fat; 2 g carbohydrate; 87 mg sodium; 0 mg cholesterol.

Melon with Prosciutto

1 medium honeydew, Persian, casaba, or Cranshaw melon
12 thin slices prosciutto (Italian ham)
6 slices lime or lemon

Halve melon and remove seeds. Cut each half into 6 slices, then remove rind. Wrap a slice of prosciutto around each melon slice. Garnish with lime slices.

Variations: Substitute 24 fresh ripe figs for the melon. Trim top of each fig and cut open diagonally to make 4 petals. Roll up each prosciutto slice. Serve 4 figs for each serving with rolled-up slices prosciutto.

Substitute 1½ cantaloupes for one of the above melons.

Yield: 6 servings

Nutrient analysis of 1 serving: 1 lean meat exchange; 1 fruit exchange; 114 Calories; 11 g protein; 2 g fat; 14 g carbohydrate; 198 mg sodium; 23 mg cholesterol.

Nachos

48 nacho chips, plain, unsalted
6 ounces shredded Monterey Jack cheese
¼ cup chopped canned Jalapeño chilies

Set oven control at broil or 550°F. Place chips on large baking sheet. Mix cheese and chilies. Top each chip with about 1 teaspoon of the cheese mixture. Broil 3 inches from heat source until cheese is melted, about 1 minute. Serve immediately.

Yield: 6 servings

Nutrient analysis of 8 nachos: 1 starch/bread exchange; 1 medium-fat meat exchange; 2 fat exchanges; 257 Calories; 9 g protein; 16 g fat; 20 g carbohydrate; 266 mg sodium; 25 mg cholesterol.

Vegetables for Dipping

Make an attractive display in a shallow basket of the following fresh vegetables:

- Asparagus, thin, peeled and uncooked or parboiled for 5 minutes and then cooled quickly under cold running water
- Green beans, uncooked if young and tender or parboiled for 5 minutes and then cooled quickly under cold running water
- Carrot spears
- Caulifloweretts
- Celery sticks
- Cucumber, pared and sliced
- Button-size mushrooms
- Peas in pod (have a dish available for empty pods)
- Red and green peppers, cut into strips
- Radishes
- Scallions
- Cherry tomatoes or large tomatoes cut into wedges
- Zucchini, sliced
- Broccoli flowerets
- Snow peas

Nutrient analysis of ½ cup: 1 vegetable exchange; 25 Calories; 2 g protein; 0 g fat; 5 g carbohydrate; 0 mg sodium; 0 mg cholesterol.

Dill Yogurt Dip

1 cup plain low-fat yogurt
⅛ teaspoon garlic powder
1 heaping teaspoon prepared white horseradish
1 heaping teaspoon prepared mustard
¼ cup snipped dill

Mix all ingredients in a small bowl. Cover and refrigerate several hours.

Yield: 1¼ cups

Nutrient analysis of 2 tablespoons: free exchange; 15 Calories; 1 g protein; 0 g fat; 2 g carbohydrate; 24 mg sodium; 1 mg cholesterol.

Favorite Dip

⅓ cup shredded Cheddar cheese
2 tablespoons Low-Calorie Mayonnaise (page 94)
1 cup plain low-fat yogurt

Process cheese and mayonnaise in blender or food processor until smooth. Remove from blender; stir in yogurt. Serve immediately.

Yield: 1½ cups

Nutrient analysis of 2 tablespoons: ¼ skim milk exchange; ½ fat exchange; 48 Calories; 3 g protein; 3 g fat; 2 g carbohydrate; 65 mg sodium; 11 mg cholesterol.

Slim Dip

1 cup low-fat cottage cheese
1 tablespoon plain low-fat yogurt

Process yogurt and cottage cheese in blender at high speed until smooth and creamy. Use as a base for dips and add your favorite flavoring such as taco sauce, mustard, Italian seasonings, etc.

Yield: 1 cup

Nutrient analysis of 1 tablespoon: free exchange.
Nutrient analysis of ¼ cup: ½ lean meat exchange; 36 Calories; 4 g protein; 0 g fat; 0 g carbohydrate; 176 mg sodium; 4 mg cholesterol.

Avocado Dip

2 cups mashed avocado (2 to 3 medium avocados)
2 tablespoons lemon juice
1 teaspoon salt
⅛ teaspoon hot pepper sauce
1 teaspoon Worcestershire sauce
1 clove garlic, crushed
1 medium tomato, peeled and minced
½ cup shredded Cheddar cheese

Mix all ingredients except cheese. Sprinkle cheese on top. Cover and refrigerate. Serve with tortilla or corn chips.

Yield: 3 cups

Nutrient analysis of 2 tablespoons: ½ vegetable exchange; 1 fat exchange; 62 Calories; 2 g protein; 6 g fat; 2 g carbohydrate; 115 mg sodium; 5 mg cholesterol.

Lobster Pâté

10 ounces cooked lobster meat (2 cooked 1-pound lobsters will yield 10 ounces of meat)
⅓ cup lemon juice
¼ teaspoon white pepper
⅛ teaspoon paprika
⅛ teaspoon salt
1 clove garlic, crushed
½ cup olive oil

Cut lobster meat into small pieces; place in bowl of food processor. Using a steel blade, process lobster until finely chopped. Add lemon juice, seasonings, and garlic; process for 1 minute. Pour oil into funnel opening while processing; process until mixture is smooth and thick. Place mixture in covered jar or bowl; refrigerate for at least 2 hours.

At serving time, dip container of pâté into hot water and invert onto serving dish. Serve as a spread.

Yield: 1¾ cups

Nutrient analysis of 2 tablespoons: ½ lean meat exchange; 1 fat exchange; 88 Calories; 4 g protein; 8 g fat; 0 g carbohydrate; 60 mg sodium; 17 mg cholesterol.

Vegetable Tempura

2 egg yolks
1 cup ice water
1 cup all-purpose flour
Green pepper, cut into 1-inch strips
Broccoli flowerets
Carrots, cut into thin rounds
Caulifowerets
Zucchini, cut into thin rounds
2 cups vegetable oil for frying
Dipping Sauce (page 65)

Heat oil to 350°F. in heavy saucepan or deep skillet.

Beat egg yolks; add water and flour and beat until flour is moistened (batter will be lumpy). Use any combination of vegetables listed above to make 4 cups. Dip them into batter. Cook in hot oil until tender and golden brown, about 2 minutes. Drain on paper towels. Serve with dipping sauce.

Yield: Approximately 5 cups

Nutrient analysis of ½ cup vegetables: 1 starch/bread exchange; ½ fat exchange; 93 Calories; 2 g protein; 3 g fat; 13 g carbohydrate; 13 mg sodium; 34 mg cholesterol.

*Dipping Sauce for Vegetable Tempura

½ cup rice wine or dry sherry
½ cup soy sauce
1 teaspoon minced fresh ginger

Mix all ingredients together.

Yield: 1 cup

Nutrient analysis of 1 tablespoon: free exchange.
Nutrient analysis of ¼ cup: ½ starch/bread exchange; 44 Calories; 4 g protein; 0 g fat; 8 g carbohydrate; 2060 mg sodium; 0 mg cholesterol.

Zucchini Antipasto

¼ cup olive oil
1 pound zucchini, cut into ¼-inch slices
Dash garlic salt
Dash freshly ground pepper
1 small onion, thinly sliced
2 teaspoons dried oregano

Preheat oven to 350°F.

Pour olive oil onto large baking sheet or jelly roll pan, 15½ x 10½ x 1 inch. Add zucchini slices and turn with spatula until all are coated with oil. Arrange slices so they overlap slightly on pan. Season with garlic salt and pepper, then sprinkle with onion slices and oregano. Bake for 20 minutes at 350°F.

Set oven control at broil or 550°F. Broil 3 inches from heat source until light brown, about 3 to 5 minutes. Cool and serve.

Variations: *Eggplant Antipasto:* Instead of zucchini, substitute 1-pound eggplant, pared, halved, and cut into ⅛- to ¼-inch slices; increase olive oil to ⅓ cup and omit oregano.

Onion Antipasto: Instead of zucchini, substitute 2 large Spanish onions, cut into 1-inch slices. Eliminate small onion slices.

Yield: 8 servings (2 ounces each)

Nutrient analysis of 2-ounce serving: ½ vegetable exchange; 1 fat exchange; 53 Calories; 1 g protein; 5 g fat; 1 g carbohydrate; 275 mg sodium; 0 mg cholesterol.

Stuffed Vine Leaves

1 jar (16 ounces) grape leaves
1 pound lean ground lamb
1 large onion, chopped
¾ cup uncooked regular white rice
1 ounce pine nuts, minced (optional)
1½ tablespoons olive oil
¼ cup snipped parsley
2 tablespoons chopped mint leaves
½ teaspoon salt
¼ teaspoon freshly ground pepper
½ teaspoon cinnamon
⅛ teaspoon ground cloves
Juice of 1 lemon
1½ cups beef bouillon
2 eggs

Preheat oven to 325°F.

Wash grape leaves well under cold running water. Place on paper towels, shiny side down, and cut off stems.

Cook and stir meat, onion, rice, and nuts in oil until meat is brown. Stir in parsley, mint leaves, salt, pepper, cinnamon, and cloves. Place 1 tablespoon of the meat mixture on each leaf. Fold up base of leaf, then fold sides to center and roll up tightly to top of leaf. Place rolls close together in baking pan, 13 x 9 x 2 inches. Sprinkle lemon juice over rolls and pour on bouillon. Bake at 325°F. for 1 hour.

Remove pan from oven and drain liquid from pan into saucepan. Beat eggs; stir into saucepan. Cook, stirring constantly, until mixture thickens and boils. Cool slightly. Pour sauce over rolls and refrigerate until serving time. Rolls will keep for 2 or 3 days.

Yield: 40 rolls

Nutrient analysis of 3 rolls: ¾ starch/bread exchange; 1 lean meat exchange; ½ fat exchange; 130 Calories; 9 g protein; 6 g fat; 9 g carbohydrate; 198 mg sodium; 70 mg cholesterol.

Broiled Scallops

2 pounds sea scallops, washed and drained
½ cup vegetable oil
½ cup olive oil
1 cup dry white wine
1 clove garlic, minced
1 teaspoon dried tarragon
½ teaspoon salt
Freshly ground pepper to taste
½ cup snipped parsley

Place scallops in deep bowl. Mix remaining ingredients and pour over scallops. Cover and refrigerate for at least 2 hours, turning scallops occasionally.

Set oven control at broil or 550°F. Arrange scallops on small skewers and place on broiler rack. Broil 3 inches from heat source, turning frequently to cook scallops on all sides, about 5 minutes.

Yield: 32 appetizer servings (1 ounce each)

Nutrient analysis of 1 appetizer serving: 1 lean meat exchange; 1/4 fat exchange; 60 Calories; 5 g protein; 4 g fat; 1 g carbohydrate; 86 mg sodium; 11 mg cholesterol.

Yield: 8 main-course servings (4 ounces each)

Nutrient analysis of 1 main-course serving: 3 medium-fat meat exchanges; 1 fat exchange; 241 Calories; 21 g protein; 15 g fat; 4 g carbohydrate; 346 mg sodium; 45 mg cholesterol.

Broiled Stuffed Mushrooms

1 pound small mushrooms
1 green pepper, seeded and finely chopped
3 scallions, chopped (include green tops)
2 tablespoons margarine
1/4 cup bread crumbs
1/4 cup snipped parsley
1/4 teaspoon dried oregano
Dash cayenne pepper
3 tablespoons shredded part-skim-milk mozzarella cheese
2 teaspoons dry white wine
3 tablespoons margarine, melted
Paprika to taste

Trim mushrooms; remove stems and reserve caps for stuffing. Chop stems. Cook and stir mushroom stems, green pepper, and scallions in 2 tablespoons margarine until mushrooms are brown. Stir in the bread crumbs, parsley, oregano, cayenne pepper, cheese, and wine and cook until heated through.

Brush mushroom caps with the 3 tablespoons melted margarine. Press stuffing into caps and place on broiler rack. Sprinkle with paprika. Set oven control at broil or 550°F. Broil mushroom caps 3 to 4 inches from heat until tender, 4 to 5 minutes.

Yield: 50–60 stuffed mushrooms

Nutrient analysis of 5 mushrooms: 1 vegetable exchange; 1 fat exchange; 76 Calories; 2 g protein; 5 g fat; 5 g carbohydrate; 85 mg sodium; 0 mg cholesterol.

Appetizer Chicken Wings

3 pounds chicken wings (about 15)
½ cup lemon juice
½ cup vegetable oil
3 cloves garlic, crushed
1 teaspoon salt
1 teaspoon freshly ground pepper

Cut bony wing tips from wings and discard. Separate chicken wings at joint. Place wing halves in shallow baking dish. Mix lemon juice, oil, garlic, salt, and pepper; pour over wing halves. Cover and refrigerate for at least 4 hours, turning occasionally.

Preheat oven to 400°F. Remove wing halves from marinade; place on rack in shallow pan. Bake for 45 minutes.

Wings can be frozen after they are baked. To serve, thaw at room temperature. Place on rack in broiler pan; broil until hot, 3 to 4 minutes.

Note: Fifteen pounds will serve 40 people.

Yield: 30 pieces

Nutrient analysis of 1 piece: ⅓ lean meat exchange; ½ fat exchange; 35 Calories; 2 g protein; 3 g fat; 0 g carbohydrate; 74 mg sodium; 9 mg cholesterol.

Asparagus Vinaigrette

1 pound asparagus, trimmed
½ cup vegetable or olive oil
2 tablespoons tarragon vinegar
1 tablespoon lemon juice
1 tablespoon chopped scallion
1½ teaspoons prepared mustard
1 clove garlic, crushed
¼ to ½ teaspoon dried tarragon, crushed
⅛ teaspoon salt

Place asparagus in a large skillet with 1 inch of salted water (½ teaspoon salt to 1 cup water). Cover and cook until just crisp-tender, 5 to 10 minutes. Drain and place asparagus in shallow dish. Mix remaining ingredients and pour over asparagus. Cover and refrigerate for 2 hours. Drain before serving. (Marinade may be used as salad dressing.)

Yield: 4 servings (3 ounces each)

Nutrient analysis of 3-ounce serving: 1 vegetable exchange; 1 fat exchange; 73 Calories; 3 g protein; 6 g fat; 5 g carbohydrate; 88 mg sodium; 0 mg cholesterol.

Tuscan Appetizer

12 ½-inch slices Italian bread
2 large tomatoes, chopped
½ red onion, chopped (optional)
¼ cup chopped fresh basil
Dash garlic salt
Dash freshly ground pepper
⅓ cup olive oil

Arrange bread slices on large platter. Stir tomatoes, onion, and basil together in bowl. Season with garlic salt and pepper. Cover bread slices with tomato mixture. Drizzle olive oil over top. Serve immediately.

Yield: 6 servings

Nutrient analysis of 1 serving: 1½ starch/bread exchanges; 2½ fat exchanges; 217 Calories; 4 g protein; 12 g fat; 24 g carbohydrate; 277 mg sodium; 0 mg cholesterol.

Beef Kebabs

1 pound lean ground beef
1 slice whole wheat bread, soaked in water and squeezed
2 onions, minced
2 cloves garlic, crushed
2 teaspoons snipped fresh coriander or ½ teaspoon ground coriander
¼ teaspoon cayenne pepper
2 teaspoons curry powder
½ teaspoon salt
1-inch piece ginger root, chopped
1 or 2 green chili peppers, thinly sliced
¼ teaspoon cloves
½ teaspoon cinnamon
¼ cup vegetable oil

Mix all ingredients except oil. Shape mixture into small balls. Heat oil in large skillet. Cook meatballs in oil until cooked through and brown. Serve as appetizers. Mixture can be shaped into larger meatballs for main dish.

Yield: 50 appetizer meatballs

Nutrient analysis of 3 meatballs: 1 lean meat exchange; ½ vegetable exchange; 72 Calories; 6 g protein; 3 g fat; 3 g carbohydrate; 81 mg sodium; 18 mg cholesterol.

Tabbouleh

1¾ cups bulgur wheat†
7 cups boiling water
1 tablespoon dried mint leaves or 3 tablespoons minced fresh mint leaves
½ cup minced scallions
2 large tomatoes, peeled, seeded, and chopped
2 cups seeded, chopped green pepper
½ teaspoon salt
½ teaspoon freshly ground pepper
2 tablespoons olive oil
2 tablespoons fresh lemon juice

Measure bulgur wheat into large bowl. Stir in boiling water, cover, and let stand until wheat is light and fluffy and water is absorbed, 2 to 3 hours.

Drain any liquid from wheat. Stir in remaining ingredients. Cover and chill for 1 to 2 hours before serving.

Variation: *Tomato Stuffed with Tabbouleh*—For each serving, cut top off tomato. Carefully remove pulp from tomato (reserve pulp for later use). Spoon ½ cup tabbouleh into tomato. Serve on lettuce.

Yield: 6 cups

Nutrient analysis of 1 cup: 1½ starch/bread exchanges; 1 vegetable exchange; 1 fat exchange; 167 Calories; 4 g protein; 5 g fat, 27 g carbohydrate; 166 mg sodium; 0 mg cholesterol.

†Bulgur wheat is sometimes called parboiled wheat. It is whole wheat that has been cooked, dried, partially debranned, and cracked into coarse fragments. It resembles whole wheat in nutritive properties and is used in place of rice in many recipes. This ancient all-wheat food originated in the Near East.

*Cream of Asparagus Soup

1 pound asparagus, trimmed and cut into 1-inch pieces
3½ cups homemade or canned chicken stock†
¼ cup margarine
¼ cup all-purpose flour
½ cup half and half cream (20%)
½ teaspoon salt
⅛ teaspoon pepper

Cook asparagus in 1 cup stock until tender, 12 to 15 minutes. Drain and set aside.

†Chicken stock also can be made by dissolving 3 chicken bouillon cubes or 3 teaspoons chicken bouillon granules in 3½ cups boiling water. Or, use canned or strained homemade stock.

Melt the margarine in a saucepan. Stir in flour. Cook, stirring constantly, until smooth and bubbly. Stir in remaining stock. Cook, stirring constantly, until mixture thickens and boils. Boil and stir for 1 minute. Stir in cream, seasonings, and asparagus and heat.

Variation: *Cream of Broccoli Soup:* Substitute 1 pound broccoli, trimmed and chopped, for the asparagus.

Yield: 6 cups

Nutrient analysis of 1 cup: 1½ vegetable exchanges; 2 fat exchanges; 126 Calories; 3 g protein; 10 g fat; 8 g carbohydrate; 440 mg sodium; 15 mg cholesterol.

*Hot and Sour Soup

4 dried black Chinese mushrooms
4 cups beef or chicken stock
¼ pound lean pork, cut into thin strips
2 bean curd cakes, cut into thin strips
2 tablespoons cornstarch
2 tablespoons water
2 tablespoons white vinegar
1 teaspoon soy sauce
½ teaspoon hot pepper sauce
2 tablespoons dry sherry
2 eggs, beaten
Dash coarse salt
Freshly ground pepper to taste
1 tablespoon sesame oil
1 scallion, chopped

Soak mushrooms in cold water for 30 minutes. Drain, reserving liquid. In a large saucepan, heat stock, reserved mushroom liquid, mushrooms, and pork strips to boiling. Reduce heat and simmer for 10 minutes. Add bean curd strips and simmer 5 minutes longer. Mix the cornstarch, water, vinegar, soy sauce and hot pepper sauce. Stir into hot stock mixture. Cook, stirring constantly, until mixture boils. Reduce heat to lowest setting; stir in sherry and eggs. Season with salt and pepper to taste. Stir in sesame oil and scallion.

Yield: 6 cups

Nutrient analysis of 1 cup: 1 medium-fat meat exchange; 1 vegetable exchange; 1 fat exchange; 141 Calories; 9 g protein; 9 g fat; 6 g carbohydrate; 456 mg sodium; 101 mg cholesterol.

*Pork and Watercress Soup

- ½ pound lean pork, cut into shreds
- 4 cups water
- 4 cups chicken stock
- 1 small onion, thinly sliced
- 1 clove garlic, crushed
- ¼ teaspoon pepper
- 1 teaspoon salt
- 1 bunch watercress, cut into 1-inch pieces

Heat meat and water to boiling in large saucepan. Reduce heat, cover, and simmer for 10 minutes. Add chicken stock, onion, garlic, pepper, and salt. Heat to boiling. Reduce heat, cover, and simmer for 10 minutes. Stir in watercress; heat to boiling and serve.

Yield: 6 cups

Nutrient analysis of ½ cup: 1 starch/bread exchange; 1 lean meat exchange; 103 Calories; 8 g protein; 1 g fat; 16 g carbohydrate; 490 mg sodium; 1 mg cholesterol.

*Split Pea Soup

- ½ cup dried split peas, soaked overnight
- 4 cups water
- 3 teaspoons instant chicken bouillon or 3 chicken bouillon cubes
- 1 clove garlic, minced
- 1 cup sliced pared potato
- 1 onion, sliced
- ½ cup sliced carrots
- 2 teaspoons dried oregano

Place all ingredients in large saucepan. Heat to boiling, stirring occasionally. Reduce heat, cover, and simmer for 1 hour. Let cool until soup can be poured into blender container or food processor; process until smooth. Heat and serve.

Yield: 6 cups

Nutrient analysis of 1 cup: 1 medium-fat meat exchange; 1 vegetable exchange; 103 Calories; 13 g protein; 5 g fat; 2 g carbohydrate; 981 mg sodium; 26 mg cholesterol.

Oyster Stew

¼ cup margarine
¼ cup diced onion
1 teaspoon paprika
1 quart fresh oysters
2 tablespoons cornstarch
½ teaspoon salt
⅛ teaspoon white pepper
4 cups milk

Melt margarine in 2-quart saucepan. Add onion and cook and stir until tender. Add paprika and oysters (with liquor). Cook over medium heat, stirring occasionally, until edges of oysters begin to curl, about 5 minutes. Blend cornstarch, salt, pepper, and milk; stir into oyster mixture. Cook, stirring constantly, *just* until mixture boils. Remove from heat and serve.

Yield: 8 cups

Nutrient analysis of 1 cup: 1 medium-fat meat exchange; ½ whole milk exchange; 127 Calories; 6 g protein; 9 g fat; 6 g carbohydrate; 211 mg sodium; 34 mg cholesterol.

**Lentil Soup*

1 pound lentils
3 quarts water
1 pound kielbasa, sliced
2 onions, chopped
1 clove garlic, minced
2 cups diced celery (with leaves)
6-ounce can tomato paste
½ teaspoon hot pepper sauce
1 teaspoon salt
1 teaspoon dry mustard
Dash freshly ground pepper
Snipped parsley to taste
Minced onion to taste

Soak lentils in water overnight as directed on package. Drain lentils and place in large soup kettle. Add the water and all the remaining ingredients except parsley and minced onion. Heat to boiling. Reduce heat, cover, and simmer until lentils are tender, 3 to 4 hours. Cool and refrigerate overnight.

To serve, heat to boiling, stirring occasionally. Serve topped with parsley and minced onion to taste.

Yield: 20 cups

Nutrient analysis of 2 cups: 2 starch/bread exchanges; 1 high-fat meat exchange; 1 vegetable exchange; 277 Calories; 16 g protein; 9 g fat; 34 g carbohydrate; 560 mg sodium; 21 mg cholesterol.

*Torsk (Cod) Chowder

1 pound torsk (cod)
2 cups water
2 cups diced pared potatoes
½ cup chopped celery
½ cup chopped onion
2 tablespoons chopped pimiento
1½ teaspoons salt
2 cups milk
1 tablespoon flour
2 slices bacon, crisply cooked and crumbled
1 tablespoon margarine
Dillweed

Skin cod if necessary and cut into ½-inch pieces. Heat water, potatoes, celery, onion, pimiento, and salt to boiling in 3-quart saucepan. Reduce heat, cover, and simmer for 10 minutes. Add fish, cover, and simmer until fish and potatoes are tender, about 5 minutes. Stir in 1¾ cups milk. Blend remaining milk and flour; stir into chowder. Heat to just below boiling, stirring constantly. Stir in bacon and margarine. Sprinkle dillweed on servings.

Yield: approximately 8 cups (6 servings)

Nutrient analysis of 1⅓ cup serving: 1½ lean meat exchanges; 1 whole milk exchange; 200 Calories; 21 g protein; 7 g fat; 12 g carbohydrate; 643 mg sodium; 51 mg cholesterol.

*Mushroom and Barley Soup

2 tablespoons margarine
1 onion, chopped
¾ pound mushrooms, chopped
2 tablespoons flour
5 cups beef stock
¼ cup plus 1 tablespoon barley
Juice of ½ lemon
Salt and freshly ground pepper to taste
Chopped fresh parsley to taste

Melt margarine in large saucepan or soup kettle. Add onion and mushrooms. Cover and cook over low heat for 10 minutes. Stir in flour until bubbly. Stir in beef stock. Heat to boiling, stirring constantly. Boil and stir for 1 minute. Stir in barley; heat to boiling. Reduce heat, cover, and simmer until barley is tender, about 30 minutes. Stir in lemon juice and season with salt and pepper. Garnish with parsley.

Yield: 8 cups

Nutrient analysis of 1 cup: 1 starch/bread exchange; 1 fat exchange; 97 Calories; 3 g protein; 4 g fat; 13 g carbohydrate; 615 mg sodium; 0 mg cholesterol.

Cockaleekie Soup

1 stewing chicken, about 3½–4 pounds
3 quarts water
4 large leeks, cut into ½-inch slices (use 2 inches of green)
3 large carrots, diced
⅓ cup barley
2 teaspoons salt
Dash white pepper
1 bay leaf
2 tablespoons snipped parsley

Remove fat from chicken. Place whole chicken in large soup kettle. Add water, and heat to boiling. Skim off foam. Add vegetables, barley, salt, pepper, and bay leaf. Heat to boiling. Reduce heat, cover, and simmer until meat begins to fall from bones, 3 to 4 hours. Remove chicken and cool slightly. Remove skin and bones and discard. Cut meat into thin shreds. Skim any fat from broth and discard bay leaf. Return meat to broth and heat. Season to taste. Sprinkle servings with parsley.

Yield: 16 cups

Nutrient analysis of 1 cup: 2 lean meat exchanges; 1 vegetable exchange; 136 Calories; 19 g protein; 5 g fat; 4 g carbohydrate; 302 mg sodium; 56 mg cholesterol.

Chilled Cantaloupe Soup

1 small (2 pound) ripe cantaloupe†
2 teaspoons fresh lemon juice
1 teaspoon curry powder
1 teaspoon minced fresh mint leaves

Halve cantaloupe. Remove seeds, pare, and cut up fruit. Place fruit, lemon juice, and curry powder in blender container or food processor. Cover and process at high speed until smooth. Refrigerate several hours. Serve in cups and garnish with mint leaves.

Yield: 2½ cups

Nutrient analysis of ½ cup: 1 fruit exchange; 54 Calories; 1 g protein; 0 g fat; 13 g carbohydrate; 14 mg sodium; 0 mg cholesterol.

†Cantaloupe should be very ripe—soft to touch.

*Minestrone Soup

4 cups water
½ cup dried navy, great Northern, or white kidney beans
¼ cup margarine
1 cup minced onion
½ cup minced leek, white part plus 1 inch of green
½ cup diced celery
2 cups diced unpared zucchini
2 cups diced carrot
1½ cups diced pared potato
28-ounce can peeled Italian plum tomatoes, drained
2½ cups chicken stock
2 bay leaves
4 sprigs parsley
1 teaspoon salt
Dash freshly ground pepper
½ cup uncooked regular rice

Heat water to boiling in medium saucepan. Add beans; heat to boiling and boil for 5 minutes, stirring frequently. Remove from heat and let beans soak in water for 3 to 4 hours. (Do not drain.)

Melt margarine in large kettle or Dutch oven. Add onion, leek, celery, and 1 cup each of the zucchini, carrot, and potato. Cook and stir until vegetables are coated, 2 to 3 minutes. Stir in tomatoes (break up tomatoes with spoon), stock, bay leaves, parsley, salt, and pepper. Heat to boiling. Reduce heat, cover, and simmer for 2 hours.

Discard bay leaves and parsley. Stir in remaining zucchini, carrot, and potato, the rice, and the beans with their liquid. Heat to boiling, stirring occasionally. Reduce heat, cover, and simmer for 1 hour.

Variation: Soup can be served with grated Parmesan cheese sprinkled on top. Count extra calories and exchanges for the cheese (2 tablespoons of grated Parmesan cheese contain 46 calories and is equal to 1 fat exchange).

Yield: 15 cups

Nutrient analysis of 1 cup: 1 starch/bread exchange; 1 fat exchange; 104 Calories; 3 g protein; 4 g fat; 15 g carbohydrate; 415 mg sodium; 0 mg cholesterol.

Gazpacho

2 medium tomatoes, peeled and chopped
1 medium zucchini, diced
1 celery stalk, finely chopped
1 small red onion, minced
1 clove garlic, crushed
4 cups canned tomato juice
Juice of 3 limes
Lime slices

Combine about ⅓ of the chopped vegetables, the garlic, and 1 cup of the tomato juice in blender container or food processor. Process until vegetables are pureed. Mix pureed vegetables and remaining vegetables in large bowl. Stir in remaining tomato juice and lime juice. Chill at least 4 hours. Garnish servings with lime slice.

Yield: 4 cups

Nutrient analysis of 1 cup: 3 vegetable exchanges; 69 Calories; 4 g protein; 1 g fat: 16 g carbohydrate; 356 mg sodium; 0 mg cholesterol.

*Vegetable Barley Soup

1 tablespoon vegetable oil
½ cup chopped onion
1 cup celery, thinly sliced
1 cup carrot, thinly sliced
1 clove garlic, minced
6 cups beef bouillon
16-ounce can tomatoes, undrained
2 tablespoons Worcestershire sauce
1 bay leaf
1 to 1½ teaspoons salt
½ teaspoon basil leaves, crushed
½ pound green beans, cut into 1½-inch pieces†
⅔ cup barley
Freshly ground pepper

Heat oil in 4-quart saucepan or kettle. Add onion, celery, carrot, and garlic; cook and stir over medium heat for 2 minutes. Add remaining ingredients; heat to boiling. Reduce heat, cover, and simmer until barley is tender, 1 to 1½ hours.

Yield: 12 cups

Nutrient analysis of 1 cup: 1 starch/bread exchange; 82 Calories; 2 g protein; 2 g fat; 14 g carbohydrate; 690 mg sodium; 0 mg cholesterol.

†A 10-ounce package of frozen cut green beans or a 16-ounce can of cut green beans, drained, can be substituted for the fresh beans. Add these beans during last 10 minutes of cooking.

SALADS AND SALAD DRESSINGS

Watercress Salad

2 cups watercress leaves
1 cup sliced Belgian endive
1 medium avocado, pared and cubed (1 cup)
¼ cup low-calorie Italian dressing†

Combine watercress leaves, endive, and avocado in salad bowl. Pour dressing over ingredients and toss.

Yield: 4 servings (1 cup each)

Nutrient analysis of 1 serving: 1 vegetable exchange; 1½ fat exchanges; 99 Calories; 1 g protein; 8 g fat; 5 g carbohydrate; 247 mg sodium; 2 mg cholesterol.

†Commercial. Usually has 2 calories per teaspoon.

Romaine Salad

1 large bunch romaine lettuce
1 tablespoon sliced scallion
2 ounces Swiss cheese, diced
1 tablespoon red wine vinegar
⅛ teaspoon garlic powder
¼ teaspoon dry mustard
⅛ teaspoon salt
Dash freshly ground pepper
3 tablespoons olive or vegetable oil

Tear lettuce into bite-size pieces and place in salad bowl. Add scallion and cheese. Shake remaining ingredients in screw-top jar; pour over ingredients in bowl and toss.

Yield: 8 servings (1½ cups each)

Nutrient analysis of 1 serving: 1½ fat exchanges; 79 Calories; 2 g protein; 7 g fat; 1 g carbohydrate; 53 mg sodium; 6 mg cholesterol.

Salad Combo

1 cup watercress leaves
1 cup sliced Belgian endive
½ cup thinly sliced zucchini
½ cup sliced plum tomato
1 cup bite-size pieces leaf lettuce
½ cup thinly sliced scallion
½ cup bite-size pieces curly endive

Combine all ingredients in salad bowl and toss. Serve with your favorite salad dressing.

Yield: 5 servings (1 cup each)

Nutrient analysis of 1 serving (without dressing): free exchange; 14 Calories; 1 g protein; 0 g fat; 3 g carbohydrate; 7 mg sodium; 0 mg cholesterol.

California Salad

½ cup alfalfa sprouts
2 cups watercress leaves
½ cup diced unpared zucchini
¼ cup sliced radish
1 cup thinly sliced carrot
6 to 8 cherry tomatoes
Salad dressing of choice (see pages 88–94)

Measure sprouts and vegetables into salad bowl and toss. Serve with dressing.

Yield: 6 servings (1 cup each)

Nutrient analysis of 1 serving (without dressing): 1 vegetable exchange; 26 Calories; 1 g protein; 0 g fat; 6 g carbohydrate; 20 mg sodium; 0 mg cholesterol.

*Caesar Salad

1 clove garlic, halved
1/3 cup olive oil
8 anchovy fillets, cut up (optional)
1 teaspoon Worcestershire sauce
1/2 teaspoon salt
1/4 teaspoon dry mustard
Freshly ground pepper
1 large or 2 small bunches romaine lettuce, washed and chilled
Coddled egg (see below)
1 lemon
Garlic croutons (see below)
1/3 cup grated Parmesan cheese

Just before serving, rub large salad bowl with cut clove of garlic. A few small slivers of garlic can be left in bowl. Add oil, anchovies, Worcestershire sauce, salt, mustard, and pepper; mix thoroughly.

Into salad bowl, tear romaine lettuce into bite-size pieces (about 12 cups). Toss until leaves glisten. Break egg onto lettuce; squeeze juice from lemon over lettuce. Toss until leaves are well coated. Sprinkle croutons and cheese over salad and toss.

Yield: 6 servings (2 cups each)

Nutrient analysis of 1 serving: 1/2 starch/bread exchange; 1/2 lean meat exchange; 1 vegetable exchange; 4 fat exchanges; 283 Calories; 8 g protein; 24 g fat; 12 g carbohydrate; 428 mg sodium; 49 mg cholesterol.

Garlic Croutons: Heat oven to 400°F. Trim crusts from 4 slices whole wheat bread. Spread both sides of bread with butter or margarine; sprinkle with 1/4 teaspoon garlic powder. Cut into 1/2-inch cubes and place in baking pan. Bake for 10 to 15 minutes, stirring occasionally, until golden brown and crisp.

Coddled Egg: Place cold egg in warm water. In separate pan place enough water to completely cover egg and heat to boiling. With a spoon, immerse egg into boiling water. Remove pan from heat; cover and let stand for 30 seconds. Immediately cool egg in cold water.

Chelese Salad

2 cups ½-inch pieces Belgian endive
3 packed cups (6 ounces) arugula pieces
¼ cup Dijon Vinaigrette (see below)

Combine all ingredients in salad bowl and toss. Serve immediately.

Yield: 5 servings (1 cup each)

Nutrient analysis of 1 serving: free exchange; 12 Calories; 0 g protein; 0 g fat; 0 g carbohydrate; trace sodium; 0 mg cholesterol.

Dijon Vinaigrette

1 cup vegetable oil
⅓ cup red wine vinegar
2 to 3 tablespoons prepared Dijon mustard
½ teaspoon freshly ground pepper
1 tablespoon dried fines herbs

Measure all ingredients into screw-top jar. Cover tightly and shake. Refrigerate for at least 2 hours.

Yield: 1½ cups

Nutrient analysis of 2 tablespoons: ½ fat exchange; 28 Calories; 0 g protein; 3 g fat; 0 g carbohydrate; 8 mg sodium; 0 mg cholesterol.

Zucchini Salad

½ pound spinach
1 cup cherry tomatoes, halved
1 cup thinly sliced unpared zucchini (1 medium)
3 thinly sliced scallions (include green tops)

Wash spinach; remove stems and tear leaves into bite-size pieces. Dry and chill. Combine spinach, tomato halves, zucchini, and scallions in salad bowl and toss. Serve with Spicy Italian Salad Dressing (page 93).

Yield: 6 servings (1 cup each)

Nutrient analysis of 1 serving (without dressing): 1 vegetable exchange; 32 Calories; 3 g protein; 0 g fat; 5 g carbohydrate; 29 mg sodium; 0 mg cholesterol.

Spinach Salad

- 10 ounces spinach (about 5 cups)
- 1 teaspoon grated onion
- 1/4 teaspoon salt
- Dash freshly ground pepper
- 1 teaspoon prepared Dijon mustard
- 1 tablespoon red wine vinegar
- 2 tablespoons olive oil
- Dash lemon juice
- 5 radishes, sliced thin

Wash spinach; remove stems and tear leaves into bite-size pieces. Dry and chill. Beat onion, salt, pepper, mustard, vinegar, and oil with fork. Stir in lemon juice (if dressing separates, beat with fork). Pour dressing over spinach in salad bowl; add radish slices and toss.

Yield: 6 servings (3/4 cup each)

Nutrient analysis of 1 serving: 1 vegetable exchange; 1 fat exchange; 67 Calories; 3 g protein; 5 g fat; 4 g carbohydrate; 152 mg sodium; 0 mg cholesterol.

Curried Fruit Salad

Arrange banana chunks, pineapple chunks or slices, seedless green grapes, apple slices, and melon wedges on platter. Serve with Curried Fruit Salad Dressing (see below).

Calculate nutrient analysis according to fruit selected.

Curried Fruit Salad Dressing

- 3/4 cup plain low-fat yogurt
- 1/4 cup low-calorie mayonnaise
- 1 teaspoon sugar
- 1 teaspoon curry powder
- 1/8 teaspoon salt
- 1 teaspoon minced fresh ginger root
- 1 teaspoon lemon juice

Mix all ingredients. Cover and refrigerate for at least 3 hours.

Yield: 1 cup

Nutrient analysis of 2 tablespoons: 1/2 fat exchange; 25 Calories; 1 g protein; 1 g fat; 2 g carbohydrate; 40 mg sodium; 5 mg cholesterol.

Citrus Salad

1 large ripe avocado
Lemon juice
2 oranges, peeled, pitted and sectioned
2 grapefruit, peeled, pitted and sectioned
Bibb lettuce

Cut avocado crosswise in half; remove pit. Peel off skin and cut into ¼-inch slices. Sprinkle slices with lemon juice. Arrange avocado slices and fruit sections on lettuce. Serve with Fruit French Dressing (page 90).

Yield: 4 servings

Nutrient analysis of 1 serving (without dressing): 1 vegetable exchange; 1 fruit exchange; 3 fat exchanges; 220 Calories; 2 g protein; 8 g fat; 16 g carbohydrate; 0 mg sodium; 0 mg cholesterol.

Sweet-'n'-Sour Fruit Slaw

1 small cabbage (14 to 15 ounces), coarsely shredded
1 medium apple, seeded and chopped
1 cup seedless grapes, halved
11-ounce can Mandarin orange sections (in natural juice or sugar-free), drained
¼ cup raisins
1 cup cottage cheese
¼ cup milk
3 tablespoons lemon juice
2 tablespoons vegetable oil
2 tablespoons honey

Combine cabbage, apple, grapes, orange sections, and raisins in a large bowl and set aside. Measure cottage cheese, milk, lemon juice, oil, and honey into blender container or food processor; process until smooth. Pour dressing over cabbage mixture and toss. Chill for 1 hour.

Yield: 10 servings (½ cup each)

Nutrient analysis of 1 serving: ½ lean meat exchange; 1 fruit exchange; 89 Calories; 3 g protein; 3 g fat; 13 g carbohydrate; 75 mg sodium; 4 mg cholesterol.

Summit Salad

1 cup thinly sliced Belgian endive
2 cups bite-size pieces leaf lettuce
1 cup watercress leaves
1 cup bite-size orange sections
½ green pepper, seeded and cut into thin strips 1 inch long
½ avocado, peeled and diced

Toss all ingredients in large bowl. Top with desired dressing. Tarragon Salad Dressing (page 92) goes well with this salad.

Yield: 6 cups

Nutrient analysis of 1 cup: 1½ vegetable exchanges; ½ fat exchange; 55 Calories; 1 g protein; 3 g fat; 7 g carbohydrate; 6 mg sodium; 0 mg cholesterol.

Salad Niçoise

1 pound romaine lettuce
1 pound fresh green beans, cooked crisp-tender†
16 cherry tomatoes, halved
¼ cup canned chick peas, drained
1 cup pitted black olives, drained
4 or 5 steamed small new potatoes, sliced (about 8 ounces)
½ cup Vinaigrette Français (page 91)
2-ounce can anchovies, drained and chopped
7-ounce can water-pack tuna, drained and flaked
3 hard-cooked eggs, cut into wedges

Line a large salad bowl with large romaine leaves and set aside; reserve smaller leaves. Combine green beans, tomatoes, chick peas, ½ cup of the olives, and the potato slices in a bowl. Reserving 2 tablespoons Vinaigrette Français, drizzle remaining dressing on ingredients in bowl and toss. Turn mixture into salad bowl. Top with small romaine leaves, anchovies, tuna, remaining olives, and egg wedges. Drizzle on remaining dressing and serve immediately.

Yield: 6 servings

Nutrient analysis of 1 serving: 1 starch/bread exchange; 1½ medium-fat meat exchanges; 1 vegetable exchange; 2 fat exchanges; 306 Calories; 14 g protein; 20 g fat; 21 g carbohydrate; 349 mg sodium; 132 mg cholesterol.

†To cook green beans crisp-tender, place beans in rapidly boiling water and cook for 5 minutes. Remove from heat and plunge beans into iced water to stop cooking. Drain.

Tomatoes with Mozzarella and Basil

4 medium tomatoes, sliced
½ pound part-skim-milk mozzarella cheese, sliced
1 tablespoon olive oil
Snipped fresh basil leaves
Freshly ground pepper

Arrange slices of tomato and cheese alternately on 4 salad plates. Drizzle olive oil over all and sprinkle with basil. Season with pepper.

Yield: 4 servings

Nutrient analysis of 1 serving: 2 lean meat exchanges; 1½ vegetable exchanges; 1 fat exchange; 210 Calories; 17 g protein; 13 g fat; 7 g carbohydrate; 299 mg sodium; 30 mg cholesterol.

Lentil Salad

3 cups cooked lentils
1 medium onion, chopped
2 stalks celery, diced
2 cups diced unpared zucchini
1 teaspoon dry mustard
¼ teaspoon garlic powder or 1 clove garlic, minced
2 teaspoons dried oregano
¼ teaspoon freshly ground pepper
2 tablespoons red wine vinegar
¼ cup plus 1 tablespoon vegetable oil
12 cherry tomatoes, halved
1 cup shredded part-skim-milk mozzarella cheese
Lettuce leaves

Combine all ingredients except tomatoes, cheese, and lettuce in large bowl. Toss until lentils and vegetables are coated with oil. Cover and refrigerate several hours to blend flavors. Mix in tomato halves and cheese; serve on lettuce leaves.

Yield: 8 servings (1¼ cups each)

Nutrient analysis of 1 serving: 1 starch/bread exchange; 2 medium-fat meat exchanges; 220 Calories; 16 g protein; 10 g fat; 17 g carbohydrate; 167 mg sodium; 15 mg cholesterol.

White Bean and Tuna Salad

- 7-ounce can water-pack tuna, drained and flaked
- 16-ounce can white beans, drained
- 1/4 cup vegetable oil
- 1 tablespoon lemon juice
- 1/4 teaspoon freshly ground pepper
- 1/4 teaspoon salt
- 1 clove garlic, minced
- 1 cup chopped onion
- Lettuce leaves
- 1/2 green pepper, seeded and cut into rings
- 1 large tomato, cut into wedges
- 3 tablespoons snipped parsley

Combine tuna, beans, oil, lemon juice, pepper, salt, garlic, and onion in bowl; toss until ingredients are coated with oil. Cover and refrigerate at least 1 hour.

Serve on lettuce leaves and garnish with green pepper rings, tomato wedges, and parsley.

Yield: 6 5-ounce or 3 10-ounce servings

Nutrient analysis of a 5-ounce serving: 1½ starch/bread exchanges; 1 lean meat exchange; 1 fat exchange; 215 Calories; 10 g protein; 10 g fat; 22 g carbohydrate; 365 mg sodium; 10 mg cholesterol.

*Pasta Salad

- 1 cup cubed cooked ham
- 1 ounce crumbled blue cheese
- 1 cup cubed cooked turkey or chicken
- 1/4 cup chopped pimiento
- 1/4 cup chopped onion
- 1/2 cup diced celery
- 1/4 cup coarsely shredded carrot
- 1/4 cup diced unpared zucchini
- 1/2 cup sour cream
- 4 tablespoons low-calorie mayonnaise
- 3 cups cold cooked pasta

Combine ham, cheese, turkey, and vegetables in a large bowl. Mix sour cream and mayonnaise; pour over ingredients in bowl and mix. Add pasta and toss. Cover and refrigerate for at least 2 hours.

Yield: 6½ cups

Nutrient analysis of 1 cup: 1 starch/bread exchange; 1 medium-fat meat exchange; 1 fat exchange; 216 Calories; 10 g protein; 11 g fat; 21 g carbohydrate; 435 mg sodium; 63 mg cholesterol.

Bean Salad

Dressing (below)
15½-ounce can chickpeas (ceci), drained
15½-ounce can red kidney beans, drained
20-ounce can white kidney beans (cannellini), drained
15-ounce can pinto beans, drained
1½ cups chopped onion
1 cup diced raw carrot
½ cup diced celery

Prepare dressing and set aside. Combine the beans, onion, carrot, and celery in a large bowl. Pour on dressing and mix well. Cover and refrigerate for at least 4 hours to blend flavors.

Yield: 16 servings (¾ cup each)

Dressing

½ cup olive oil
¼ cup red wine vinegar
2 teaspoons dry mustard
Dash freshly ground pepper
1 teaspoon salt

Measure all ingredients into screw-top jar. Cover tightly and shake until well mixed.

Yield: ¾ cup

Nutrient analysis of 1 serving: 1 starch/bread exchange; ½ lean meat exchange; 1 vegetable exchange; 1 fat exchange; 174 Calories; 7 g protein; 8 g fat; 20 g carbohydrate; 386 mg sodium; 0 mg cholesterol.

Brown Rice and Cucumber Salad

3 cups cooked brown rice, cooled
¼ pound mushrooms, sliced
¼ cup chopped scallions (include green)
1 large cucumber, seeded and diced
¼ cup chopped celery
1 tomato, cut up
1 cup cooked peas
¼ cup snipped fresh parsley
⅓ cup Oil and Vinegar Dressing (below)

Combine rice, mushrooms, scallions, cucumber, celery, tomato, peas, and parsley in a large bowl. Toss with enough dressing to coat ingredients. Cover and refrigerate for at least 2 hours.

Yield: 8 servings (1 cup each)

Nutrient analysis of 1 serving: 1 starch/bread exchange; 1 vegetable exchange; ½ fat exchange; 111 Calories; 3 g protein; 3 g fat; 19 g carbohydrate; 93 mg sodium; 0 mg cholesterol.

Oil and Vinegar Dressing

2 tablespoons red wine vinegar
¼ cup plus 2 tablespoons olive oil
½ teaspoon salt
2 drops hot pepper sauce
¼ teaspoon freshly ground pepper
⅛ teaspoon dry mustard

Measure all ingredients into tightly closed screw-top jar. Cover and shake. Refrigerate until needed and shake before using.

Yield: ½ cup

Nutrient analysis of 2 tablespoons: 3 fat exchanges; 149 Calories; 0 g protein; 17 g fat; 0 g carbohydrate; 283 mg sodium; 0 mg cholesterol.

French Dressing

- ½ cup vegetable oil
- 3 tablespoons red wine vinegar
- 2 tablespoons lemon juice
- 1 tablespoon chopped onion or snipped chives
- 2 teaspoons snipped parsley
- 1¾ teaspoons paprika
- ½ teaspoon dried basil
- ⅛ teaspoon pepper
- 1½ cloves garlic, peeled

Shake all ingredients in tightly closed screw-top jar. Refrigerate for at least 12 hours to blend flavors. Remove garlic and shake before using.

Yield: about ¾ cup

Nutrient analysis of 1 tablespoon: 2 fat exchanges; 85 Calories; 0 g protein; 9 g fat; 0 g carbohydrate; 0 mg sodium; 0 mg cholesterol.

Zesty French Dressing

- ⅔ cup vegetable oil
- ⅓ cup lemon juice or white wine vinegar
- 1 teaspoon hot pepper sauce
- 1 teaspoon paprika
- 1 teaspoon dry mustard
- 1 teaspoon sugar

Shake all ingredients in tightly closed screw-top jar. Refrigerate until ready to use.

Yield: 1 cup

Nutrient analysis of 1 tablespoon: 2 fat exchanges; 83 Calories; 0 g protein; 9 g fat; 0 g carbohydrate; 0 mg sodium; 0 mg cholesterol.

Fruit French Dressing

- ½ cup vegetable oil
- 2 tablespoons white wine vinegar
- 2 tablespoons lemon juice
- ½ teaspoon salt
- ¼ teaspoon dry mustard
- ¼ teaspoon paprika
- 1 tablespoon confectioners' sugar

Shake all ingredients in tightly closed screw-top jar. Refrigerate for at least 1 hour. Shake before serving.

Yield: ¾ cup

Nutrient analysis of 2 tablespoons: 4 fat exchanges; 180 Calories; 0 g protein; 20 g fat; 0 g carbohydrate; 162 mg sodium; 0 mg cholesterol.

Vinaigrette Dressing

- ¾ cup olive oil
- ½ cup tarragon or red wine vinegar
- ¼ teaspoon hot pepper sauce
- 1 tablespoon snipped chives
- 1 tablespoon snipped dill or 1 teaspoon dried dillweed

Beat all ingredients thoroughly in small bowl. Use as a marinade for cooked vegetables or as dressing for tossed salads.

Yield: about 1⅓ cups

Nutrient analysis of 1 tablespoon: 2 fat exchanges; 95 Calories; 0 g protein; 10 g fat; 0 g carbohydrate; trace sodium; 0 mg cholesterol.

Vinaigrette Français

¼ cup red wine vinegar
¾ cup vegetable oil
1 teaspoon salt
Dash freshly ground pepper
1 clove garlic, split
1 teaspoon dried salad herbs
1 teaspoon dry mustard

Shake all ingredients in tightly closed screw-top jar. Refrigerate for at least 1 hour. Discard garlic and shake before using.

Yield: 1 cup

Nutrient analysis of 1 tablespoon: 2 fat exchanges; 98 Calories; 0 g protein; 10 g fat; 0 g carbohydrate; 121 mg sodium; 0 mg cholesterol.

Herb Salad Dressing

1 cup vegetable oil
⅓ cup white wine vinegar
1 scallion, minced (include 1 inch of green top)
1 tablespoon snipped parsley or 1 teaspoon dried parsley flakes
1 teaspoon dry mustard
1 teaspoon dried thyme leaves
1 teaspoon dried tarragon leaves
1 clove garlic, split

Shake all ingredients in tightly closed screw-top jar. Refrigerate for at least 4 hours. Remove garlic clove before using.

Yield: 1⅓ cups

Nutrient analysis of 1 tablespoon: 2 fat exchanges; 98 Calories; 0 g protein; 11 g fat; 0 g carbohydrate; 0 mg sodium; 0 mg cholesterol.

Tarragon Salad Dressing

¾ cup vegetable oil
¼ cup tarragon or white wine vinegar
1 teaspoon snipped parsley
½ teaspoon dried tarragon, crushed
1 clove garlic, split
⅛ teaspoon salt
1 teaspoon dry mustard
2 teaspoons minced onion
Dash freshly ground pepper

Shake all ingredients in tightly closed screw-top jar. Refrigerate for at least 4 hours. Remove garlic and shake before using.

Yield: 1 cup

Nutrient analysis of 1 tablespoon: 2 fat exchanges; 98 Calories; 0 g protein; 10 g fat; 0 g carbohydrate; 16 mg sodium; 0 mg cholesterol.

Italian Salad Dressing

¾ cup vegetable oil
¼ cup red wine vinegar
⅛ teaspoon salt
⅛ teaspoon freshly ground pepper
½ teaspoon dry mustard
¼ teaspoon paprika
⅛ teaspoon cayenne pepper
½ teaspoon dried oregano
½ teaspoon dried marjoram
1 clove garlic, split
¼ teaspoon dried basil

Shake all ingredients in tightly closed screw-top jar. Refrigerate for at least 4 hours. Remove garlic and shake before using.

Yield: about 1 cup

Nutrient analysis of 1 tablespoon: 2 fat exchanges; 98 Calories; 0 g protein; 10 g fat; 0 g carbohydrate; 16 mg sodium; 0 mg cholesterol.

Spicy Italian Salad Dressing

1 cup vegetable oil
⅓ cup red wine vinegar
⅛ teaspoon crushed dried red pepper
1 clove garlic, split
¼ teaspoon garlic powder
2 teaspoons dry mustard
1 tablespoon minced onion
¼ teaspoon salt
3 peppercorns
¾ teaspoon dried oregano
½ teaspoon dried basil
¼ teaspoon dried marjoram
3 or 4 drops hot pepper sauce

Shake all ingredients in tightly closed screw-top jar. Refrigerate for at least 4 hours. Remove garlic clove and peppercorns and shake before using.

Yield: 1⅓ cups

Nutrient analysis of 1 tablespoon: 2 fat exchanges; 98 Calories; 0 g protein; 11 g fat; 0 g carbohydrate; 28 mg sodium; 0 mg cholesterol.

Lemon Dressing

¼ cup vegetable oil
2 tablespoons lemon juice
1 tablespoon plus 1½ teaspoons tarragon vinegar
1 teaspoon snipped parsley
¼ teaspoon freshly ground pepper

Shake all ingredients in tightly closed screw-top jar.

Yield: about ¾ cup

Nutrient analysis of 2 tablespoons: 2 fat exchanges; 83 Calories; 0 g protein; 9 g fat; 0 g carbohydrate; 0 mg sodium; 0 mg cholesterol.

Mustard Dressing

1½ cups buttermilk
½ cup prepared yellow mustard
1 tablespoon frozen apple juice concentrate

Measure all ingredients into blender container or food processor; process until smooth. Refrigerate until ready to use.

Yield: about 2 cups

Nutrient analysis of 2 tablespoons: free exchange; 11 Calories; 1 g protein; 0 g fat; 1 g carbohydrate; 24 mg sodium; 1 mg cholesterol.

Herbed Mayonnaise

1 cup low-calorie mayonnaise
2 teaspoons lemon juice
1 tablespoon snipped parsley
1 tablespoon snipped chives
½ teaspoon dried tarragon
½ teaspoon dried chervil

Mix all ingredients in a small bowl. Cover and refrigerate for 1 to 2 hours. Serve with fish.

Yield: 1 cup

Nutrient analysis of 2 tablespoons: 1 fat exchange; 44 Calories; 0 g protein; 4 g fat; 2 g carbohydrate; 38 mg sodium; 16 mg cholesterol.

Low-Calorie Mayonnaise

2 cups creamed cottage cheese
¼ cup plain low-fat yogurt
1 egg
1 to 2 teaspoons dry mustard, according to taste
1 tablespoon lemon juice
2 tablespoons olive oil
1 tablespoon white pepper
Dash hot pepper sauce

Place cottage cheese, yogurt, and egg into blender container or food processor. Process until smooth. Add remaining ingredients and process until smooth. Refrigerate until ready to use. This mayonnaise will keep for 5 days in refrigerator.

Yield: 2¼ cups

Nutrient analysis of 2 tablespoons: ½ fat exchange; 34 Calories; 2 g protein; 2 g fat; 1 g carbohydrate; 6 mg sodium; 14 mg cholesterol.

VEGETABLES

Asparagus

To prepare asparagus, break or cut off white stem ends. (Ends can be peeled and sliced and used in salads for extra crunch.) Carefully wash asparagus and remove scales with a knife or vegetable peeler.

Asparagus can be cooked by tying trimmed stalks together and standing them upright in a deep pot. Add one inch boiling water and a dash of salt. Cover and cook until crisp-tender, 15 to 20 minutes.

Asparagus also can be cooked horizontally, by placing stalks flat in a wide pan or skillet. Cover with boiling salted water. Cover pan and simmer until crisp-tender, 10 to 15 minutes.

To cook asparagus in microwave oven, place 1 pound asparagus in small, nonmetallic dish. Add ¼ cup water. Cover dish; cook on high for 8 minutes, then test with fork for tenderness. Continue cooking if necessary.

Nutrient analysis of 1 serving (½ cup): 1 vegetable exchange; 25 Calories; 2 g protein; 0 g fat; 5 g carbohydrate; 31 mg sodium; 0 mg cholesterol.

Asparagus with Lemon

20 thick asparagus stalks
1 cup boiling water
¼ cup plus 2 tablespoons unsalted margarine
Juice of 1 lemon
Dash each salt and freshly ground pepper

Peel asparagus from bottom to within 3 inches of tip. Place in shallow skillet; pour in boiling water. Cover and cook over high heat until crisp-tender, 10 to 12 minutes. Drain and arrange on warm platter. Melt margarine; stir in lemon juice and pour over asparagus. Season with salt and pepper.

Yield: 4 servings

Nutrient analysis of 1 serving: 1 vegetable exchange; 2 fat exchanges; 123 Calories; 2 g protein; 11 g fat; 4 g carbohydrate; 114 mg sodium; 0 mg cholesterol.

Asparagus Stir-Fry

1 tablespoon vegetable oil
1 tablespoon margarine
2 pounds asparagus, cut diagonally into 1-inch pieces
1 tablespoon sesame seeds

Heat wok or 10-inch skillet over high heat for 30 seconds. Add oil and margarine and heat an additional 30 seconds. Rotate pan to coat with oil. Reduce heat to medium. Add asparagus and sesame seeds; stir-fry until asparagus is crisp-tender, 4 to 5 minutes.

Yield: 6 servings (½ cup each)

Nutrient analysis of 1 serving: 1 vegetable exchange; 1 fat exchange; 69 Calories; 3 g protein; 6 g fat; 4 g carbohydrate; 12 mg sodium; 0 mg cholesterol.

Broccoli

1 bunch broccoli (about 2 pounds)
2 tablespoons vegetable oil
½ cup chicken stock
12 canned small white onions, well drained
6 cherry tomatoes

Trim large leaves from broccoli and remove tough ends of lower stems. Wash broccoli; separate flowerets. If stems are thicker than 1 inch, make lengthwise gashes in each stem.

Heat oil in medium saucepan or wok. Stir-fry broccoli in oil for 2 to 3 minutes. Pour in chicken stock, cover, and reduce heat to medium. Steam for 4 minutes. Add onions and tomatoes. Cover and cook until heated through, 2 minutes.

Note: Fresh small white onions can be used. In small saucepan, heat 1 inch of chicken stock to boiling. Add onions, cover, and cook for 5 minutes. Drain, reserving broth for use later in recipe.

Yield: 6 servings (1 cup each)

Nutrient analysis of 1 serving: 1 vegetable exchange; 1 fat exchange; 69 Calories; 2 g protein; 5 g fat; 5 g carbohydrate; 241 mg sodium; 0 mg cholesterol.

*Broccoli and Carrots

- 2 tablespoons olive oil
- 5 to 6 cups broccoli flowerets
- 2 large carrots, sliced thinly on diagonal
- ¼ cup beef stock
- ¼ cup soy sauce
- Salt and freshly ground pepper to taste

Heat wok or large skillet over high heat for 30 seconds. Add oil to pan and heat another 30 seconds. Rotate pan to coat with oil. Reduce heat; add broccoli and carrots. Cook and stir vegetables until broccoli is bright green. Stir in stock and soy sauce; cover and cook for 1 to 2 minutes. Season with salt and pepper to taste.

Yield: 6 servings (1 cup each)

Nutrient analysis of 1 serving: 1 vegetable exchange; 1 fat exchange; 68 Calories; 3 g protein; 5 g fat; 4 g carbohydrate; 760 mg sodium; 0 mg cholesterol.

Broccoli Casserole

- 10-ounce package frozen chopped broccoli
- ½ 10½-ounce can condensed cream of mushroom soup
- ½ cup (2 ounces) shredded sharp Cheddar cheese
- ¼ cup minced onion
- ¼ cup low-calorie mayonnaise
- ½ teaspoon dry mustard
- 1 egg, beaten
- Freshly ground pepper to taste
- 4 unsalted whole wheat soda crackers, crumbled
- ¼ cup unprocessed bran

Preheat oven to 350°F.

Cook broccoli as directed on package, but decrease cooking time 2 minutes. Drain broccoli and turn into large bowl. Stir in soup, cheese, onion, mayonnaise, mustard, and egg. Season with pepper to taste. Pour into greased 1-quart casserole. Mix cracker crumbs and bran; sprinkle over top.

Bake for 45 minutes at 350°F., until golden brown.

Yield: 6 servings (1 cup each)

Nutrient analysis of 1 serving: ½ lean meat exchange; 1½ vegetable exchanges; 1 fat exchange; 110 Calories; 6 g protein; 8 g fat; 8 g carbohydrate; 317 mg sodium; 59 mg cholesterol.

*Broccoli Stir-Fry

1 large bunch broccoli (about 2 pounds)
2 teaspoons vegetable oil
½ cup chicken stock
2 tablespoons soy sauce

Trim large leaves from broccoli; remove tough ends of lower stems. Separate into flowerets. If stems are thicker than 1 inch in diameter, make lengthwise gashes in each stem.

Heat wok or large skillet over high heat for 30 seconds. Add oil; heat another 30 seconds. Rotate pan to coat with oil. Reduce heat to medium and add broccoli. Stir-fry until broccoli is bright green, 1 to 2 minutes. Stir in stock and soy sauce. Reduce heat, cover, and cook 2 minutes longer. Remove broccoli from liquid to warm serving dish.

Yield: 4 servings (1 cup each)

Nutrient analysis of 1 serving: 1 vegetable exchange; ½ fat exchange; 44 Calories; 3 g protein; 3 g fat; 3 g carbohydrate; 582 mg sodium; 0 mg cholesterol.

Broccoli with Garlic

1 bunch broccoli (about 2½ pounds)
3 tablespoons olive oil
3 cloves garlic, crushed
½ cup beef stock
1 lemon, thinly sliced

Trim large leaves from broccoli; remove tough ends of lower stem. Wash broccoli and divide into flowerets. If stems are thicker than 1 inch in diameter, make lengthwise gashes in each stem.

Heat wok or large skillet over high heat for 30 seconds. Add the oil and heat another 30 seconds. Rotate pan to coat with oil. Add garlic and stir until brown. Remove garlic and reduce heat to medium. Add broccoli and cook, stirring occasionally, until broccoli is bright green, 3 to 4 minutes. Add beef stock, cover and simmer for 3 to 4 minutes. Remove broccoli from liquid and garnish with lemon slices.

Yield: 6 servings (scant ¾ cup each)

Nutrient analysis of 1 serving: 1 vegetable exchange; 1 fat exchange; 65 Calories; 1 g protein; 5 g fat; 4 g carbohydrate; 76 mg sodium; 0 mg cholesterol.

Broccoli Soufflé

10-ounce package frozen chopped broccoli
3 eggs, separated
1 tablespoon flour
1 cup low-calorie mayonnaise
¼ teaspoon salt

Preheat oven to 350°F.

Cook broccoli as directed on package. Drain and set aside. Beat egg yolks until fluffy. Beat in flour, mayonnaise, and salt, then stir in broccoli.

Beat egg whites until stiff peaks form. Pour broccoli mixture onto egg whites and fold together carefully. Pour into greased 1½-quart casserole. Bake for 30 minutes at 350°F. Serve immediately.

Variation: Substitute 10-ounce package frozen chopped spinach or cut-up asparagus for the broccoli.

Yield: 6 servings (½ cup each)

Nutrient analysis of 1 serving: ½ medium-fat meat exchange; 1 vegetable exchange; 1 fat exchange; 111 Calories; 5 g protein; 8 g fat; 5 g carbohydrate; 117 mg sodium; 153 mg cholesterol.

Steamed Carrots with Dillweed

3 cups diagonally sliced carrots
2 tablespoons margarine
Dash freshly ground pepper
1 teaspoon dry mustard
1 teaspoon dried dillweed

Heat ½ inch water in saucepan to boiling. Place steamer basket with carrots in saucepan. Cover and steam until carrots are crisp-tender, 10 to 12 minutes. Turn into warm bowl.

Melt margarine in small skillet or saucepan. Mix in pepper, mustard, and dillweed. Pour over carrots and toss.

Yield: 4 servings (½ cup each)

Nutrient analysis of 1 serving: 1½ vegetable exchanges; 1 fat exchange; 89 Calories; 1 g protein; 6 g fat; 8 g carbohydrate; 108 mg sodium; 0 mg cholesterol.

Carrots with Water Chestnuts and Orange Sections

1 pound carrots, cut into 3-inch narrow strips
Salt and freshly ground pepper to taste
2 tablespoons margarine
8-ounce can whole water chestnuts, drained and halved
2 oranges, peeled, pitted, sectioned, and cut up

Heat ½ inch water in saucepan to boiling. Place steamer basket with carrots in pan. Cover and steam until carrots are crisp-tender, 10 to 15 minutes. Turn carrots into warm bowl; season with salt and pepper. Add margarine, water chestnuts, and orange pieces, and toss.

Yield: 4 servings (1 cup each)

Nutrient analysis of 1 serving: 1 vegetable exchange; 2 fruit exchanges; 1 fat exchange; 138 Calories; 2 g protein; 6 g fat; 20 g carbohydrate; 174 mg sodium; 0 mg cholesterol.

Carrots and Zucchini

4 cups sliced carrot
¼ cup snipped fresh dill
4 cups sliced unpared zucchini
3 tablespoons margarine
Salt and freshly ground pepper to taste

Heat ½ inch water in saucepan to boiling. Place steamer basket with carrots and dill in saucepan. Cover and steam for 8 minutes. Add zucchini, cover, and steam 5 minutes longer. Turn vegetables into heated serving bowl; add margarine and toss until vegetables are coated. Season with salt and pepper to taste.

Yield: 6 servings (¾ cup each)

Nutrient analysis of 1 serving: 2 vegetable exchanges; 1 fat exchange; 101 Calories; 2 g protein; 6 g fat; 11 g carbohydrate; 227 mg sodium; 0 mg cholesterol.

Cauliflower with Cheese and Bacon

- 1 medium head cauliflower (about 2 pounds)
- 1 cup shredded Cheddar cheese
- 2 slices bacon, cut into ¼-inch pieces, fried until crisp, and drained

Remove outer leaves and stalk of cauliflower. Cut off any discoloration on flowerets. Wash cauliflower and leave whole. Heat ½ inch water in large saucepan to boiling. Place steamer basket with cauliflower in saucepan. Cover and steam until tender, 30 to 40 minutes. Place cauliflower in warm serving dish; sprinkle cheese and bacon on top.

Yield: 6 servings (¾ cup each)

Nutrient analysis of 1 serving: 1 lean meat exchange; 1 fat exchange; 92 Calories; 6 g protein; 7 g fat; 1 g carbohydrate; 156 mg sodium; 21 mg cholesterol.

*Sautéed Cucumbers

- 2 unwaxed large hothouse cucumbers
- ½ cup margarine
- 1 teaspoon salt
- ¼ teaspoon pepper
- Dash hot pepper sauce

Cut cucumbers crosswise into ¼-inch slices. Melt margarine in skillet. Add cucumber slices, salt, pepper, and pepper sauce. Cook and stir until cucumbers are crisp-tender, about 5 minutes. Remove from pan with slotted spoon to drain off cooking fat.

Yield: 4 servings

Nutrient analysis of 1 serving: 1 vegetable exchange; 1 fat exchange; 82 Calories; 1 g protein; 6 g fat; 7 g carbohydrate; 567 mg sodium; 0 mg cholesterol.

Eggplant

1 large eggplant (about 2 pounds)
2 cups sliced onion (2 medium)
2 cloves garlic, minced
¼ cup olive oil
¼ cup vegetable oil
Salt and freshly ground pepper to taste
2 tablespoons grated Parmesan cheese

Wash eggplant, cut off stem ends, and, if desired, pare. Cut into ½-inch cubes. There should be about 8 cups.

Cook and stir eggplant, onion, and garlic in combined oils over medium heat until vegetables are tender but not brown. Season with salt and pepper to taste. Turn vegetables into ungreased 1½-quart casserole dish. Sprinkle cheese on top. Bake in 325°F. oven for 30 minutes.

Yield: 6 servings (1 cup each)

Nutrient analysis of 1 serving: 1½ vegetable exchanges; 2 fat exchanges; 122 Calories; 3 g protein; 10 g fat; 8 g carbohydrate; 315 mg sodium; 2 mg cholesterol.

Eggplant Provençale

4 large or 6 medium tomatoes, peeled, seeded, chopped, and drained
2 small cloves garlic, crushed
1 tablespoon olive oil
Salt and freshly ground pepper to taste
3 tablespoons (additional) olive oil
1 eggplant (about 1 pound), peeled and cut into ¾-inch cubes
Snipped parsley

Cook and stir tomatoes and garlic in 1 tablespoon oil until tomatoes are tender, about 4 minutes. Season with salt and pepper to taste. Remove from heat and keep warm.

Heat 3 tablespoons oil in large skillet over medium heat. Add eggplant; cook and stir until eggplant is tender, 5 to 10 minutes. Stir in tomato mixture and cook 3 minutes longer. Garnish with parsley before serving.

Yield: 8 servings (½ cup each)

Nutrient analysis of 1 serving: 1 vegetable exchange; 1½ fat exchanges; 85 Calories; 1 g protein; 7 g fat; 5 g carbohydrate; 275 mg sodium; 0 mg cholesterol.

Green Beans

1 pound green beans
½ cup chopped shallots
1 cup diced tomato
4 ounces (about 1 cup) sliced mushrooms
2 tablespoons margarine
2 tablespoons olive oil
Salt and freshly ground pepper to taste

Remove ends from beans. Leave beans whole or cut crosswise into 1-inch pieces. Place beans in 1 inch salted water (½ teaspoon salt to 1 cup water). Bring to a boil and cook uncovered for 5 minutes. Cover and cook until tender, 5 to 10 minutes longer. Drain beans, turn into a warm bowl, and set aside.

Cook and stir shallots, tomato, and mushrooms in margarine and oil until mushrooms are tender, about 4 minutes. Season with salt and pepper to taste. Add vegetable mixture to beans and toss.

Yield: 6 servings (½ cup each)

Nutrient analysis of 1 serving: 1 vegetable exchange; 1 fat exchange; 63 Calories; 2 g protein; 4 g fat; 6 g carbohydrate; 345 mg sodium; 0 mg cholesterol.

Sesame Stir-Fried Green Beans

1 pound green beans
3 tablespoons vegetable oil
1 clove garlic, crushed
2 teaspoons grated fresh ginger root
½ teaspoon salt
2 tablespoons sesame seeds

Halve beans lengthwise. Heat wok or large frying pan. Add oil and rotate pan to coat. Add garlic, ginger root, and beans; stir-fry until beans are crisp-tender, 3 to 4 minutes. Stir in salt and sesame seeds and serve.

Yield: 4 servings (½ cup each)

Nutrient analysis of 1 serving: 1 vegetable exchange; 1 fat exchange; 57 Calories; 2 g protein; 6 g fat; 4 g carbohydrate; 245 mg sodium; 0 mg cholesterol.

Green Beans Milano

- **1 medium onion, chopped fine**
- **1 clove garlic, minced**
- **3 tablespoons vegetable oil**
- **2 cups coarsely chopped, peeled tomatoes**
- **1½ pounds green beans, trimmed**
- **½ cup water**
- **¼ teaspoon salt**
- **½ teaspoon pepper**
- **½ teaspoon dried oregano**

Cook and stir onion and garlic in oil in large skillet until onion is tender, 3 to 4 minutes. Add remaining ingredients and heat to boiling. Reduce heat, cover, and simmer until beans are crisp-tender, about 10 to 12 minutes.

Yield: 6 servings

Nutrient analysis of 1 serving: 1½ vegetable exchanges; 1 fat exchange; 91 Calories; 2 g protein; 7 g fat; 7 g carbohydrate; 84 mg sodium; 0 mg cholesterol.

Steamed Green Beans and Tomato

- **1 pound green beans**
- **1 cup cherry tomatoes**
- **Salt and freshly ground pepper to taste**
- **2 tablespoons margarine**

Cut ends from beans. Leave beans whole or cut crosswise into 1-inch pieces. Heat ½ inch water in saucepan to boiling. Place steamer basket with beans in saucepan. Cover and steam until beans are crisp-tender, 7 to 10 minutes. Place tomatoes in basket with beans. Cover and steam 1 to 2 minutes longer. Turn vegetables into warm bowl. Season with salt and pepper to taste. Add margarine and toss until vegetables are coated.

Yield: 5 servings (½ cup each)

Nutrient analysis of 1 serving: 1 vegetable exchange; 1 fat exchange; 60 Calories; 1 g protein; 5 g fat; 4 g carbohydrate; 340 mg sodium; 0 mg cholesterol.

Cooked Greens

2 pounds greens (kale, mustard, turnip, or dandelion)
2 cloves garlic, minced
¼ cup olive oil
Dash salt
½ teaspoon pepper

Place washed greens in saucepan with just the water that clings to leaves. Cover and cook for 15 to 20 minutes for dandelion and mustard greens; 15 to 25 minutes for turnip greens and kale. Drain. Cook and stir garlic in oil until brown. Stir in greens, salt, and pepper; heat through.

Yield: 5 servings

Nutrient analysis of 1 serving: 1 vegetable exchange; 1 fat exchange; 75 Calories; 3 g protein; 5 g fat; 4 g carbohydrate; 192 mg sodium; 0 mg cholesterol.

Petits Pois

1 small head Boston lettuce, shredded
4 cups shelled fresh peas or 2 10-ounce packages frozen green peas
4 sprigs parsley, tied together
½ teaspoon salt
¼ teaspoon sugar
1 teaspoon dried thyme
¼ cup margarine
2 tablespoons water
1 tablespoon minced onion

Place lettuce in saucepan. Add remaining ingredients. Heat to boiling, stirring once or twice. Reduce heat, cover, and simmer for 10 minutes. Remove parsley sprigs before serving.

Yield: 6 servings

Nutrient analysis of 1 serving: 1 starch/bread exchange; 1 fat exchange; 145 Calories; 6 g protein; 8 g fat; 13 g carbohydrate; 379 mg sodium; 0 mg cholesterol.

Green and Red Peppers

1 cup sliced onion
1 tablespoon vegetable oil
1 tablespoon margarine
2 medium green peppers, seeded and cut into strips ½ inch wide
2 medium red peppers, seeded and cut into strips ½ inch wide
Salt and freshly ground pepper to taste

Cook and stir onion in oil and margarine over medium heat until tender. Stir in peppers. Reduce heat, cover, and simmer to desired doneness, 5 to 10 minutes. Season with salt and pepper.

Yield: 4 servings (1 cup each)

Nutrient analysis of 1 serving: 1 vegetable exchange; 1½ fat exchanges; 86 Calories; 1 g protein; 7 g fat; 6 g carbohydrate; 287 mg sodium; 0 mg cholesterol.

**Spinach with Tomatoes*

1 pound spinach, washed
2 cloves garlic, crushed
2 tablespoons olive oil
16-ounce can whole tomatoes, drained and chopped (reserve juice for future use)
Salt and freshly ground pepper to taste

Place spinach in saucepan with just the water that clings to leaves. Cover and cook about 3 minutes. Drain well and chop.

Cook and stir garlic in oil over medium heat, 1 to 2 minutes (do not overcook). Stir in tomatoes. Season with salt and pepper to taste. Reduce heat and simmer for 2 to 3 minutes. Stir in spinach; simmer until hot, about 10 minutes.

Yield: 4 servings (½ cup each)

Nutrient analysis of 1 serving: 1½ vegetable exchanges; 1½ fat exchanges; 99 Calories; 3 g protein; 7 g fat; 7 g carbohydrate; 485 mg sodium; 0 mg cholesterol.

Acorn Squash with Zucchini

2 acorn squash (1 pound each)
4 ounces unpared zucchini, diced
2 tablespoons minced onion
1 tablespoon margarine
Salt and freshly ground pepper to taste

Halve each acorn squash; discard seeds and fibers. Place in ungreased baking dish, 13½ x 9 x 2 inches. Pour water into dish to ¼-inch depth and cover with aluminum foil. Bake in 400°F. oven until tender, about 30 minutes.

Cook and stir zucchini and onion in margarine until tender. Season with salt and pepper. Remove foil from acorn squash and fill halves with zucchini mixture. Bake uncovered until filling is hot, about 15 minutes.

Yield: 4 servings

Nutrient analysis of 1 serving: 1 starch/bread exchange; ½ fat exchange; 100 Calories; 3 g protein; 3 g fat; 18 g carbohydrate; 375 mg sodium; 0 mg cholesterol.

Yellow Summer Squash

1 yellow summer squash (about 1 pound)
1 bunch scallions, sliced thin (include green tops)
Salt and freshly ground pepper to taste

Slice squash; remove rind and cut into 1-inch pieces (there should be about 4 cups). Heat ½ inch water in saucepan to boiling. Place steamer basket with squash and scallions in saucepan. Cover and steam until squash is tender, 6 to 8 minutes. Season with salt and pepper to taste. Turn into warm serving dish.

Yield: 4 servings (½ cup each)

Nutrient analysis of 1 serving: 2 vegetable exchanges; 57 Calories; 2 g protein; 0 g fat; 11 g carbohydrate; 275 mg sodium; 0 mg cholesterol.

Puree of Turnips

2 pounds turnips, pared and cut into cubes
3 tablespoons skim milk
1 tablespoon margarine
1/8 teaspoon nutmeg
Salt and white pepper to taste

Heat 1 inch salted water in saucepan (1/2 teaspoon salt to 1 cup water) to boiling. Add turnips, cover, and bring to boil. Reduce heat and cook until tender, 15 to 20 minutes. Drain. Mash turnips with fork or electric beater. Add milk, margarine, and nutmeg, and beat until smooth. Season with salt and white pepper.

Yield: 4 servings (1 cup each)

Nutrient analysis of 1 serving: 1 1/2 vegetable exchanges; 1/2 fat exchange; 65 Calories; 4 g protein; 4 g fat; 7 g carbohydrate; 388 mg sodium; 0 mg cholesterol.

Ratatouille

1 medium eggplant (about 1 1/2 pounds), pared and cut into 1-inch cubes
3 medium zucchini, cut into quarters lengthwise and sliced 3/4 inch thick
1 large Bermuda onion, cut into quarters and sliced 3/4 inch thick
1/4 cup olive oil
15-ounce can tomato sauce
1/2 cup shredded processed American cheese

Cook and stir eggplant, zucchini, and onion in oil in large skillet over medium heat for 10 minutes. Stir in tomato sauce and heat to boiling. Reduce heat, cover, and simmer for 30 minutes, stirring occasionally, until vegetables are tender. Sprinkle cheese on top and continue to cook for 5 minutes.

Yield: 8 servings

Nutrient analysis of 1 serving: 2 vegetable exchanges; 1 fat exchange; 101 Calories; 5 g protein; 4 g fat; 10 g carbohydrate; 393 mg sodium; 5 mg cholesterol.

Red and Green Stir-Fry

1 pound zucchini (about 4 small)
1 medium red pepper
1 large onion
2 tablespoons olive oil
2 tablespoons margarine
Salt and freshly ground pepper to taste

Cut unpared zucchini into 2- to 3-inch-long narrow strips. Seed red pepper and cut into 2-inch-long narrow strips. Cut onion into thin slices and separate into rings.

Heat oil and margarine in large skillet. Add vegetables; cook and stir until vegetables are tender, about 5 minutes. Season with salt and pepper to taste.

Yield: 4 servings (1 cup each)

Nutrient analysis of 1 serving: 2 vegetable exchanges; 1 fat exchange; 100 Calories; 3 g protein; 6 g fat; 9 g carbohydrate; 348 mg sodium; 0 mg cholesterol.

Steamed Summer Vegetables

2 cups sliced, unpared zucchini
1 cup diagonally sliced carrot
Salt and freshly ground pepper to taste
2 tablespoons margarine
2 tablespoons minced scallions
2 tablespoons minced tomato

Heat ½ inch water in saucepan to boiling. Place steamer basket with zucchini and carrot slices in saucepan. Cover and steam until carrots are crisp-tender, about 10 minutes.

Turn vegetables into warm serving dish; season with salt and pepper to taste. Add margarine and toss until vegetables are coated. Sprinkle scallions and tomato on top.

Yield: 6 servings (½ cup each)

Nutrient analysis of 1 serving: 1 vegetable exchange; 1 fat exchange; 53 Calories; 1 g protein; 4 g fat; 4 g carbohydrate; 57 mg sodium; 0 mg cholesterol.

*Vegetable Platter

- 1 medium bunch celery
- 1 medium cauliflower (about 2 pounds)
- 3 cups beef stock
- ¾ teaspoon salt
- 2 cups sliced carrot
- 3 cups broccoli flowerets
- 1 tablespoon margarine
- 2 tablespoons toasted sesame seeds†
- 2 tablespoons snipped chives
- 2 tablespoons lemon juice

Cut off root end of celery and remove coarse outer stalks. Wash celery. Cut celery bunch crosswise once so bottom section is 5 inches long (reserve top section for other uses). Cut 5-inch portion crosswise into four sections, each 1¼ inches long, and tie each section into a bundle with string.

Remove outer leaves and stalk of cauliflower. Cut off any discoloration on flowerets; wash cauliflower thoroughly. Heat beef stock and salt to boiling in a 3-quart saucepan. Add the cauliflower and heat to boiling. Reduce heat, cover, and simmer for 10 minutes. Place celery bundles under cauliflower; cover and simmer until cauliflower is tender, 15 to 20 minutes. Drain.

Heat 1 inch salted water to boiling. Add carrot slices and heat to boiling. Cover and simmer until crisp-tender, 12 to 15 minutes. Drain.

Heat ½ inch salted water to boiling. Place broccoli flowerets in steam basket. Steam for 10 minutes, until crisp-tender. Remove from basket.

Heat margarine in small skillet. Cook and stir sesame seeds, chives, and lemon juice until heated through, about 5 minutes.

Place cauliflower in center of large serving platter. Arrange carrot slices, broccoli, and celery around it. Drizzle lemon-sesame seed sauce on vegetables.

Yield: 8 servings (1¼ cups each)

Nutrient analysis of 1 serving: 3 vegetable exchanges; 1 fat exchange; 122 Calories; 7 g protein; 6 g fat; 15 g carbohydrate; 547 mg sodium; 0 mg cholesterol.

†To toast sesame seeds, place in 350°F. oven for 10 to 15 minutes until golden.

Winter Vegetable Platter

- 2 cups shredded cabbage
- 1 cup diced turnip
- 1 cup diced parsnip
- 1 cup pared and diced sweet potato or yam
- 1 cup diagonally sliced carrot
- ¼ cup margarine
- 1 tablespoon snipped parsley
- 1 tablespoon dried dillweed
- Dash each salt and pepper

Layer vegetables, in order listed, in steamer. Steam until vegetables are tender, 15 to 20 minutes. Arrange vegetables on heated platter. Melt margarine in small skillet, stir in parsley and dillweed, season with salt and pepper, and pour over vegetables.

Yield: 6 servings (1 cup each)

Nutrient analysis of 1 serving: 1 starch/bread exchange; 1½ fat exchanges; 135 Calories; 2 g protein; 9 g fat; 14 g carbohydrate; 375 mg sodium; 0 mg cholesterol.

Zucchini Stir-Fry

- 4 slices lean bacon, cut into ½-inch pieces
- ¼ cup olive oil
- 1 bunch scallions (white part only), sliced thin (about 1 cup)
- 4 to 6 unpared medium zucchini, cut into 3-inch-long narrow strips
- ¼ cup grated Parmesan cheese

Fry bacon in large skillet until crisp. Drain on paper towels. Drain fat from skillet and wipe skillet clean with paper towels.

Heat oil in skillet until hot. Rotate pan to coat with oil. Add scallions; stir-fry until tender (do not brown). Add zucchini and bacon; cook and stir over medium heat until zucchini is crisp-tender, 3 to 4 minutes. Stir in cheese and serve.

Yield: 4 servings (1 cup each)

Nutrient analysis of 1 serving: 1 vegetable exchange; 2 fat exchanges; 124 Calories; 4 g protein; 12 g fat; 2 g carbohydrate; 205 mg sodium; 10 mg cholesterol.

*Zucchini and Tomatoes

4 small zucchini (about 1 pound)
Soy sauce
Salt and freshly ground pepper
Garlic salt
1 medium onion, sliced and separated into rings
2 large tomatoes, peeled and cut into wedges
¾ cup shredded sharp Cheddar cheese

Slice unpared zucchini into greased 2½-quart casserole dish. Sprinkle with a few drops soy sauce; season with salt, pepper, and garlic salt. Arrange onion rings on zucchini and top with tomato wedges. Sprinkle with a few drops additional soy sauce and season with dash each salt, pepper, and garlic salt. Sprinkle on cheese. Bake in 350°F. oven for 40 minutes.

Yield: 8 servings

Nutrient analysis of 1 serving: ½ medium-fat meat exchange; 1 vegetable exchange; 65 Calories; 4 g protein; 4 g fat; 5 g carbohydrate; 416 mg sodium; 11 mg cholesterol.

RICE, STUFFING, POTATOES, AND BEANS

Chinese Boiled Rice

1 cup uncooked long-grain rice
1½ cups water

Wash rice by rubbing it between hands in large bowl of water. Drain and repeat this process 4 or 5 times, until water is no longer milky.

Place washed rice in medium saucepan. Add 1½ cups water, or until water is 1 inch above rice. (Chinese grandmothers measure the water by adding enough water to reach first joint of index finger above surface of rice.) Cover pan and heat to boiling. Reduce heat and cook until water is absorbed. Turn heat to lowest setting and steam rice for 15 to 20 minutes.

Yield: 3 cups

Nutrient analysis of ⅓ cup: 1 starch/bread exchange; 60 Calories; 2 g protein; 0 g fat; 14 g carbohydrate; 1 mg sodium; 0 mg cholesterol.

Brown and Wild Rice

¾ cup wild rice
1 cup brown rice
6 cups chicken stock
¼ cup snipped parsley

Wash wild rice by placing in wire strainer; run cold water through it while lifting rice with fingers to clean thoroughly. Place rice in large saucepan. Add brown rice and stock. Heat to boiling, stirring once or twice. Reduce heat to simmer; cover pan tightly and cook until all liquid is absorbed and rice is tender, 50 to 60 minutes. Fluff rice with fork and mix in parsley.

Yield: 10 servings (½ cup each)

Nutrient analysis of ½ cup: 1 starch/bread exchange; 70 Calories; 3 g protein; 1 g fat; 13 g carbohydrate; 361 mg sodium; 1 mg cholesterol.

*Rice Italiano

4 cups chicken stock
2 teaspoons Italian herb seasoning
1 teaspoon Worcestershire sauce
1 tablespoon dry mustard
2 cups uncooked regular rice
1 ounce pine nuts

Heat chicken stock, herb seasoning, Worcestershire sauce, mustard, and rice to boiling in large saucepan, stirring once or twice. Reduce heat, cover pan tightly, and cook for 14 minutes. Fluff rice with fork and stir in nuts. Cover and let steam for 5 to 10 minutes.

Yield: 8 servings (½ cup each)

Nutrient analysis of 1 serving: 2 starch/bread exchanges; ½ fat exchange; 180 Calories; 7 g protein; 3 g fat; 32 g carbohydrate; 488 mg sodium; 1 mg cholesterol.

Brown Rice Pilaf

1 medium onion, chopped
1 green pepper, seeded and diced
1 red pepper, seeded and diced
1 tablespoon vegetable oil
1 cup chopped fresh mushrooms
1 cup brown rice
3 cups chicken stock

Cook and stir onion and green and red peppers in oil in large saucepan over medium heat just until vegetables are soft, 2 to 3 minutes. Stir in mushrooms; cook and stir 2 minutes longer.

Stir in rice and chicken stock. Heat to boiling, stirring frequently. Reduce heat, cover, and simmer until liquid is absorbed, about 45 minutes.

Yield: 6 servings (¾ cup each)

Nutrient analysis of 1 serving: 1½ starch/bread exchanges; 1 vegetable exchange; 1 fat exchange; 168 Calories; 6 g protein; 4 g fat; 28 g carbohydrate; 326 mg sodium; 1 mg cholesterol.

**Brown and Wild Rice Pilaf*

½ cup uncooked brown rice
½ cup uncooked wild rice
½ cup finely chopped onion
½ cup diced celery
¼ cup margarine
½ cup sliced mushrooms
¼ teaspoon dried sage
¼ teaspoon dried marjoram
¼ teaspoon dried thyme
3½ cups chicken stock

Cook and stir brown rice, wild rice, onion, and celery in margarine until onion is tender. Stir in mushrooms, sage, marjoram, thyme, and stock. Heat to boiling, stirring occasionally. Pour into ungreased 1½-quart casserole dish. Cover tightly. Bake in 350°F. oven until all liquid is absorbed, about 1 hour.

Yield: 12 servings (½ cup each)

Nutrient analysis of 1 serving: 1 starch/bread exchange; 1 fat exchange; 109 Calories; 4 g protein; 5 g fat; 13 g carbohydrate; 459 mg sodium; 1 mg cholesterol.

**Yellow Rice Pilaf*

½ cup shredded carrot
½ cup minced onion
½ cup celery, sliced thin
2 tablespoons margarine
1 cup brown rice
2½ cups water
1½ teaspoons salt

Cook and stir carrot, onion, and celery in margarine in medium saucepan until vegetables are tender. Stir in rice, water, and salt. Heat to boiling. Reduce heat, cover, and simmer until all liquid is absorbed, about 50 minutes.

Yield: 4 cups

Nutrient analysis of ½ cup: 1 starch/bread exchange; 1 vegetable exchange; ½ fat exchange; 118 Calories; 2 g protein; 4 g fat; 20 g carbohydrate; 412 mg sodium; 0 mg cholesterol.

*Stuffing

1 cup chopped onion
1 cup diced celery
2 medium apples, pared, cored and diced
1 cup chopped pecans
8-ounce package herb stuffing mix
½ cup margarine, melted

Combine onion, celery, apples, pecans, and stuffing mix in large bowl. Pour margarine over ingredients and mix lightly.

Yield: 5 cups; enough stuffing for 10-pound turkey or 2 roasting chickens

Nutrient analysis of ½ cup: 1 starch/bread exchange; 1 fruit exchange; 3 fat exchanges; 262 Calories; 4 g protein; 18 g fat; 24 g carbohydrate; 505 mg sodium; 0 mg cholesterol.

Potato-Onion Bake

2½ pounds potatoes
½ pound onions, sliced
4 tablespoons margarine
Salt and freshly ground pepper to taste

Spray 2½-quart casserole dish with vegetable spray. Cut unpared potatoes into ½-inch slices. Alternate layers of potatoes and onions. Dot each layer with margarine, and season with salt and pepper. Bake in 325°F. oven until potatoes are tender, about 40 minutes.

Yield: 8 servings (¾ cup each)

Nutrient analysis of 1 serving: 1½ starch/bread exchanges; 1 vegetable exchange; 1 fat exchange; 169 Calories; 4 g protein; 6 g fat; 26 g carbohydrate; 278 mg sodium; 0 mg cholesterol.

New Potatoes

12 small new red potatoes
2 tablespoons margarine
1 tablespoon snipped parsley

Pare narrow strip around middle of each potato. Place in steamer; steam until just tender, about 20 minutes (do not overcook). Melt margarine in medium skillet; add potatoes and coat with margarine. Sprinkle with parsley.

Yield: 4 servings

Nutrient analysis of 1 serving: 1½ starch/bread exchanges; 1 fat exchange; 168 Calories; 3 g protein; 6 g fat; 26 g carbohydrate; 75 mg sodium; 0 mg cholesterol.

Black Beans

8 ounces dried black beans
2 cups chopped onion
2 tablespoons vegetable oil
4-ounce jar pimiento, drained and chopped
1 teaspoon salt
½ teaspoon dried oregano
1 teaspoon parsley flakes
4 to 5 drops hot pepper sauce
¼ cup reserved bean liquid

Soak beans in 4 cups water for 2 hours. Drain and place beans in 2-quart saucepan. Add 4 cups fresh water and heat to boiling. Reduce heat, cover, and simmer until tender, about 4 hours. Add water to beans during cooking if necessary. Drain beans, reserving liquid.

Cook and stir onion in oil until tender, about 5 minutes. Stir in beans and remaining ingredients. Heat to boiling. Reduce heat, cover, and simmer for 1 hour. Stir occasionally, adding more reserved bean liquid if necessary.

Yield: 8 servings (½ cup each)

Nutrient analysis of 1 serving: 1 starch/bread exchange; ½ fat exchange; 88 Calories; 3 g protein; 3 g fat; 12 g carbohydrate; 246 mg sodium; 0 mg cholesterol.

*White Beans and Tomatoes

16-ounce can whole tomatoes
20-ounce can white kidney beans, drained
2 cups zucchini, sliced thin
Salt and freshly ground pepper to taste

Empty tomatoes into saucepan; break up tomatoes with fork. Stir in beans and zucchini. Heat to boiling. Reduce heat, cover, and simmer until zucchini is crisp-tender, 10 to 15 minutes. Season with salt and pepper to taste.

Yield: 8 servings (¾ cup each)

Nutrient analysis of 1 serving: ½ starch/bread exchange; 1½ vegetable exchanges; 75 Calories; 5 g protein; 0 g fat, 14 g carbohydrate; 548 mg sodium; 0 mg cholesterol.

BREADS AND SANDWICHES

Baking Powder Biscuits

¾ cup whole wheat flour
1¼ cups all-purpose flour
3 teaspoons baking powder
¼ teaspoon salt
½ cup vegetable oil
⅔ cup skim milk
Margarine

Preheat oven to 450°F.

Measure flours, baking powder, and salt into a mixing bowl. Pour oil and milk into measuring cup (do not stir); pour into flour mixture. Stir with fork until mixture cleans side of bowl and forms a ball.

To knead dough, turn onto waxed paper. Lift paper by one corner and fold dough in half; press down firmly and pull paper back. Repeat until dough looks smooth. Pat or roll dough ½ inch thick between 2 sheets of waxed paper. Cut with unfloured 2-inch biscuit cutter. Place on ungreased baking sheet.

Bake at 450°F. until golden brown, 10 to 12 minutes. Serve hot with margarine.

Variations:

Drop Biscuits: Increase milk to 1 cup. Omit kneading and drop dough, 1 teaspoon at a time, onto baking sheet sprayed with vegetable spray.

Baking Powder Biscuits (no salt): Substitute 1 tablespoon plus 1½ teaspoons low-sodium baking powder for the baking powder and omit salt.

Herb Biscuits: Add 1¼ teaspoons caraway seed, ½ teaspoon dried, crumbled leaf sage, and ¼ teaspoon dry mustard to flour mixture.

Yield: 16 biscuits

Nutrient analysis of 1 biscuit: 1 starch/bread exchange; 1 fat exchange; 120 Calories; 2 g protein; 7 g fat; 12 g carbohydrate; 116 mg sodium; 0 mg cholesterol.

Bran Scones

1½ cups buttermilk
2 cups dry bran bud cereal
2 cups all-purpose flour
1 teaspoon baking soda
2 teaspoons baking powder
⅛ teaspoon salt
½ cup margarine

Preheat oven to 350°F.

Pour buttermilk over cereal in bowl and set aside. Measure the flour, baking soda, baking powder, and salt into mixing bowl. Cut in margarine with pastry blender or fork. Stir in the buttermilk mixture. Turn dough onto lightly floured cloth-covered board and roll to ½-inch thickness. Cut with floured 2-inch round cutter. Bake at 350°F. on greased baking sheet until golden brown, 30 to 35 minutes.

Yield: 24 scones

Nutrient analysis of 1 scone: 1 starch/bread exchange; 1 fat exchange; 104 Calories; 2 g protein; 4 g fat; 14 g carbohydrate; 192 mg sodium; 1 mg cholesterol.

Zucchini Muffins

¾ cup whole wheat flour
1 cup all-purpose flour
2 tablespoons unprocessed bran
3 teaspoons baking powder
½ teaspoon salt
¼ cup brown sugar, packed
1 cup shredded unpared zucchini
2 teaspoons grated lemon peel
1 egg
1 cup skim milk
¼ cup molasses
½ cup vegetable oil

Preheat oven to 400°F. Grease bottoms of 12 medium muffin cups (2¾ inches in diameter) and set aside.

In the large bowl of an electric mixer, stir together the whole wheat flour, all-purpose flour, bran, baking powder, and salt. Add remaining ingredients; mix at low speed, scraping bowl frequently, *just* until all flour is moistened. Do not beat. Fill muffin cups three-fourths full.

Bake at 400°F. for 25 minutes. Remove from cups immediately.

Variation: Substitute shredded carrot and orange peel for the zucchini and lemon peel.

Yield: 12 muffins

Nutrient analysis of 1 muffin: 1 starch/bread exchange; 2 fat exchanges; 178 Calories; 3 g protein; 10 g fat; 19 g carbohydrate; 208 mg sodium; 22 mg cholesterol.

Ever-Ready Bran Muffins

1 cup boiling water
3 cups unprocessed wheat bran
½ cup margarine or vegetable oil
1 cup brown sugar, packed
2 eggs
1½ cups whole wheat flour
1 cup all-purpose flour
2½ teaspoons baking soda
1 teaspoon salt
2 cups skim milk

Pour boiling water over 1 cup of the bran; set aside to steep.

Cream margarine and sugar thoroughly. Beat in eggs, one at a time. Mix in flours, soda, salt, and milk. Stir remaining bran into steeped bran; mix into the flour mixture.

Pour batter into a plastic container. Cover tightly and store in refrigerator at least 12 hours before baking. Batter will keep in refrigerator for 6 weeks.

To bake, preheat oven to 400°F. Grease desired number of muffin cups and fill them half full with batter. Bake for 18 to 20 minutes.

Variations: Cored, unpared, chopped apple, cranberries, cut-up dates, or raisins can be added to batter. Be sure to add the extra calories and fruit exchange.

Yield: 32 muffins

Nutrient analysis of 1 muffin: 1½ starch/bread exchanges; 1 fat exchange; 150 calories; 2 g protein; 5 g fat; 23 g carbohydrate; 140 mg sodium; 16 mg cholesterol.

Country-Style Rolls

- **1 package active dry yeast**
- **1 cup warm water (105 to 115°F.)**
- **2 tablespoons sugar**
- **½ teaspoon salt**
- **¼ cup egg substitute**
- **2 tablespoons vegetable oil**
- **1¼ cups all-purpose flour**
- **1 cup whole wheat flour**

Soften yeast in warm water in large bowl of an electric mixer. Add sugar, salt, egg substitute, oil, and 1 cup of the all-purpose flour; beat until smooth. Mix in remaining flour until smooth, scraping batter from side of bowl. Cover and let rise in a warm place until doubled in bulk, about 30 minutes.

Grease 16 muffin cups. Stir down batter and spoon into muffin cups, filling each about half full. Let rise, uncovered, for 20 minutes.

Preheat oven to 400°F. Place muffin tins in oven and bake until golden brown, about 15 minutes.

Yield: 16 rolls

Nutrient analysis of 1 roll: 1 starch/bread exchange; ½ fat exchange; 89 Calories; 2 g protein; 2 g fat; 14 g carbohydrate; 68 mg sodium; 0 mg cholesterol.

High-Fiber Bread or Rolls

- **3 packages active dry yeast**
- **4 cups warm water (105 to 115°F.)**
- **2 tablespoons sugar**
- **1 cup unprocessed wheat bran**
- **1 cup untoasted wheat germ**
- **1 cup uncooked regular rolled oats**
- **1 cup rye flour**
- **2 tablespoons salt**
- **¼ cup plus 2 tablespoons vegetable oil**
- **¾ cup honey**
- **4 cups all-purpose flour**
- **4 cups whole wheat flour**

Soften yeast in warm water in a large bowl. Stir in sugar, wheat bran, wheat germ, rolled oats, rye flour, salt, oil, honey, and 2 cups of the all-purpose flour. Beat until smooth. Cover and let rise in a warm place until bubbly, about 30 minutes.

Stir in the whole wheat flour. Mix in enough remaining all-purpose flour to make dough easy to handle. Turn onto floured cloth-covered board; knead until smooth and elastic, about 10 minutes. Cover and let rise in a warm place until doubled in bulk, about 1 hour. Dough is ready if an indentation remains when touched.

Punch down dough; divide into four equal parts. Shape each fourth into a loaf or 12 rolls. Place each loaf seam side down in greased loaf pan, 9 x 5 x 3 or 8½ x 4½ x 2½ inches. Place rolls on greased baking pan. Let rise until doubled in bulk, about 1 hour for loaves or 40 to 45 minutes for rolls.

Preheat oven to 350°F. Place pans in oven and bake loaves until they are a deep golden brown and sound hollow when tapped, 45 to 60 minutes. Bake rolls until a deep golden brown, 20 to 25 minutes.

Yield: 4 loaves (12 slices each) or 48 rolls

Nutrient analysis of 1 slice or 1 roll: 2 starch/bread exchanges; 149 Calories; 5 g protein; 3 g fat; 27 g carbohydrate; 244 mg sodium; 0 mg cholesterol.

Colonial Bread

- **½ cup yellow cornmeal**
- **⅓ cup brown sugar, packed**
- **1 tablespoon salt**
- **2 cups boiling water**
- **¼ cup vegetable oil**
- **2 packages active dry yeast**
- **½ cup warm water (105 to 115°F.)**
- **¾ cup whole wheat flour**
- **½ cup rye flour**
- **4¼ to 4½ cups all-purpose flour**

Measure cornmeal, sugar, and salt into large mixing bowl. Stir in boiling water; cover and let stand for 30 minutes.

Stir yeast into the warm water, then stir yeast mixture and oil into cornmeal mixture. Add the whole wheat and rye flours and mix until smooth. Stir in enough all-purpose flour to make dough easy to handle. Turn dough onto lightly floured cloth-covered board. Cover and let rest for 10 minutes.

Knead until smooth and elastic, about 10 minutes. Place in greased bowl; turn greased side up. Cover and let rise until double in bulk, about 1 hour. Dough is ready if indentation remains when touched.

Punch down dough; divide in half. Shape each half into loaf. Place loaves, seam side down, in 2 greased loaf pans, 9 x 5 x 3 inches. Let rise until double in bulk, about 1 hour.

Preheat oven to 375°F. Place pans in oven and bake until loaves sound hollow when tapped, 40 to 45 minutes. Remove from pans and cool on wire racks.

Yield: 2 loaves (16 slices per loaf)

Nutrient analysis of 1 slice: 1 starch/bread exchange; ½ fat exchange; 102 Calories; 3 g protein; 2 g fat; 18 g carbohydrate; 182 mg sodium; 0 mg cholesterol.

Oatmeal Currant Bread

1¼ cups skim milk
¼ cup margarine
1 cup quick-cooking oats
1 package active dry yeast
¼ cup warm water (105 to 115°F.)
⅓ cup maple syrup
1 egg
1½ teaspoons salt
¾ cup whole wheat flour
2 cups all-purpose flour
½ cup currants

Heat milk and margarine to boiling; pour over oats in bowl. Let cool to lukewarm.

Dissolve yeast in warm water in large bowl of electric mixer. Add the syrup, egg, salt, whole wheat flour, ¾ cup all-purpose flour, and the oat mixture. Beat at medium speed for 3 minutes, scraping bowl frequently. Mix in remaining flour and the currants with a spoon. Grease 2 loaf pans, 8½ x 3½ x 2½ inches, and sprinkle with oats. Divide dough between pans. Let rise in warm place until double in bulk.

Preheat oven to 350°F. Place pans in oven and bake for 45 to 50 minutes. (If loaves brown too quickly, cover with foil during part of the baking time.) Cool loaves on wire racks.

Yield: 2 loaves (12 slices per loaf)

Nutrient analysis of 1 slice: 1 starch/bread exchange; 1 fat exchange; 101 Calories; 3 g protein; 3 g fat; 17 g carbohydrate; 155 mg sodium; 11 mg cholesterol.

Beer Bread

3 cups self-rising flour
3 tablespoons sugar
12-ounce can beer (at room temperature)
Margarine

Preheat oven to 375°F.

Spray a 9 x 5 x 3-inch loaf pan with vegetable spray. Measure the flour, sugar, and beer into a mixing bowl. Mix until dough cleans side of bowl. Turn dough into pan. Bake at 375°F. for 40 to 45 minutes. Remove from pan and coat top of loaf with margarine.

Yield: 1 loaf (12 slices)

Nutrient analysis of 1 slice: 2 starch/bread exchanges; 134 Calories; 3 g protein; 1 g fat; 27 g carbohydrate; 382 mg sodium; 0 mg cholesterol.

Beer Rye Bread

- 2 packages active dry yeast
- ¼ cup warm water (105 to 115°F.)
- 2 cups beer
- ¼ cup margarine
- ⅓ cup molasses
- ½ cup wheat germ
- 1 tablespoon grated orange peel
- 2 teaspoons salt
- 2 cups rye flour
- 4 to 5 cups all-purpose flour
- Cornmeal
- 1 egg
- 1 tablespoon water

Dissolve yeast in warm water and set aside.

Heat beer, margarine, and molasses together until lukewarm. Pour into mixing bowl; blend in wheat germ, orange peel, salt, and yeast mixture. Mix in rye flour and enough all-purpose flour to make dough easy to handle.

Turn dough onto lightly floured cloth-covered board; knead until smooth and elastic, about 10 minutes. Place in greased bowl; turn greased side up. Cover and let rise in a warm place until double in bulk, 1½ to 2 hours.

Punch down dough and knead lightly. Cover and let rest for 10 minutes.

Grease baking sheet and sprinkle with cornmeal. Shape dough into 2 rounds and place on baking sheet. Cover and let rise until double in bulk, about 1 hour.

Preheat oven to 350°F. Mix egg and 1 tablespoon water; brush up to half the mixture on loaves. Bake for 25 minutes. Remove from oven and brush again with remaining egg glaze. Bake until loaves sound hollow when tapped, 15 to 20 minutes longer. Remove from baking sheet and cool on wire racks.

Yield: 2 loaves (12 slices per loaf)

Nutrient analysis of 1 slice: 2 starch/bread exchanges; 152 Calories; 4 g protein; 3 g fat; 26 g carbohydrate; 189 mg sodium; 11 mg cholesterol.

Swedish Rye Bread

2 packages active dry yeast
1½ cups warm water (105 to 115°F.)
¼ cup molasses
¼ cup sugar
1 tablespoon salt
2 tablespoons shortening
Grated peel of 1 orange
2½ cups medium rye flour
2¼ to 2¾ cups all-purpose flour

Soften yeast in warm water in large bowl of electric mixer. Add molasses, sugar, salt, shortening, orange peel, and rye flour; beat at medium speed until smooth. Remove beater; stir in enough all-purpose flour to make dough easy to handle (dough will be sticky).

Turn dough onto lightly floured cloth-covered board. Cover and let rest for 10 minutes. Knead until smooth and elastic, about 5 minutes. Place in greased bowl; turn greased side up. Cover and let rise in a warm place until double in bulk, about 1 hour. Dough is ready if an indentation remains when touched.

Punch down dough. Round up and let rise until double in bulk, about 40 minutes.

Punch down dough again and divide in half. Shape each half into a loaf. Place in 2 greased loaf pans, 8½ x 4 x 2¾ inches. Cover and let rise for 1 hour.

Preheat oven to 375°F. Place pans in oven and bake until loaves sound hollow when tapped, 30 to 35 minutes. Cool on wire racks.

Yield: 2 loaves (16 slices per loaf)

Nutrient analysis of 1 slice: ¾ starch/bread exchange; 57 Calories; 1 g protein; 1 g fat; 11 g carbohydrate; 193 mg sodium; 0 mg cholesterol.

Easy Whole Wheat Bread

3 packages active dry yeast
1 cup warm water (105 to 115°F.)
3 cups lukewarm water
¼ cup plus 1 tablespoon honey
2 eggs, beaten
1 tablespoon plus 1 teaspoon salt
½ cup unprocessed bran
8 cups whole wheat flour

Soften yeast in warm water. Stir in lukewarm water, honey, eggs, salt, bran, and 4 cups of the flour. Beat until smooth. Mix in remaining flour until smooth. (Dough will be sticky.) Spoon dough into 2 greased loaf pans, 9 x 5 x 3 inches. Cover and let rise in a warm place until dough is above edges of pans, about 1 hour.

Preheat oven to 400°F. Place pans in oven and bake for 50 to 60 minutes. Cool loaves in pans for 10 minutes, then remove to wire racks o cool.

Yield: 2 loaves (16 slices per loaf)

Nutrient analysis of 1 slice: 2 starch/bread exchanges; 132 Calories; 5 g protein; 1 g fat; 28 g carbohydrate; 248 mg sodium; 16 mg cholesterol.

Honey Wheat Bread

2 packages active dry yeast
½ cup warm water (105 to 115°F.)
⅓ cup honey
1 tablespoon salt
¼ cup vegetable oil
1¾ cups warm water (additional)
3 cups stone-ground whole wheat flour
3 to 4 cups all-purpose flour

Dissolve yeast in ½ cup warm water in a large mixing bowl. Stir in the honey, salt, oil, 1¾ cups warm water, and the whole wheat flour. Beat until smooth. Stir in enough all-purpose flour to make dough easy to handle.

Turn dough onto lightly floured cloth-covered board; knead until smooth and elastic, about 10 minutes. Place in greased bowl; turn greased side up. Cover and let rise in warm place until double in bulk, about 1 hour. Dough is ready if an indentation remains when touched.

Punch down dough; divide in half. Shape each half into loaf. Place loaves, seam side down, in 2 greased loaf pans, 9 x 5 x 3 inches. Let rise until double in bulk, about 1 hour.

Preheat oven to 375°F. Place loaf pans in oven and bake until loaves are golden brown and sound hollow when tapped, 40 to 45 minutes. Remove from pans; cool on wire rack.

Yield: 2 loaves (16 slices per loaf)

Nutrient analysis of 1 slice: 1⅓ starch/bread exchanges; 102 Calories; 3 g protein; 1 g fat; 20 g carbohydrate; 189 mg sodium; 0 mg cholesterol.

*Broiled Swiss Crabmeat Sandwich

- 7½-ounce can crabmeat, drained and cartilage removed
- 2 tablespoons olive oil
- ½ teaspoon cumin
- 1 tablespoon grated onion
- 1 tablespoon snipped parsley
- 1 teaspoon lemon juice
- Dash salt
- 4 slices bread
- 4 slices Swiss cheese

Place crabmeat, olive oil, cumin, onion, parsley, lemon juice, and salt in blender container or food processor. Process until smooth. Spread mixture on bread slices; top each with cheese slice.

Set oven control at broil or 550°F. Broil 3 inches from heat source until cheese is melted.

Yield: 4 open sandwiches

Nutrient analysis of 1 sandwich: 1 starch/bread exchange; 2 medium-fat meat exchanges; 1 fat exchange; 276 Calories; 20 g protein; 17 g fat; 13 g carbohydrate; 782 mg sodium; 80 mg cholesterol.

*Pita Sandwich

- 2 16-ounce cans white kidney beans, drained
- 5 tablespoons vegetable oil
- 2 tablespoons lemon juice
- 1 teaspoon dried oregano
- ½ teaspoon salt
- ½ teaspoon cumin
- ¼ teaspoon pepper
- 2 ounces Swiss cheese, cut into ¼-inch cubes
- 2 medium tomatoes, peeled and diced
- 1 cucumber, pared and diced
- ½ cup shredded carrot
- 4 small whole wheat pita breads, halved
- 2 tablespoons snipped parsley

Combine beans, oil, lemon juice, oregano, salt, cumin, and pepper in a bowl. Stir in the cheese, tomatoes, cucumber, and carrot. Cover and refrigerate for 2 hours. Drain.

Spoon ⅔ cup mixture into each pita bread pocket and sprinkle with parsley.

Yield: 4 sandwiches (2 halves per serving)

Nutrient analysis of 1 standwich: 2 starch/bread exchanges; 1 medium-fat meat exchange; 2 vegetable exchanges; 2 fat exchanges; 333 Calories; 13 g protein; 15 g fat; 39 g carbohydrate; 769 mg sodium; 14 mg cholesterol.

Open Sandwiches

Open sandwiches are attractive and easy to prepare. It is important that they be served fresh. Choose the type of bread preferred; the bread slices should be about ¼ inch thick. The bread can be toasted if desired. The spreads (margarine and dressings), accompaniments, and garnishes should be ready for the assembly of the sandwich. Here are a few suggestions:

*Slices of soft processed cheese on chopped radishes
Lettuce leaf with rolled cheese slices
Apple and banana, sliced thin, prepared mustard, and parsley
Lettuce leaf, cabbage salad, and tomato wedge
Small meatballs, with slices of cucumber and tomato
Tomato slices, chopped onion
Roast beef, sliced thin, pickled onions, and parsley
Shredded carrot, banana slices, and parsley
*Cheese slices with rings of green pepper
Cold sliced potato, snipped chives, herring tidbits, and sour cream
*Sliced hard-cooked egg, anchovy fillets, and dill sprig
Lettuce, Jellied Veal (page 160), sliced thin, lemon wedge, and dill sprig

Use instructions on page 23 to calculate the nutrient content of the sandwich.

Margarine Spreads

Mix ½ cup unsalted margarine, softened, and any one of the following:

Garlic—1 medium clove garlic, minced
Tarragon—1 teaspoon dried tarragon and ¼ teaspoon paprika
Onion—2 tablespoons minced onion or snipped chives
Seeded—1 to 2 teaspoons dill or sesame seeds
Basil—1 teaspoon dried basil
Italian—1 teaspoon Italian seasoning

Yield: ½ cup

Nutrient analysis of 1 teaspoon: 1 fat exchange; 36 Calories; 0 g protein; 4 g fat; 0 g carbohydrate; 1 mg sodium; 0 mg cholesterol.

PASTA

Tomato Sauce

2 cups minced onion
2 garlic cloves, crushed
¼ cup vegetable oil
½ teaspoon freshly ground pepper
1 teaspoon dried oregano
½ teaspoon basil
6-ounce can tomato paste
2 28-ounce cans Italian plum tomatoes, pureed and undrained
¾ cup water
Salt to taste

Cook and stir onion and garlic in oil until onion is tender. Stir in remaining ingredients, except salt. Heat to boiling. Reduce heat and simmer over very low flame for 2 hours, stirring occasionally. Add salt to taste.

Yield: 6 cups

Nutrient analysis of ¼ cup: 1 vegetable exchange; 1 fat exchange; 66 Calories; 1 g protein; 5 g fat; 5 g carbohydrate; 122 mg sodium; 0 mg cholesterol.

Thick Tomato Sauce

1 cup chopped onion
¼ cup vegetable oil
2 cups finely chopped, drained, canned Italian plum tomatoes
15-ounce can tomato puree
1 clove garlic, crushed
1 teaspoon dried oregano
Dash freshly ground pepper

Cook and stir onion in oil until tender. Stir in remaining ingredients. Heat to boiling, stirring frequently. Reduce heat and simmer for 1 hour, stirring occasionally. (Sauce becomes smoother the longer it simmers.) If desired, sauce can be pureed in blender or food processor for smoother consistency.

Yield: 4 cups

Nutrient analysis of ⅔ cup: 2 vegetable exchanges; 2 fat exchanges; 129 Calories; 3 g protein; 9 g fat; 11 g carbohydrate; 135 mg sodium; 0 mg cholesterol.

Fresh Tomato Sauce

1 medium onion, minced
1 clove garlic, minced
1 carrot, diced
1 stalk celery, diced
¼ cup margarine
¼ cup olive oil
4 pounds tomatoes, peeled and coarsely chopped (preferably plum tomatoes)
1 tablespoon sugar
¼ teaspoon salt
1 teaspoon dried oregano
1 teaspoon dried basil
1 tablespoon snipped parsley
Freshly ground pepper to taste

Cook and stir onion, garlic, carrot, and celery in margarine and oil until vegetables are tender. Stir in tomatoes, sugar, salt, oregano, basil, and parsley. Season with pepper. Heat to boiling, stirring occasionally. Reduce heat, cover, and simmer, stirring occasionally and breaking up tomatoes, for 2 to 3 hours. (For thicker sauce, remove cover during last 1½ hours of cooking.) If desired, strain sauce.

Note: Two cans (28 ounces each) Italian plum tomatoes can be substituted for the fresh tomatoes, but this will raise the sodium content considerably. This recipe can be doubled. Cooled sauce can be frozen in plastic containers and then thawed and heated at serving time.

Yield: 8 servings (3½–4 cups sauce, enough for 1 pound of pasta)

Nutrient analysis of 1 serving: 3 vegetable exchanges; 3 fat exchanges; 177 Calories; 3 g protein; 14 g fat; 14 g carbohydrate; 330 mg sodium; 0 mg cholesterol.

Pesto

- **2 cups coarsely chopped fresh basil† or 2 cups coarsely chopped Italian (flat-leaf) parsley and 2 tablespoons dried basil**
- **½ teaspoon freshly ground black pepper**
- **1 to 2 teaspoons minced garlic**
- **½ teaspoon salt**
- **3 tablespoons chopped pine nuts (pignola), or use walnuts**
- **1 cup olive oil**
- **½ cup fresh-grated Parmesan cheese**

Measure all ingredients except cheese and pasta into blender container or food processor. Process until smooth. Pour sauce into saucepan and heat over low flame. Remove from heat; stir in cheese until blended. Pour over pasta and toss. (Include the pasta in your meal plan.)

Yield: 8 servings (approximately 2 cups)

Nutrient analysis of ½ cup serving of pesto: 1 medium-fat meat exchange; 4 fat exchanges; 270 Calories; 3 g protein; 27 g fat; 3 g carbohydrate; 180 mg sodium; 6 mg cholesterol.

†Strip leaves from stems of basil. Chop coarsely and pack tightly in measuring cup. Pesto is best when it is freshly made, but it can be partially prepared, excluding the cheese, and frozen.

**White Clam Sauce*

- **3 cloves garlic, crushed**
- **1 cup snipped parsley**
- **½ cup olive oil**
- **1 teaspoon hot pepper sauce**
- **2 6½-ounce cans minced clams, undrained**
- **1½ cups bottled clam juice**
- **3 pounds clams in shells ("steamers")**

Cook and stir garlic and parsley in oil for 5 minutes. Stir in pepper sauce, minced clams with their liquid, and clam juice. Heat to boiling. Reduce heat and simmer for 30 minutes.

Wash clams thoroughly, discarding any broken shell or opened clams. Add clams to sauce. Cover and cook until clams open, 5 to 10 minutes. Serve on hot pasta. (Be sure to include the pasta in your meal plan.)

Yield: 6 servings

Nutrient analysis of 1 serving of sauce: 4 medium-fat meat exchanges; 316 Calories; 27 g protein; 22 g fat; 5 g carbohydrate; 564 mg sodium; 97 mg cholesterol.

Mushroom-Almond Pasta

- 1 cup uncooked pasta (about 5 ounces)
- 8 ounces mushrooms, sliced thin (4 cups)
- 4 ounces toasted sliced almonds† (1 cup)
- 2 tablespoons margarine
- Salt and freshly ground pepper to taste
- ½ cup grated Parmesan cheese
- 4 tablespoons snipped parsley

Cook pasta as directed on package; drain and keep warm. Cook and stir mushrooms and almonds in margarine over medium-high heat until mushrooms are soft, 4 to 5 minutes. Season with salt and pepper.

Divide warm pasta into four ½-cup servings and top each with ¾ cup of the mushroom-almond mixture. Sprinkle each with 2 tablespoons Parmesan cheese and 1 tablespoon parsley.

Yield: 4 servings

Nutrient analysis of 1 serving: 1 starch/bread exchange; 1½ medium-fat meat exchanges; 2 vegetable exchanges; 3 fat exchanges; 372 Calories; 16 g protein; 22 g fat; 28 g carbohydrate; 324 mg sodium; 10 mg cholesterol.

†To toast almond slices, spread slices on baking sheet. Toast in 350°F. oven until golden, about 5 minutes.

Pasta with Vegetables

- 1½ cups uncooked pasta (7 ounces)
- 4 ounces sliced onion
- 2 tablespoons margarine
- 4 ounces unpared zucchini slices
- 4 ounces chopped green pepper
- 4 ounces chopped red pepper
- 4 ounces broccoli flowerets
- ¼ cup grated Parmesan cheese

Cook pasta as directed on package; drain and keep warm.

Cook and stir onion in margarine just until soft, about 3 minutes. Add zucchini, green pepper, red pepper, and broccoli. Cook and stir until crisp-tender and heated through, about 5 minutes. Combine warm pasta and vegetable mixture in a large bowl; sprinkle with Parmesan cheese and toss.

Yield: 4 servings (1½ cups each)

Nutrient analysis of 1 serving: 2 starch/bread exchanges; 2 vegetable exchanges; 2 fat exchanges; 296 Calories; 10 g protein; 9 g fat; 38 g carbohydrate; 174 mg sodium; 5 mg cholesterol.

*Paglia e Fieno (Straw and Hay)

½ pound white linguine
½ pound green linguine†
2 teaspoons olive oil
½ cup margarine
12 medium mushrooms, sliced and cut into ¼-inch strips
¼ pound prosciutto, thinly sliced and cut into ¼-inch strips
¼ cup chicken stock
1 cup whipping cream
4 ounces Parmesan cheese, freshly grated
Salt and freshly ground pepper to taste

Cook linguine separately in boiling salted water. Follow package directions, and add 1 teaspoon olive oil to the water in each pot. Drain quickly, allowing some water to remain on pasta. Combine linguines in one pot and place over low heat.

Stir in margarine, mushrooms, and prosciutto with wooden spoon or fork. Add chicken stock and cream and toss. Sprinkle with Parmesan cheese and season with salt and pepper. Serve in heated bowls with additional grated Parmesan cheese if desired.

Yield: 6 servings

Nutrient analysis of 1 serving: 4 starch/bread exchanges; 2 medium-fat meat exchanges; 1 vegetable exchange; 2 fat exchanges; 585 Calories; 16 g protein; 20 g fat; 61 g carbohydrate; 564 mg sodium; 11 mg cholesterol.

†Green linguine takes about 1 minute longer to cook.

*Spaghetti Primavera

8-ounce package spaghetti
4 cups chopped fresh broccoli
2 cups fresh cauliflowerets
2 tablespoons margarine
1 pint cherry tomatoes
2 cloves garlic, minced
2 tablespoons vegetable oil
2 tablespoons margarine (additional)
½ teaspoon salt
1 teaspoon dried basil
Dash freshly ground pepper
½ cup grated Parmesan cheese
¼ cup snipped parsley
½ to 1 cup chicken stock

Begin to cook spaghetti as directed on package; add the broccoli and cauliflowerets for the last 5 minutes of cooking. Drain; return spaghetti and vegetables to pot and add 2 tablespoons margarine. Toss to coat ingredients. Cook and stir tomatoes and garlic in combination of oil and margarine for 6 minutes. Stir in the salt, basil, and pepper. Add tomatoes to spaghetti mixture. Stir in the cheese, parsley, and enough chicken stock for desired consistency of sauce. Heat, stirring frequently, until warmed through, and serve.

Yield: 8 servings

Nutrient analysis of 1 serving: 2 starch/bread exchanges; 2 vegetable exchanges; 2 fat exchanges; 279 Calories; 12 g protein; 12 g fat; 37 g carbohydrate; 421 mg sodium; 4 mg cholesterol.

Asparagus and Noodles

¾ pound asparagus, washed and scaled
6-ounce package whole wheat ribbon noodles
¼ cup margarine
¼ cup grated Parmesan cheese

Cut asparagus diagonally into 1-inch pieces. Heat 1 inch water in saucepan with vegetable steamer. Place asparagus stalk pieces in steamer and steam for 10 to 15 minutes. Add asparagus tip pieces and steam 5 minutes longer.

Cook noodles as directed on package, except omit salt. Stir in margarine and cheese; toss until noodles are coated. Add asparagus and mix. Serve immediately.

Yield: 4 servings

Nutrient analysis of 1 serving: 1 starch/bread exchange; 2 vegetable exchanges; 3 fat exchanges; 274 Calories; 10 g protein; 17 g fat; 23 g carbohydrate; 330 mg sodium; 34 mg cholesterol.

*Lasagna

6 cups Tomato Sauce (page 130)
16-ounce package lasagna noodles, cooked according to package directions and drained
1 pound lean ground beef, browned and drained on paper towels
15-ounce carton shredded part-skim-milk ricotta cheese
¾ cup grated Romano cheese
2 tablespoons snipped parsley
3 eggs, beaten
½ teaspoon salt
½ teaspoon freshly ground pepper
1 teaspoon dried oregano
¾ cup grated Romano cheese (additional)
8 ounces shredded part-skim-milk mozzarella cheese

Preheat oven to 350°F.

Pour thin layer of tomato sauce into greased baking pan 13 x 9 x 2 inches. Arrange ⅓ of lasagna noodles on sauce.

Mix meat, ricotta cheese, ¾ cup grated Romano cheese, parsley, eggs, salt, pepper, and oregano together well. Spoon half this mixture on noodles. Mix remaining Romano cheese and mozzarella cheese; sprinkle half cheese mixture on top. Repeat layers, using half remaining tomato sauce, remaining meat mixture, and half remaining cheese mixture. Top with remaining noodles, tomato sauce, and cheese mixture.

Cover baking pan with aluminum foil and bake at 350°F. for 20 minutes. Remove foil and bake 10 minutes longer.

Yield: 9 servings

Nutrient analysis of 1 serving: 2 starch/bread exchanges; 4 medium-fat meat exchanges; 443 Calories; 35 g protein; 19 g fat; 28 g carbohydrate; 640 mg sodium; 201 mg cholesterol.

*Spinach Lasagna

10-ounce package frozen chopped spinach, thawed and drained
15-ounce carton part-skim-milk ricotta cheese
2 cups shredded part-skim-milk mozzarella cheese
1 egg, beaten
½ teaspoon salt
⅛ teaspoon pepper
¾ teaspoon dried oregano
32-ounce jar spaghetti sauce†
½ package (8 ounces) lasagna noodles
1 cup water

Preheat oven to 350°F. Grease a baking pan, 13 x 9 x 2 inches, and set aside.

†4 cups Tomato Sauce (page 130) can be used in this recipe.

Mix spinach, ricotta cheese, 1 cup of mozzarella cheese, egg, salt, pepper, and oregano. Pour ⅓ of the spaghetti sauce in baking pan. Top with ⅓ of the uncooked noodles, and ½ the cheese mixture. Repeat. Top with remaining noodles and remaining sauce. Sprinkle 1 cup mozzarella cheese on top. Pour water around edges of pan. Cover pan tightly with aluminum foil. Bake at 350°F. for 1 hour and 15 minutes. Let stand for 15 minutes before serving.

Yield: 8 servings

Nutrient analysis of 1 serving: 3½ starch/bread exchanges; 2 medium-fat meat exchanges; 2 vegetable exchanges; 1½ fat exchanges; 518 Calories; 24 g protein; 18 g fat; 63 g carbohydrate; 1,003 mg sodium; 167 mg cholesterol.

**Cheese Manicotti*

15-ounce carton part-skim-milk ricotta cheese
¼ pound part-skim-milk mozzarella cheese, diced
2 eggs, beaten
¾ cup grated Parmesan cheese
2 tablespoons snipped parsley
½ teaspoon salt
Dash freshly ground pepper
¼ cup wheat germ
8-ounce package manicotti tubes
15-ounce can tomato sauce
¼ cup grated Parmesan cheese (additional)
¼ cup shredded part-skim-milk mozzarella cheese (additional)

Mix ricotta cheese, diced mozzarella cheese, eggs, ¾ cup Parmesan cheese, parsley, salt, pepper, and wheat germ thoroughly. Set aside.

Preheat oven to 350°F. Cook manicotti tubes as directed on package and drain.

Fill tubes with cheese filling, using butter knife or teaspoon. Place filled tubes in greased baking dish, 11¾ x 7½ x 1½ inches. Pour tomato sauce over tubes. Cover with aluminum foil and bake at 350°F. for 15 to 20 minutes. Remove foil; sprinkle the ¼ cup Parmesan cheese and shredded mozarella cheese on top. Bake uncovered 10 minutes longer.

Yield: 7 servings

Nutrient analysis of 1 serving (2 tubes plus 2 tablespoons sauce): 2 starch/bread exchanges; 3 medium-fat meat exchanges; ½ fat exchange; 389 Calories; 25 g protein; 18 g fat; 30 g carbohydrate; 894 mg sodium; 117 mg cholesterol.

NON-MEAT MAIN DISHES

Cheese Soufflé

3 tablespoons margarine
3 tablespoons flour
2 teaspoons dry mustard
Dash cayenne pepper
1 cup milk
2 cups shredded sharp Cheddar cheese (8 ounces)
6 eggs, separated

Melt margarine in saucepan over low heat. Stir in flour, mustard, and cayenne pepper. Cook over low heat until smooth and bubbly. Remove from heat and stir in milk. Heat to boiling, stirring constantly. Boil, stirring constantly, for 1 minute. Stir in cheese; simmer over low heat until cheese is melted. Remove from heat and cool slightly.

Beat egg yolks until thick. Slowly blend into cheese mixture. Cool mixture about 15 minutes.

Preheat oven to 350°F. Grease soufflé dish, 10 x 5½ inches, or use a 2-quart casserole dish.

Beat egg whites just until stiff peaks form. Stir about half the egg whites into the cheese mixture. (Mixture will be foamy.) Carefully fold in remaining whites. Pour mixture into prepared soufflé dish. Bake until golden and puffed, about 25 minutes. Serve immediately.

Yield: 6 servings

Nutrient analysis of 1 serving: 2 medium-fat meat exchanges; ½ whole milk exchange; 2 fat exchanges; 309 Calories; 17 g protein; 24 g fat; 6 g carbohydrate; 389 mg sodium; 302 mg cholesterol.

Fresh Vegetable Soufflé

¼ cup all-purpose flour
⅛ teaspoon freshly ground pepper
½ teaspoon dried dillweed
½ teaspoon dry mustard
½ cup low-fat mayonnaise
¼ cup milk
1 cup finely chopped cooked vegetables (carrot, green beans, green pepper, or corn)
4 egg whites

Preheat oven to 325°F. Spray 1½-quart soufflé dish or casserole dish with vegetable spray.

Mix flour, pepper, dillweed, mustard, and mayonnaise. Stir in milk and vegetables.

Beat egg whites until stiff peaks form. Fold vegetable mixture into egg whites. Pour into prepared soufflé dish. Bake at 325°F. until knife inserted in center comes out clean, about 40 minutes. Serve immediately.

Yield: 4 servings

Nutrient analysis of 1 serving: 1 lean meat exchange; 2 vegetable exchanges; 104 Calories; 5 g protein; 4 g fat; 11 g carbohydrate; 96 mg sodium; 16 mg cholesterol.

**Asparagus Quiche*

Pastry for 9-inch one-crust pie (page 210)
¼ cup grated Parmesan cheese
½ pound asparagus, trimmed and sliced thin
4 ounces shredded Swiss cheese
¼ cup sliced scallions (include tops)
3 eggs
⅔ cup chicken stock
½ cup light cream (20% fat)
½ teaspoon salt
¼ teaspoon hot pepper sauce

Prepare pastry and chill.

Preheat oven to 450°F.

Prick bottom and sides of pastry-lined pie pan with fork and bake for 5 minutes. Remove from oven and sprinkle 2 tablespoons Parmesan cheese in pastry shell. Place half the asparagus in pastry shell. Top with half the Swiss cheese and scallions. Layer the remaining asparagus, Swiss cheese, and scallions in pastry. Beat eggs, chicken stock, cream, and seasonings; pour over layers. Sprinkle remaining 2 tablespoons Parmesan cheese on top. Bake for 10 minutes at 450°F. Reduce oven temperature to 325°F. and bake until knife inserted in center comes out clean, 20 to 25 minutes. Let stand for 10 minutes before cutting.

Yield: 12 appetizer servings or 6 entrée servings

Nutrient analysis of 1 entrée serving: 2 starch/bread exchanges; 1 high-fat meat exchange; 2 vegetable exchanges; 3 fat exchanges; 411 Calories; 13 g protein; 25 g fat; 42 g carbohydrate; 719 mg sodium; 37 mg cholesterol.

Tomato-Zucchini Whole Wheat Pie

Pastry for 9-inch one-crust whole wheat pie (page 210)
3 cups sliced unpared zucchini (2 to 4 small)
2 medium onions, sliced thin and separated into rings
2 tablespoons vegetable oil
¼ teaspoon garlic salt
Freshly ground pepper
1 medium tomato, sliced
1 egg
1 cup skim milk
1 tablespoon Italian herb seasoning
1 teaspoon dry mustard
¼ teaspoon salt
½ cup shredded part-skim-milk mozzarella cheese
Freshly ground pepper (additional)
¼ cup grated Parmesan cheese

Prepare pastry and set aside.

In a large skillet, cook and stir zucchini and onion in oil until onion is tender and zucchini is light brown, about 5 minutes. Season with garlic salt and pepper.

Preheat oven to 350°F.

Place zucchini-onion mixture in pastry-lined pie pan; top with tomato slices.

Beat egg, milk, Italian seasoning, mustard, and ¼ teaspoon salt. Stir in mozzarella cheese; season with pepper and pour over vegetables. Sprinkle Parmesan cheese on top. Bake at 350°F. for 40 to 45 minutes, until filling is set and top is brown.

Yield: 6 servings

Nutrient analysis of 1 serving: 1 starch/bread exchange; 1 medium-fat meat exchange; 2 vegetable exchanges; 3 fat exchanges; 323 Calories; 10 g protein; 22 g fat; 23 g carbohydrate; 374 mg sodium; 52 mg cholesterol.

*Eggplant Parmigiana

½ cup minced onion
1 clove garlic, minced
2 tablespoons vegetable oil
8-ounce can tomatoes, with liquid
8-ounce can tomato sauce
½ teaspoon salt
1 teaspoon dried oregano
½ teaspoon dried basil
¼ teaspoon pepper
1½ pounds eggplant
1½ pounds lean ground beef
¼ cup unprocessed bran
1 tablespoon wheat germ
½ teaspoon salt (additional)
⅛ teaspoon pepper (additional)
¼ cup grated Parmesan cheese
8 ounces part-skim-milk mozzarella cheese, sliced

Cook and stir onion and garlic in oil in saucepan until onion is tender, about 5 minutes. Stir in tomatoes and then liquid (breaking up tomatoes with fork), tomato sauce, ½ teaspoon salt, oregano, basil, and ¼ teaspoon pepper. Heat to boiling, stirring occasionally. Reduce heat and simmer uncovered for 30 minutes.

Preheat oven to 350°F. Spray baking sheet with vegetable spray.

Trim ends and cut eggplant into ½-inch-thick slices. Arrange in 1 layer on baking sheet and bake for 20 minutes.

Mix the ground beef, bran, wheat germ, ½ teaspoon salt, and ⅛ teaspoon pepper. Shape mixture into 8 patties, about ½ inch thick. Set oven control at broil or 550°F. Broil patties 3 inches from heat source, 3 to 4 minutes per side.

Pour half the tomato sauce into a baking pan, 13 x 9 x 2 inches. Layer the eggplant slices over the bottom of pan, then top with a layer of meat patties. Pour on remaining tomato sauce. Sprinkle with Parmesan cheese and arrange slices of mozzarella cheese on top. Bake in 350°F. oven for 30 minutes.

Yield: 8 servings

Nutrient analysis of 1 serving: 4 lean meat exchanges; 2 vegetable exchanges; 1 fat exchange; 314 Calories; 29 g protein; 17 g fat; 12 g carbohydrate; 675 mg sodium; 75 mg cholesterol.

Zucchini Casserole

2 egg whites
1/3 cup skim milk
4 medium unpared zucchini, diced (2 pounds)
1/2 cup bran
1 cup chopped onion
1/4 teaspoon garlic salt
Dash freshly ground pepper
2 cups shredded Cheddar cheese (8 ounces)

Preheat oven to 325°F. Spray a 1½-quart casserole dish with vegetable spray.

Beat egg whites and skim milk in a large bowl until blended. Stir in remaining ingredients. Pour into casserole. Bake at 325°F. for 40 minutes.

Yield: Six servings (1 cup each)

Nutrient analysis of 1 serving: 1 medium-fat meat exchange; 1 vegetable exchange; 1 low-fat milk exchange; ½ fat exchange; 208 Calories; 14 g protein; 13 g fat; 14 g carbohydrate; 258 mg sodium; 39 mg cholesterol.

Ratatouille Pie

Pastry for 9-inch one-crust pie (page 210)
1 large onion, sliced thin
2 cups diced pared eggplant
1 cup diced unpared zucchini
1 green pepper, seeded and chopped
2 tablespoons olive oil
Dash garlic salt
Freshly ground pepper
1 large or 2 medium tomatoes, peeled and sliced
1½ cups shredded Swiss cheese (6 ounces)

Prepare pastry and set aside.

Preheat oven to 350°F.

Cook and stir onion, eggplant, zucchini, and green pepper in olive oil in large skillet until eggplant is tender, 8 to 10 minutes. Season with garlic salt and pepper. Turn into pastry-lined pie pan. Place tomato slices on top and sprinkle with cheese.

Bake at 350°F. for 30 minutes, until cheese is melted.

Yield: 12 appetizer servings or 6 entrée servings

Nutrient analysis of 1 entrée serving: 1 starch/bread exchange; 1 medium-fat meat exchange; 1 vegetable exchange; 3 fat exchanges; 332 Calories; 10 g protein; 23 g fat; 22 g carbohydrate; 207 mg sodium; 4 mg cholesterol.

FISH AND SHELLFISH

Oven-Baked Haddock

Zucchini-Leek Sauté (see below)
2 pounds haddock
½ cup bread crumbs
¼ cup grated Parmesan cheese
1 teaspoon dried oregano
1 teaspoon snipped parsley
¼ teaspoon garlic powder
1 tablespoon sesame seeds
¼ cup all-purpose flour
1 egg, beaten

Prepare zucchini-leek sauté; keep warm. Preheat oven to 400°F.

Cut fish into 6 serving pieces. Mix bread crumbs, cheese, oregano, parsley, garlic powder, and sesame seeds. Dip fish into flour, then into egg, and then coat with bread crumb mixture. Place on greased baking sheet.

Bake at 400°F. until fish flakes easily with fork, 10 to 12 minutes. Remove fish to warm platter and surround with Zucchini-Leek Sauté.

Zucchini-Leek Sauté

3 tablespoons olive oil
1 leek, cut into ¼-inch slices (include green top)
3 small unpared zucchini, cut into ½-inch slices
1 red pepper, cut into 1-inch strips

Heat oil in large skillet. Cook and stir vegetables in skillet until tender, 8 to 10 minutes.

Yield: 6 servings

Nutrient analysis of 1 serving: 4 lean meat exchanges; 2 vegetable exchanges; 275 Calories; 34 g protein; 10 g fat; 12 g carbohydrate; 217 mg sodium; 47 mg cholesterol.

*Celestial Steamed Fish

2 pounds any lean fish in 1 piece
½ teaspoon salt
2-inch piece ginger, cut into slivers
3 tablespoons vegetable oil
3 tablespoons soy sauce
4 scallions, slivered
Sesame oil

Clean fish and wipe dry. Place in steamer; sprinkle with salt and ginger. Bring water to a boil in saucepan, add steamer basket, cover, and steam for 20 minutes. (If you do not have a steamer, place a rack in a skillet or heavy pot large enough to hold a plate with fish on it. Place fish on plate; sprinkle with salt and ginger. Place plate on rack in skillet. Pour in enough boiling water to cover the rack. Cover and steam fish for 20 minutes.) Remove fish to serving dish. Heat vegetable oil; pour over fish. Sprinkle on soy sauce and top fish with scallion slivers. Drizzle sesame oil on top.

Yield: 4 servings

Nutrient analysis of 1 serving: 3 medium-fat meat exchanges; ½ fat exchange; 250 Calories; 20 g protein; 18 g fat; 2 g carbohydrate; 1,280 mg sodium; 101 mg cholesterol.

*Herb-Baked Flounder

1 pound flounder fillets†
1 teaspoon snipped parsley
¼ teaspoon dried thyme
Salt and freshly ground pepper to taste
¾ cup chicken stock
½ pound mushrooms, sliced
2 teaspoons margarine
Lemon wedges
1 tomato, sliced thin

Place fish in a greased shallow baking dish. Sprinkle with parsley, thyme, salt, and pepper. Pour stock over fish. Bake in 450°F. oven until fish flakes easily with fork, 15 to 20 minutes. Remove fish to warm platter.

Cook and stir mushrooms in margarine until tender and all liquid is absorbed. Surround fish with mushrooms and garnish with lemon wedges and tomato slices.

Yield: 4 servings

Nutrient analysis of 1 serving: 3 lean meat exchanges; 1 vegetable exchange; 149 Calories; 21 g protein; 5 g fat; 5 g carbohydrate; 454 mg sodium; 76 mg cholesterol.

†Any firm lean fish fillets can be used in this recipe.

Poached Whole Fish

Court Bouillon (see below)

3- to 4-pound lake trout or similar fish, cleaned (with head and tail on)

Prepare Court Bouillon. Wash fish quickly in cold water, then pat dry. Wrap in double-thickness dampened cheesecloth (cheesecloth should be 12 inches wider than length of fish). Leave 6 inches of cheesecloth at each end of fish; twist ends and tie with string. Place fish in warm bouillon. If liquid is not 1½ to 2 inches above fish, add water. Cover and simmer 15 minutes. Remove pan from heat, but let fish sit in the bouillon an additional 15 minutes.

Using the tied ends, lift fish to cutting board. Open cloth and skin fish with a sharp knife, beginning at tail end. Pull skin from tail to gill. Using the cloth, turn fish and skin other side. Serve fish hot or cold. If fish is to be glazed, wrap in plastic wrap and then in aluminum foil and chill.

Court Bouillon

8 cups water
2 cups dry white wine
¼ cup white wine vinegar
3 onions, sliced
2 carrots, cut into 1-inch pieces
4 celery stalks, cut into 1-inch pieces
2 bay leaves
½ teaspoon dried tarragon
½ teaspoon dried thyme
1 tablespoon salt
10 peppercorns

Place all ingredients in a large saucepan and bring to a boil. Reduce heat and simmer for 30 minutes. Strain through a sieve. Cool to lukewarm. Do not place fish in boiling liquid to poach.

Yield: 6 to 8 servings

Nutrient analysis of 1 3-ounce serving: 3 medium-fat meat exchanges; 226 Calories; 22 g protein; 9 g fat; 0 g carbohydrate; 160 mg sodium; 46 mg cholesterol.

Baked Snapper in Sour Cream

1 lemon or medium onion, sliced thin
1 pound red snapper fillets, 1 inch thick
Salt and freshly ground pepper to taste
⅔ cup dairy sour cream
Paprika

Preheat oven to 400°F.

Arrange lemon slices in greased shallow baking pan. Place fish on slices and season with salt and pepper. Cover pan with aluminum foil. Bake at 400°F. until fish flakes easily with fork, 14 to 20 minutes.

Remove foil and spread sour cream on fish. Sprinkle with paprika. Set oven control at broil or 550°F. Broil fish 3 inches from heat source until golden.

Variation: Mix 1 teaspoon minced onion and ½ teaspoon prepared brown mustard into sour cream before spreading on fish.

Yield: 4 servings

Nutrient analysis of 1 serving: 3 lean meat exchanges; 1 vegetable exchange; 168 Calories; 24 g protein; 6 g fat; 4 g carbohydrate; 157 mg sodium; 77 mg cholesterol.

**Curried Fish Fillets*

1 pound fresh or defrosted lean fish fillets (flounder, sole, cod, halibut, or haddock)
½ teaspoon salt
¼ teaspoon white pepper
1 cup tomato, peeled, seeded, and chopped
⅓ cup sliced scallions
1 cup skim milk
2 teaspoons cornstarch
2 teaspoons snipped parsley
1 clove garlic, minced
2 teaspoons curry powder
½ teaspoon dried basil

Preheat oven to 400°F.

Arrange fish in single layer in baking dish, 10 x 10 x 2 inches. Sprinkle with salt and pepper. Spread tomato and scallions evenly on fish. Blend milk and cornstarch; stir in remaining ingredients and pour mixture over fish. Cover with aluminum foil. Bake at 400°F. until fish flakes easily with fork, 20 to 25 minutes.

Yield: 4 servings

Nutrient analysis of 1 serving: 3 lean meat exchanges; 1½ vegetable exchanges; 142 Calories; 23 g protein; 2 g fat; 8 g carbohydrate; 472 mg sodium; 76 mg cholesterol.

*Italian Baked Fish Fillets

- 1½ pound fish fillets
- 1 cup bread crumbs
- ¼ teaspoon pepper
- ¼ teaspoon salt
- ½ teaspoon dried oregano or Italian herb seasoning
- ½ cup grated Parmesan or Romano cheese
- 2 tablespoons snipped parsley
- ¼ teaspoon garlic powder
- 2 eggs
- ¼ cup all-purpose flour
- Parsley sprigs
- Lemon wedges

Preheat oven to 350°F. Grease a baking sheet and set aside. If fillets are large, cut into serving-size pieces.

Mix bread crumbs, pepper, salt, oregano, cheese, parsley, and garlic powder in pie pan. Beat eggs in flat bowl. Dip fish into flour, then into eggs, and then coat with crumb mixture. Place on prepared baking sheet. Bake at 350°F. until fish flakes easily with fork, 10 to 15 minutes. Remove to heated platter and garnish with parsley sprigs and lemon wedges.

Yield: 6 servings

Nutrient analysis of 1 serving: 1 starch/bread exchange; 3 lean meat exchanges; 204 Calories; 26 g protein; 4 g fat; 16 g carbohydrate; 545 mg sodium; 171 mg cholesterol.

Broiled Sole

- 1½ pounds sole fillets
- Salt and freshly ground pepper to taste
- 1 lemon, halved
- 1 medium tomato, peeled and chopped
- 1 tablespoon margarine
- 1 tablespoon snipped parsley

Set oven control at broil or 550°F. Place fish in 1 layer on sheet of lightly oiled heavy-duty aluminum foil. Turn up edges to form a low edge. Place on baking sheet. Season fish with salt and pepper. Squeeze juice from 1 lemon half onto fish. Top with tomato and dot with margarine.

Broil fish 3 inches from heat source until fish flakes easily with fork, 3 to 4 minutes. Remove fish to warm platter and sprinkle with parsley. Cut remaining half lemon into thin slices and arrange around fish.

Yield: 6 servings

Nutrient analysis of 1 serving: 2½ lean meat exchanges; 118 Calories; 19 g protein; 4 g fat; 1 g carbohydrate; 170 mg sodium; 86 mg cholesterol.

Fillet of Sole Pedro

1½ pounds sole fillets
Juice of 1 lemon
Salt and freshly ground pepper to taste
1 medium tomato, peeled and sliced
1 tablespoon margarine
Lemon wedges
Snipped parsley

Cover baking sheet with aluminum foil; spray with vegetable spray. Arrange fish in 1 layer on foil. Sprinkle lemon juice onto fish. Season fish with salt and pepper. Arrange tomato slices on fish and dot with margarine. Bake in 325°F. oven until fish flakes easily with fork, 10 to 15 minutes. Remove fish to heated platter and garnish with lemon wedges and parsley.

Yield: 6 servings

Nutrient analysis of 1 serving: 3 lean meat exchanges; 130 Calories; 20 g protein; 5 g fat; 1 g carbohydrate; 127 mg sodium; 86 mg cholesterol.

Herbed Sole

½ teaspoon freshly ground pepper
¼ teaspoon dried fines herbes
2 pounds sole or flounder fillets
½ cup dry white wine or apple juice
2 tablespoons lemon juice
¼ pound mushrooms, sliced
2 tablespoons margarine
1 small onion, thinly sliced
Snipped parsley
Lemon wedges

Preheat oven to 350°F. Grease shallow baking dish, 11¾ x 7½ x 1¾ inches. Set aside.

Mix pepper and fines herbes; season both sides of fish and arrange in baking dish. Combine wine and lemon juice; pour over fish. Cook and stir mushrooms in margarine for 5 minutes. Place mushrooms and onion slices around fish.

Bake at 350°F. until fish flakes easily with fork, about 20 minutes. Sprinkle parsley on fish and serve with lemon wedges.

Yield: 8 to 10 servings (3 ounces each)

Nutrient analysis of 1 serving: 2 lean meat exchanges; 118 Calories; 17 g protein; 5 g fat; 1 g carbohydrate; 186 mg sodium; 60 mg cholesterol.

Sole Amandine

- 3 tablespoons margarine
- 1½ pounds sole fillets
- ¼ cup sliced unsalted almonds
- 1 teaspoon grated lemon peel
- 2 teaspoons lemon juice
- Parsley sprigs
- Lemon wedges

Melt 2 tablespoons margarine in a large skillet over medium heat. Place as many fillets as will fit in 1 layer in skillet and cook until golden brown, about 2 minutes per side. Two or more batches may be needed. Remove fish to serving platter and keep warm.

Melt remaining tablespoon of margarine in skillet. Cook and stir almonds, lemon peel, and juice for 1 minute. Pour over fish and garnish with parsley and lemon wedges.

Yield: 6 servings (3 ounces each)

Nutrient analysis of 1 serving: 3 medium-fat meat exchanges; 1 fat exchange; 299 Calories; 23 g protein; 23 g fat; 0 g carbohydrate; 107 mg sodium; 86 mg cholesterol.

Grilled Salmon

- ¼ cup unsalted margarine, softened
- 1 tablespoon prepared yellow mustard
- Juice of half lemon
- Dash cayenne pepper
- 1 tablespoon snipped parsley
- 4 salmon steaks (4 ounces each)
- Salt and freshly ground pepper to taste
- Olive oil

Mix margarine, mustard, lemon juice, cayenne pepper, and parsley in small bowl. Cover and refrigerate 1 hour.

Set oven control at broil or 550°F. Season steaks with salt and freshly ground pepper. Brush oil on steaks. Broil steaks 4 inches from heat source, turning once, until fish flakes easily with fork, about 7 minutes. Serve with sauce.

Yield: 4 servings

Nutrient analysis of 1 serving: 4 medium-fat meat exchanges; 324 Calories; 27 g protein; 23 g fat; 0 g carbohydrate; 228 mg sodium; 47 mg cholesterol.

*Salmon Loaf

16-ounce can red salmon
Skim milk (approximately 4 ounces)
3 tablespoons margarine
3 tablespoons flour
½ teaspoon salt
Dash freshly ground pepper
2 tablespoons minced onion
1 cup whole wheat bread crumbs
½ cup unprocessed bran
1 egg, beaten

Preheat oven to 350°F.

Drain salmon and flake, reserving liquid. Remove large bones and skin from salmon and discard. Measure reserved liquid; add enough milk to make 1 cup.

Melt margarine in saucepan over low heat. Blend in flour, salt, and pepper. Cook over low heat, stirring constantly, until mixture is smooth and bubbly. Remove from heat. Stir in salmon liquid-milk mixture. Heat to boiling, stirring constantly. Boil and stir for 1 minute. Mix in salmon, onion, bread crumbs, bran, and egg. Turn into a greased loaf pan, 9 x 5 x 4 inches. Bake at 350°F. for 35 to 40 minutes.

Yield: 8 servings

Nutrient analysis of 1 serving: 1 starch/bread exchange; 2 lean meat exchanges; 1 fat exchange; 220 Calories; 16 g protein; 11 g fat; 12 g carbohydrate; 550 mg sodium; 335 mg cholesterol.

Cold Poached Salmon with Dill Mayonnaise

4- to 5-pound salmon, whole or filleted
8 cups water
½ cup white vinegar
1 onion, sliced
2 or 3 sprigs parsley
1½ teaspoons salt
1 teaspoon peppercorns
1 bay leaf
Dill Mayonnaise (page 151)
Fresh dill sprigs
Lemon slices

If using whole salmon, have head and tail removed. Wrap salmon in cheesecloth and set aside. Heat water, vinegar, onion, parsley, salt, peppercorns, and bay leaf to boiling in large saucepan. Reduce heat, cover, and simmer for 30 minutes. Carefully place salmon in liquid. Liquid should cover salmon; if necessary, add boiling water. Cover, and simmer until fish flakes easily with fork. (Allow 10 minutes per inch of thickness measured at thickest part.) Remove salmon from liquid and refrigerate. When cold, unwrap salmon and carefully remove skin. Serve with Dill Mayonnaise and garnish with sprigs of dill and slices of lemon.

Variation: Salmon can be served hot. Remove salmon from liquid; unwrap and carefully remove skin. Serve with Hollandaise Sauce (page 198).

Yield: 6 servings

Nutrient analysis of 3 ounces salmon without mayonnaise: 3 lean meat exchanges; 158 Calories; 23 g protein; 6 g fat; 0 g carbohydrate; 250 mg sodium; 39 mg cholesterol.

Dill Mayonnaise

- **1 tablespoon plus 1½ teaspoons lemon juice**
- **1 teaspoon prepared Dijon mustard**
- **3 tablespoons snipped parsley**
- **1 tablespoon snipped dill**
- **2 teaspoons snipped chives**
- **½ teaspoon salt**
- **1 egg**
- **⅓ cup olive oil**
- **⅔ cup vegetable oil**

Measure all ingredients except vegetable oil into blender container or food processor. Cover and process at high speed for 30 seconds. Continuing to process at high speed, slowly add vegetable oil. Continue blending until mixture is the consistency of mayonnaise. Cover and refrigerate until ready to use.

Note: All olive oil (1 cup) or all vegetable oil (1 cup) can be used in this recipe.

Yield: 1½ cups

Nutrient analysis of 2 tablespoons: 4 fat exchanges; 171 Calories; 1 g protein; 19 g fat; 0 g carbohydrate; 86 mg sodium; 22 mg cholesterol.

Broiled Trout with Dill

4 4-ounce trout fillets
½ lemon
½ teaspoon garlic salt
Freshly ground pepper
½ cup Italian-style bread crumbs
2 teaspoons snipped dill
1 teaspoon Worcestershire sauce
2 teaspoons margarine

Line broiler tray with aluminum foil. Arrange fish in 1 layer on foil. Squeeze juice from lemon onto fish. Mix garlic salt, pepper, bread crumbs, dill, and Worcestershire sauce. Sprinkle over fish, then dot each fish with ½ teaspoon margarine.

Set oven control at broil or 550°F. Broil fish 4 inches from heat source until fish flakes easily with fork, 6 to 8 minutes.

Yield: 4 servings

Nutrient analysis of 1 serving: 1 starch/bread exchange; 4 lean meat exchanges; 294 Calories; 31 g protein; 13 g fat; 12 g carbohydrate; 761 mg sodium; 62 mg cholesterol.

Trout with Mushrooms

4 6- to 7-ounce rainbow trout, cleaned (heads removed)
Salt and freshly ground pepper to taste
1 tablespoon dried chervil
4 teaspoons margarine
1 cup scallions, sliced thin (include green tops)
2 tablespoons margarine
8 ounces mushrooms, sliced thin
Salt and pepper to taste
Hot pepper sauce (optional)
Lemon wedges

Line broiler pan with aluminum foil. Arrange fish in pan; season with salt and pepper, and sprinkle with chervil. Dot each fish with 1 teaspoon margarine.

Set oven control at broil or 550°F. Broil fish 3 inches from heat source until fish flakes easily with fork, 8 to 10 minutes.

Cook and stir scallions in 2 tablespoons margarine for 1 minute. Add mushrooms; cook and stir until mushrooms are soft, 2 to 3 minutes. Season with salt and pepper and, if desired, a few drops of hot pepper sauce. Top fish with mushroom mixture and garnish with lemon wedges.

Yield: 4 servings

Nutrient analysis of 1 serving: 2½ medium-fat meat exchanges; 1 vegetable exchange; 2 fat exchanges; 317 Calories; 17 g protein; 25 g fat; 4 g carbohydrate; 276 mg sodium; 62 mg cholesterol.

Trout à la Summit

6 6- to 7-ounce whole rainbow trout, heads and backbones removed
½ lemon
Freshly ground pepper
3 tablespoons margarine
2 ounces sliced almonds
4 scallions, sliced thin (include green tops)
2 tablespoons margarine (additional)
1 cup seedless ruby grapes, halved

Line broiler pan with aluminum foil. Spread fish flat, skin side down, in pan in 1 layer. Squeeze juice from lemon on fish; season with pepper. Dot fish with the 3 tablespoons margarine.

Set oven control at broil or 550°F. Broil fish 3 inches from heat source until fish flakes easily with fork, 5 to 7 minutes.

While fish is broiling, cook and stir almonds and scallions in 2 tablespoons margarine until scallions are soft. Stir in grapes and heat through. Serve fish topped with grape mixture.

Yield: 6 servings

Nutrient analysis of 1 serving: 3 medium-fat meat exchanges; 2 fat exchanges; 310 Calories; 19 g protein; 26 g fat; 2 g carbohydrate; 211 mg sodium; 62 mg cholesterol.

Swordfish Steaks

4 6-ounce swordfish steaks†
Juice of 2 limes or lemons
1 teaspoon freshly shredded ginger or 2 teaspoons powdered ginger
4 teaspoons margarine
Dash salt and freshly ground pepper
Snipped parsley
Lime or lemon wedges

Arrange fish in baking dish, 11¾ x 7½ x 1¾ inches. Mix lime juice and ginger; pour over fish. Marinate for 30 to 40 minutes, turning fish several times.

Set oven control at broil or 550°F. Spray broiler tray with vegetable spray. Arrange fish on tray and dot each steak with 1 teaspoon margarine. Broil 3 inches from heat source for 5 minutes. Turn and broil until fish flakes easily with fork, about 5 minutes more. Garnish with parsley and lime wedges.

Yield: 4 servings

Nutrient analysis of 1 serving: 4½ lean meat exchanges; 255 Calories; 32 g protein; 14 g fat; 0 g carbohydrate; 279 mg sodium; 101 mg cholesterol.

†Any firm fish steaks can be used in this recipe.

Scallops Provençal

1 pound bay scallops
2 cloves garlic, minced
2 tablespoons vegetable oil
2 tablespoons margarine
¼ cup all-purpose flour
½ teaspoon salt
¼ teaspoon freshly ground pepper
Snipped parsley
Lemon wedges

Rinse scallops and drain. (If using large sea scallops, cut each into quarters.) Cook and stir garlic in oil and margarine in skillet for 2 to 3 minutes. Mix flour, salt, and pepper; coat scallops with flour mixture.

Add scallops to skillet and cook over medium heat for 3 to 5 minutes. Stir often, making sure all sides are browned. Remove to heated platter and garnish with parsley and lemon wedges.

Yield: 4 servings

Nutrient analysis of 1 serving: ½ starch/bread exchange; 3 lean meat exchanges: 169 Calories; 20 g protein; 7 g fat; 8 g carbohydrate; 356 mg sodium; 45 mg cholesterol.

Crab Norfolk

¼ cup margarine
4 cloves garlic, crushed
1⅓ cups cooked or frozen crabmeat
Dash freshly ground pepper
½ cup snipped parsley
Lemon wedges

Melt margarine in skillet. Add garlic; cook and stir over low heat for 5 minutes. Add crabmeat; cook and stir over medium heat for 3 to 5 minutes. Remove crabmeat to warm platter. Season with pepper and garnish with parsley and lemon wedges.

Yield: 4 servings

Nutrient analysis of 1 serving: 2½ lean meat exchanges; 150 Calories; 16 g protein; 9 g fat; 1 g carbohydrate; 220 mg sodium; 92 mg cholesterol.

*Zuppa di Pesce

2-pound whole red snapper or bass
8-ounce bottle clam juice
6 cups water
1½ teaspoons salt
½ teaspoon peppercorns
1 onion, sliced
1 leek, split (optional)
1 stalk celery
1 bay leaf
½ teaspoon fennel seeds
½ teaspoon dried thyme
¼ teaspoon hot pepper sauce
28-ounce can Italian tomatoes
2 cloves garlic, split
Small bunch parsley
¼ teaspoon saffron filaments
2 tablespoons vegetable oil
1 large onion, chopped (additional)
2 cloves garlic, minced (additional)
8 ounces shrimp, shelled
8 ounces scallops, cut up if large
3 pounds mussels
12 small clams
1 cup dry white wine
Slices Italian bread, spread with garlic butter and toasted

Cut snapper into 1½-inch pieces, reserving heads and tails. Refrigerate fish pieces, and place fish heads and tails in a large kettle. Add the clam juice, water, salt, peppercorns, sliced onion, leek, celery, bay leaf, fennel, thyme, hot pepper sauce, tomatoes, split garlic, and parsley. Heat to boiling. Reduce heat and simmer, partially covered, for 2 hours. Strain fish stock into large bowl. Stir in saffron and set aside.

Heat vegetable oil in Dutch oven or large flameproof casserole. Cook and stir chopped onion and minced garlic in oil until onion is tender. Add snapper pieces and brown on both sides. Add the shrimp, scallops, mussels, clams, wine, and reserved fish stock and stir once. Heat to boiling, cover, and steam until shellfish have opened, 10 to 15 minutes. Serve with toasted Italian bread.

Yield: 10 servings

Nutrient analysis of 1 serving (not including bread): 5 lean meat exchanges; 2 vegetable exchanges; 243 Calories; 35 g protein; 6 g fat; 12 g carbohydrate; 1,022 mg sodium; 148 mg cholesterol.

**Seafood Marinara*

24 cleaned mussels (see note below)
24 cleaned clams (see note below)
1 pound scallops
2 tablespoons flour
¼ cup minced onion
1 teaspoon dried oregano
½ teaspoon dried thyme
¼ cup vegetable oil
¼ cup snipped parsley
15-ounce can tomato sauce
6-ounce can tomato paste
Hot cooked linguine

Steam mussels and clams in 1 cup water until shells open. Discard any that do not open. Drain, reserving liquid.

Coat scallops with flour. Cook and stir onion, oregano, and thyme in oil in large saucepan until onion is tender. Stir in scallops and parsley; cook and stir until scallops are golden. Stir in tomato sauce, tomato paste, mussels, and clams. Heat to boiling, stirring occasionally. Reduce heat, and simmer for 10 minutes. Serve over hot linguine.

Note: To clean clams and mussels, soak in water, then scrub shells well and remove beards from mussels.

Yield: 6 servings

Nutrient analysis of 1 serving (without linguine): 1 starch/bread exchange; 4 lean meat exchanges: 1 vegetable exchange; 345 Calories; 37 g protein; 12 g fat; 22 g carbohydrate; 885 mg sodium; 108 mg cholesterol.

MEATS

Veal Piccata

1½ pounds veal scallops
Freshly ground pepper
2 tablespoons margarine
1½ teaspoons dried tarragon
8 thin lemon slices
¼ cup white wine or vermouth
2 tablespoons snipped parsley

Place veal scallops between sheets of waxed paper and pound carefully to ½-inch thickness. (A rolling pin or mallet can be used.) Season veal scallops with pepper. Melt margarine in large skillet. Brown veal scallops, 3 or 4 at a time, over medium-high heat. Turn and brown other side. Remove veal scallops to warm platter. Add lemon slices and wine to skillet and heat through. Pour over veal scallops and sprinkle parsley on top.

Yield: 6 servings (3 ounces each)

Nutrient analysis of 1 serving of veal plus sauce: 3 lean meat exchanges; 1 fat exchange; 216 Calories; 21 g protein; 15 g fat; 0 g carbohydrate; 93 mg sodium; 70 mg cholesterol.

Dilled Veal Burgers

1 pound lean ground veal
1 pound lean ground beef
2 tablespoons snipped dill
1 tablespoon Worcestershire sauce
1 teaspoon garlic salt
1 tablespoon spicy brown mustard
2 tablespoons wheat germ
3 drops hot pepper sauce

Mix all ingredients together thoroughly. Shape mixture into 8 patties, each about 3 inches in diameter and 1 inch thick.

Set oven control at broil or 550°F. Broil patties 3 inches from heat source, turning once, until done as desired. Can be served with Béarnaise Sauce (page 199) and snipped dill.

Yield: 8 servings

Nutrient analysis of 1 serving: 3 lean meat exchanges; 1 vegetable exchange; 194 Calories; 22 g protein; 10 g fat; 4 g carbohydrate; 250 mg sodium; 69 mg cholesterol.

Osso Buco à la Romana

8 pounds veal shanks
¾ cup all-purpose flour
¼ cup bran
1 teaspoon salt
Dash freshly ground pepper
½ cup vegetable oil
½ cup margarine
2 cups chopped onion
1 cup chopped carrot
1 cup chopped celery
1 leek or 4 scallions, chopped
2 teaspoons minced garlic
1 cup white wine
35-ounce can Italian tomatoes, drained and tomatoes broken apart
1 teaspoon dried basil
1 teaspoon dried thyme
½ teaspoon dried oregano
1 cup chicken stock
6 sprigs parsley
2 bay leaves, crumbled
¼ cup snipped parsley
2 teaspoons shredded orange peel

Have butcher saw veal shanks into 3-inch pieces and tie each piece with string.

Preheat oven to 350°F.

Mix flour, bran, salt, and pepper; coat meat with flour mixture. Heat the oil in a large skillet. Sauté meat until browned and remove to a large shallow casserole.

Melt margarine in skillet. Cook and stir onion, carrot, celery, leek, and garlic in skillet until onion is tender. Spoon vegetables around and under veal. Mix wine, tomatoes, basil, thyme, oregano, and stock; pour over meat. Place parsley sprigs and bay leaves between meat pieces. Cover and bake at 350°F. for 45 minutes. Reduce heat to 325°F. and bake 2 hours more, basting often, until meat is tender. Remove meat to ovenproof platter.

Cool slightly and then pour vegetables and liquid into blender container or food processor. Process until smooth. Pour into saucepan and heat to boiling. Reduce heat and cook uncovered until liquid is reduced by one half.

Set oven control at broil or 550°F. Broil meat 3 inches from heat source until brown, 5 to 7 minutes. Pour sauce on meat and sprinkle top with snipped parsley and orange peel.

Yield: 8 to 10 servings (4 ounces each)

Nutrient analysis of 1 serving veal plus ½ cup sauce: ¾ starch/bread exchange; 4 medium-fat meat exchanges; 357 Calories; 30 g protein; 20 g fat; 10 g carbohydrate; 398 mg sodium; 97 mg cholesterol.

Lemon-Dilled Veal Scallops

6 boneless veal cutlets (4 ounces each)
3 tablespoons flour
¼ teaspoon salt
Dash freshly ground pepper
3 tablespoons olive oil
½ cup white wine
1 lemon, cut into thin slices
3 tablespoons snipped dill

Pound meat to ½ inch thickness. Mix flour, salt, and pepper. Heat oil in large skillet. Coat meat with flour mixture and brown quickly on both sides. Pour ¼ cup wine into skillet and simmer for 2 minutes. Sprinkle lemon slices and 2 tablespoons dill on meat; simmer 1 minute more.

Remove meat to heated platter. Pour remaining wine into skillet. Cook, stirring constantly, until heated through, 1 to 2 minutes. Pour over meat and garnish with remaining snipped dill.

Yield: 6 servings

Nutrient analysis of 1 serving: 4 lean meat exchanges; 1 fat exchange; 277 Calories; 28 g protein; 17 g fat; 3 g carbohydrate; 127 mg sodium; 70 mg cholesterol.

Lemon Ginger Veal

2½ pounds boneless veal scallops
Salt and freshly ground pepper to taste
2 tablespoons flour
¼ cup margarine
1½ teaspoons fresh ginger
½ teaspoon dried tarragon
⅓ cup snipped parsley
½ cup dry white wine
3 tablespoons lemon juice
½ lemon, sliced thin
1 clove garlic, crushed

Cut veal steak into 8 serving pieces; pound each until ½ inch thick. Season with salt and pepper and coat with flour. Melt margarine in large skillet. Cook meat, 2 or 3 pieces at a time, until golden brown. Remove from skillet and keep warm. When all pieces are browned, return meat to skillet. Sprinkle with ginger, tarragon, and half the parsley. Add wine, lemon juice, lemon slices, and garlic; heat to boiling. Reduce heat, cover, and cook for 5 minutes. Serve meat with sauce and garnish with remaining parsley.

Yield: 8 servings (3 ounces each)

Nutrient analysis of 1 serving: 3 lean meat exchanges; 161 Calories; 21 g protein; 6 g fat; 3 g carbohydrate; 268 mg sodium; 70 mg cholesterol.

Jellied Veal

3 pounds veal shank, split
1 pound pork loin roast
1 tablespoon salt
1 large onion, cut up
3 bay leaves
10 whole allspice
2 teaspoons white pepper
1 tablespoon white vinegar
1 envelope (1/4 ounce) unflavored gelatin
1/4 cup cold water

Place veal and pork in large kettle. Cover meat with water, and then add salt, onion, bay leaves, and allspice. Cover and cook until meat falls off bones, about 2 hours. Cool.

Remove meat from bones. Grind meat with coarse blade on grinder. Strain stock; stir in pepper and vinegar. (More salt can be added if needed.) Soften gelatin in 1/4 cup water. Heat stock to boiling. Stir in gelatin until dissolved. Stir in meat; pour into 2 loaf pans, 8 1/2 x 4 1/2 x 3 inches. Refrigerate until firm. Serve in thin slices with wedges of lemon.

Yield: 2 loaves, 12 slices each

Nutrient analysis of 1 slice: 2 lean meat exchanges; 109 Calories; 12 g protein; 6 g fat; 0 g carbohydrate; 265 mg sodium; 41 mg cholesterol.

Scaloppine con Funghi

4 boneless veal cutlets (4 ounces each)
Salt and freshly ground pepper to taste
2 tablespoons flour
2 tablespoons olive oil
1/2 cup white vermouth or Italian white wine
2 cups thinly sliced mushrooms
Snipped parsley
Lemon wedges

Pound meat with mallet or edge of saucer until 1/4 inch thick. Season with salt and pepper. Coat meat with flour. Heat oil in large skillet; brown meat over medium-high heat, 3 to 4 minutes per side. Pour wine into skillet and heat to boiling. Reduce heat, cover, and simmer for 2 to 3 minutes. Spread mushrooms over meat in skillet. Cover and simmer 2 to 3 minutes more. Remove meat and mushrooms to warm platter. Pour sauce in skillet over meat. Garnish with parsley and lemon wedges.

Yield: 4 servings

Nutrient analysis of 1 serving: 4 lean meat exchanges; 1 vegetable exchange; 1 fat exchange; 295 Calories; 29 g protein; 17 g fat; 6 g carbohydrate; 111 mg sodium; 70 mg cholesterol.

Veal Marsala with Prosciutto

1½ pounds boneless veal scallops
2 tablespoons flour
¼ cup olive oil
¼ cup margarine
⅓ cup minced onion
1 clove garlic, crushed
½ pound mushrooms, sliced thin
1 teaspoon fresh lemon juice
¾ cup Marsala wine
¼ cup snipped parsley
1 tablespoon fresh or 1 teaspoon dried basil
¼ pound prosciutto, sliced thin and cut into ½-inch strips
Salt and pepper to taste

Cut veal into 6 serving pieces. Pound with mallet or saucer edge until ½ inch thick; coat with flour. Heat oil and margarine in large skillet. Cook veal until tender and brown, about 4 minutes per side. Remove to warm platter and keep warm.

Cook and stir onion and garlic in skillet until onion is tender, 3 to 4 minutes. Add mushrooms and lemon juice; cook and stir over medium heat until mushrooms are soft. Stir in wine, parsley, basil, and prosciutto. Heat to boiling. Reduce heat and simmer for 1 minute. Season with salt and pepper. Return meat to sauce and heat through, 2 to 3 minutes.

Yield: 6 servings (3 ounces each)

Nutrient analysis of 1 serving of veal plus sauce: 4 lean meat exchanges; 1½ vegetable exchanges; 1 fat exchange; 327 Calories; 27 g protein; 17 g fat; 7 g carbohydrate; 332 mg sodium; 93 mg cholesterol.

High-Fiber Meat Loaf

1 pound lean ground beef
1 cup tomato juice
½ cup regular rolled oats
2 tablespoons bran
½ cup carrot, finely diced
1 egg white, beaten
¼ cup chopped onion
½ teaspoon salt
Dash freshly ground pepper
¼ teaspoon dry mustard

Preheat oven to 350°F.

Measure all ingredients into bowl and mix. Press mixture into loaf pan, 8½ x 4½ x 2¾ inches. Bake at 350°F. for 1 hour. Allow loaf to stand for 5 minutes before slicing.

Yield: 8 servings

Nutrient analysis of 1 serving: 1 starch/bread exchange; 2 lean meat exchanges; 198 Calories; 16 g protein; 6 g fat; 22 g carbohydrate; 240 mg sodium; 40 mg cholesterol.

All-Day Oven Stew

2½ pounds boneless lean stew meat, cubed
2 cups 1½-inch pieces celery
6 medium carrots, cut into 1½-inch pieces
10 small white onions, whole, or 3 or 4 yellow onions, quartered
6 medium potatoes, peeled and quartered
28-ounce can tomato puree
1 tablespoon salt
Dash freshly ground pepper
1 tablespoon cornstarch

Preheat oven to 250°F.

Combine meat, celery, carrots, onions, and potatoes in 3-quart casserole. Mix tomato puree, salt, pepper, and cornstarch. Pour into casserole. Stir, cover, and bake at 250°F. for 5 hours.

Note: One tablespoon Italian seasoning or other favorite herbs can be added to this stew.

Yield: 6 servings

Nutrient analysis of 1 serving: 2 starch/bread exchanges; 3 medium-fat meat exchanges; 1 vegetable exchange; 412 Calories; 29 g protein; 14 g fat; 33 g carbohydrate; 709 mg sodium; 127 mg cholesterol.

Beef Wellington

5- to 6-pound fillet of beef
½ cup sliced onion
½ cup carrot, sliced thin
½ cup celery, sliced thin
¼ teaspoon dried thyme
¼ teaspoon dried sage
1 bay leaf
3 allspice berries or whole cloves
5 peppercorns
⅓ cup olive oil
1 teaspoon salt
1 cup white vermouth
⅓ cup cognac
Mushroom Stuffing (see below)
17¾-ounce package frozen puff pastry or pastry for Lattice Crust Pie (page 210)
1 egg white
1 tablespoon water

Have butcher trim fat and gristle from beef fillet and tie thin strips of fat salt pork or beef suet around it.

Cook and stir vegetables and seasonings in olive oil until vegetables are tender, about 10 minutes. Place meat in casserole or baking dish and season with salt. Cover meat with vegetable mixture and pour on vermouth and cognac. Cover and refrigerate. Turn and baste meat every several hours for at least 24 hours. (This stiffens the meat so that it holds its shape in the crust.)

Prepare mushroom stuffing (see below). Remove meat from marinade and pat dry with paper towels.

Place meat on rack in shallow baking pan. Roast in 425°F. oven for 1 hour, or until meat thermometer registers 140° for rare. Cool meat slightly. Remove salt pork covering.

Prepare puff pastry as directed on package, except roll into rectangle 18 x 24 inches, or large enough to enclose meat. Trim edges of pastry evenly. Place meat along edge of long side of pastry; spread mushroom stuffing over remaining surface, leaving a 1-inch margin on each side. Roll up meat and pastry. Seal seam and ends securely, moistening with water if necessary. Beat egg white and water slightly; brush over pastry. Cut any remaining pastry into decorative shapes; arrange on top and brush with egg white mixture.

Place pastry-covered meat, seam side down, on baking sheet. Roast in 425°F. oven until pastry is golden brown, 40 minutes. Use 2 broad spatulas to remove meat to warm serving platter.

Mushroom Stuffing

2½ pounds fresh mushrooms, minced
1 pound shallots, minced
½ cup margarine
2-ounce can pâté

Cook and stir mushrooms and shallots in margarine in large skillet over low heat until all liquid is absorbed. Remove from heat and mix in pâté.

Yield: 16 slices (3-ounce slice meat plus pastry and stuffing)

Nutrient analysis of 1 slice (including pastry and stuffing): 1 starch/bread exchange; 3 medium-fat meat exchanges; 1 vegetable exchange; 3 fat exchanges; 475 Calories; 28 g protein; 30 g fat; 19 g carbohydrate; 465 mg sodium; 112 mg cholesterol.

Flank Steak and Peppers

1 pound lean flank steak, scored
1 teaspoon garlic salt
Dash freshly ground pepper
½ cup vegetable oil
2 tablespoons red wine vinegar
½ teaspoon garlic powder
½ teaspoon dry mustard
1 teaspoon dried thyme
Pepper Topping (see below)

Season steak with garlic salt and pepper. Place in shallow bowl. Mix oil, vinegar, garlic powder, mustard, and thyme. Pour over steak. Cover and marinate in refrigerator, turning occasionally, 3 to 4 hours or overnight.

Prepare Pepper Topping and keep warm.

Set oven control at broil or 550°F. Broil steak about 3 inches from heat source for 5 minutes. Turn meat and broil about 5 minutes more, or until done as desired. Remove to heated platter. Cut meat across grain at a slanted angle into thin slices. Spoon on Pepper Topping and serve.

Pepper Topping

1 large onion, sliced thin
1 green pepper, seeded and cut into thin slices
1 red pepper, seeded and cut into thin slices
¼ cup vegetable oil

Cook and stir vegetables in oil over medium heat until onion is tender.

Yield: 4 servings (3 ounces each)

Nutrient analysis of 1 serving: 3 medium-fat meat exchanges; 1 vegetable exchange; 1 fat exchange; 341 Calories; 26 g protein; 25 g fat; 4 g carbohydrate; 220 mg sodium; 79 mg cholesterol.

Beef Fillet with Vegetable Topping

1 medium red onion, sliced thin
¼ green pepper, seeded and sliced thin
3 tablespoons olive oil
1 cup sliced mushrooms
Dash garlic salt
Dash freshly ground pepper
2 beef tenderloin fillets (2 inches thick and approximately 2½ pounds)

Cook and stir onion and green pepper in oil until tender. Add mushrooms. Cook and stir until mushrooms are heated through, about 1 minute. Season with garlic salt and pepper. Remove from heat and keep warm.

Set oven control at broil or 550°F. Broil meat, turning once, to desired doneness—10 to 15 minutes for rare, 15 to 20 minutes for medium. Remove meat to warm platter; top with vegetables and, if desired, 1 tablespoon Béarnaise Sauce (page 199).

Yield: 8 to 10 servings

Nutrient analysis (3-ounces beef plus ½ cup topping): 3 medium-fat meat exchanges; 1 vegetable exchange; 261 Calories; 23 g protein; 16 g fat; 5 g carbohydrate; 245 mg sodium; 79 mg cholesterol.

Steak with Tomato-Garlic Sauce

3 tablespoons olive oil
3 cloves garlic, minced
16-ounce can whole tomatoes, drained and quartered (reserve juice for future use)
1 tablespoon snipped fresh basil or 1 teaspoon dried basil
¼ cup snipped parsley
Salt and pepper to taste
3 to 4 pounds boneless sirloin steak (1½ inches thick)
Freshly ground pepper
2 cloves garlic, slivered
3 tablespoons olive oil (additional)
2 tablespoons capers
¼ cup snipped parsley (additional)

Heat 3 tablespoons oil in saucepan over high heat. Remove from heat and add minced garlic, tomatoes, basil, and ¼ cup parsley. Season with salt and pepper. Heat to boiling and boil for 1 minute. Reduce heat and simmer for 10 minutes. Remove from heat and keep warm.

Season both sides of meat with pepper. Insert slivers of garlic on one side of meat. Heat 3 tablespoons oil just to smoking in large heavy skillet. Add meat and cook for 1 minute. Turn and cook 1 minute longer. Pour sauce over meat. Reduce heat, cover, and cook over medium heat for 5 minutes (for well-done, cook 10 minutes). Scrape sauce from meat back into skillet. Remove meat to heated platter and carve across grain into ¼-inch slices. Stir capers into sauce and heat for 1 minute. Spoon sauce over meat and sprinkle with ¼ cup parsley.

Yield: 8 to 10 servings (3 ounces each)

Nutrient analysis of 1 serving: 3 medium-fat meat exchanges; ½ vegetable exchange; 3 fat exchanges; 382 Calories; 19 g protein; 33 g fat; 3 g carbohydrate; 247 mg sodium; 76 mg cholesterol.

London Broil

2¾-pound very lean flank steak, scored

Set oven control at broil or 550°F. Broil steak 2 to 3 inches from heat source for about 10 minutes, or until browned. Turn meat; broil about 10 minutes more, or until browned. Remove to heated platter. Cut meat across grain at a slanted angle into thin slices.

Yield: 8 servings (3 ounces)

Nutrient analysis of 1 serving: 3 medium-fat meat exchanges; 226 Calories; 24 g protein; 14 g fat: 0 g carbohydrate; 62 mg sodium; 109 mg cholesterol.

**Mock Steak Béarnaise*

1 pound lean ground beef
4 slices whole wheat bread
1½ tablespoons margarine
1 medium tomato, sliced
4 tablespoons Béarnaise Sauce (page 199)
Parsley sprigs

Shape meat into 4 patties, each about 3 inches in diameter and 1 inch thick. Set oven control at broil or 550°F. Broil patties 3 inches from heat source, 3 to 4 minutes per side for rare, 5 to 7 minutes for medium.

Remove crusts from bread and cut into 4 3-inch circles. Spread with margarine; toast in large skillet. Place tomato slice on each toast round, then top with meat patty and 1 tablespoon Béarnaise Sauce. Garnish with parsley sprig.

Yield: 4 servings

Nutrient analysis of 1 serving: 1 starch/bread exchange; 3 medium-fat meat exchanges; 2½ fat exchanges; 407 Calories; 25 g protein; 30 g fat; 12 g carbohydrate; 446 mg sodium; 148 mg cholesterol.

Hamburgers Deluxe

- 2 pounds lean ground beef
- 1 egg
- 1 tablespoon capers
- 1 tablespoon Worcestershire sauce
- 1 teaspoon garlic salt
- Freshly ground pepper
- 6 teaspoons blue cheese, softened

Mix all ingredients except blue cheese. Shape mixture into 6 patties, each about 3 inches in diameter and 1 inch thick. Make indentation in center of each patty; place 1 teaspoon blue cheese in each and cover with meat.

Set oven control at broil or 550°F. Broil patties 3 inches from heat source, 3 to 4 minutes per side for rare, 5 to 7 minutes for medium.

Yield: 6 servings

Nutrient analysis of 1 serving: 4 medium-fat meat exchanges; 293 Calories; 34 g protein; 16 g fat; 1 g carbohydrate; 245 mg sodium; 156 mg cholesterol.

**Skillet Dinner*

- 2 tablespoons vegetable oil
- 1 pound flank steak, scored
- ½ cup chopped onion
- ½ cup beef stock
- 2 cloves garlic, crushed
- 1 teaspoon hot pepper sauce
- ½ teaspoon dried oregano
- ½ teaspoon salt
- 1 bay leaf
- 2 cups green beans, cut into 1-inch pieces (½ pound)
- 3 medium potatoes, pared and quartered
- 4 carrots, cut into 2- to 3-inch pieces

Heat oil in large skillet; brown meat on both sides over medium heat. Add onions; cook and stir until tender. Stir in stock, garlic, pepper sauce, oregano, salt, and bay leaf. Heat to boiling, reduce heat, cover, and simmer for 1 hour. Add more water or stock if necessary. Add beans, potatoes, and carrots. Cover and cook over medium heat until potatoes are tender, about 30 minutes. Remove bay leaf before serving.

Yield: 4 servings (3 ounces each)

Nutrient analysis of 1 serving: 1 starch/bread exchange; 3 medium-fat meat exchanges; 2 vegetable exchanges; 348 Calories; 30 g protein; 14 g fat; 27 g carbohydrate; 446 mg sodium; 79 mg cholesterol.

Steak Diane

1 cup sliced mushrooms
2 tablespoons minced onion
1 clove garlic, crushed
⅛ teaspoon salt
1 teaspoon lemon juice
1 teaspoon Worcestershire sauce
3 tablespoons margarine
2 tablespoons snipped parsley
2 tablespoons margarine (additional)
1 pound tenderloin, cut into 8 slices

Cook and stir mushrooms, onion, and seasonings in 3 tablespoons margarine until mushrooms are tender. Stir in parsley and keep sauce warm.

Melt the 2 tablespoons margarine in a large skillet. Cook meat in margarine, turning once, over medium-high heat to medium doneness, 3 to 4 minutes per side. Serve with mushroom sauce.

Yield: 4 servings (3 ounces each)

Nutrient analysis of 1 serving: 3 medium-fat meat exchanges; 1 vegetable exchange; 1 fat exchange; 301 Calories; 23 g protein; 22 g fat; 2 g carbohydrate; 295 mg sodium; 79 mg cholesterol.

Curried Beef

1 tablespoon curry powder
½ cup water
¼ cup unsalted margarine
3 medium onions, chopped or sliced thin
½ clove garlic, minced
1½ pounds beef chuck or round, cut into 1-inch cubes
1 tablespoon cornstarch
Freshly ground pepper
3 cups water

Soak curry powder in ½ cup water for 1 hour.

Melt margarine in large skillet. Cook and stir onions, garlic, and meat in margarine until meat is browned. Stir in curry mixture. Cook over medium heat, stirring constantly, for 10 minutes. Mix cornstarch, pepper, and 3 cups water; stir into meat mixture. Heat to boiling, stirring frequently. Reduce heat, cover, and simmer until meat is tender, about 2 hours.

Yield: 8 servings

Nutrient analysis of 1 serving: 2 medium-fat meat exchanges; 1 vegetable exchange; 176 Calories; 19 g protein; 9 g fat; 4 g carbohydrate; 49 mg sodium; 57 mg cholesterol.

Beef with Broccoli

1 pound flank steak, trimmed of all fat and shredded†
2 cloves garlic, minced
1 teaspoon grated fresh ginger root
⅓ cup vegetable oil
1 pound broccoli, separated into small flowerets and thinly sliced stems
1½ teaspoons cornstarch
3 tablespoons water
1 tablespoon plus 1½ teaspoons soy sauce

Combine shredded meat, garlic, and ginger root in bowl and toss. Let stand for 30 minutes.

Heat wok or large fry pan; add oil and rotate pan to coat. Add meat and stir-fry until meat is browned, 2 to 3 minutes. Add broccoli and stir-fry until crisp-tender, 1 to 2 minutes. Mix cornstarch, water, and soy sauce; stir into meat mixture. Cook, stirring constantly, until mixture boils and thickens. Continue to cook and stir for 1 minute.

Yield: 6 servings

Nutrient analysis of 1 serving: 2 medium-fat meat exchanges; 1 vegetable exchange; 150 Calories; 19 g protein; 7 g fat; 3 g carbohydrate; 293 mg sodium; 53 mg cholesterol.

†Cut meat with grain into long strips about 2 inches wide. Cut each strip across grain into ⅛-inch slices. Stack slices and cut into thin strips.

Brisket with Apples and Caraway

3 cups cored, sliced, unpared tart apples
3 cups sliced onion
1 slice rye bread
2 teaspoons caraway seeds
3 pounds trimmed beef brisket
2 tablespoons flour
1/4 teaspoon black pepper
1 tablespoon red wine vinegar

Arrange half the apple slices, half the onion slices, the bread, and 1 teaspoon caraway seeds in a 2-quart casserole. Sear meat in its own fat and place in casserole; sprinkle with flour and pepper. Cover meat with remaining apple and onion slices and caraway seeds. Cover tightly and bake in 350°F. oven until meat is tender, about 2 hours.† Remove meat to warm platter. Skim any fat from liquid. Pour apple-onion mixture into food mill, blender, or food processor and process until smooth. Stir in vinegar and, if desired, season with pepper. If necessary, thin sauce with water.

Cut meat into thin slices; arrange slices on serving platter. Heat pureed sauce to boiling and pour over meat. Nice served with steamed new potatoes and fresh green beans.

Yield: 8 to 10 servings

Nutrient analysis of 1 serving (3 ounces meat plus 1/8 of sauce): 3 medium-fat meat exchanges; 1 fruit exchange; 279 Calories; 25 g protein; 12 g fat; 17 g carbohydrate; 102 mg sodium; 70 mg cholesterol.

†This recipe can be made a day ahead to this point. Refrigerate overnight. Skim fat from liquid. Remove meat and puree apple-onion mixture. Replace meat in casserole; pour puree over it and reheat at 325°F. for 1 hour.

Country-Boiled Short Ribs

8 lean short ribs (approximately 3 pounds)
½ cup diced onion
1 cup diced carrot
1 cup diced celery
½ bay leaf
2 whole cloves
¼ teaspoon peppercorns, crushed
Salt
8 small potatoes, pared
1 small cabbage, cut into wedges
Horseradish Sauce (see below)

Place meat in 2½-quart saucepan. Add water to 2-inch depth around meat. Heat to boiling; remove scum as it comes to top. Add onion, carrot, celery, bay leaf, cloves, and peppercorns. Heat to boiling. Reduce heat, cover, and simmer until meat is tender, about 2½ hours.

Heat 1 inch water and ½ teaspoon salt to boiling in saucepan. Add potatoes, cover, and heat to boiling. Reduce heat and cook until tender, 30 to 35 minutes. Drain.

Heat 1 inch water and ½ teaspoon salt to boiling in another saucepan. Add cabbage, cover, and heat to boiling. Reduce heat and cook until cabbage is crisp-tender, 10 to 12 minutes. Drain.

Arrange meat, potatoes, and cabbage on serving platter. Serve with Horseradish Sauce.

Horseradish Sauce

Mix 1 cup plain low-fat yogurt and ½ cup well-drained prepared white horseradish.

Yield: 8 servings (1 rib, 1 potato, and ½ cup cabbage)

Nutrient analysis of 1 serving: 1 starch/bread exchanges; 3 high-fat meat exchanges; 1 vegetable exchange; 2 fat exchanges; 496 Calories; 24 g protein; 32 g fat; 28 g carbohydrate; 347 mg sodium; 81 mg cholesterol.

Beef or Lamb Shish Kebabs

Meat-Basting Sauce (see below)
6 ounces beef or lamb cubes
2 small onions, quartered
6 cherry tomatoes
6 fresh mushroom caps
1 medium green pepper, seeded and cut into 1-inch pieces

Prepare Meat-Basting Sauce. Place meat in deep bowl; pour sauce on meat and refrigerate for at least 3 hours, turning meat occasionally. (Can be refrigerated up to 24 hours.)

Drain meat, reserving sauce. Alternate meat, onion quarters, tomatoes, mushrooms, and green pepper pieces on skewers.

Set oven control at broil or 550°F. Broil kebabs 3 inches from heat source, turning kebabs and basting occasionally with reserved sauce, until done as desired. Kebabs can also be grilled over hot coals.

Yield: 3 servings

Nutrient analysis of 1 serving: 2 medium-fat meat exchanges; 2½ vegetable exchanges; 218 Calories; 12 g protein; 12 g fat; 13 g carbohydrate; 32 mg sodium; 39 mg cholesterol.

Meat-Basting Sauce

1 cup red wine
1 cup vegetable oil
¼ cup red wine vinegar
2 medium onions, chopped
2 cloves garlic, peeled
⅛ teaspoon rosemary leaves
⅛ teaspoon cayenne pepper

Shake all ingredients in tightly covered screw-top jar.

Yield: About 2¼ cups

Nutrient analysis of 1 teaspoon: 1 fat exchange; 57 Calories; 0 g protein; 6 g fat; 1 g carbohydrate; 1 mg sodium; 0 mg cholesterol.

Crown Roast of Lamb

24-rib crown roast of lamb (approximately 5 pounds)
Brown Rice Pilaf (page 114)
Dilled Carrots (page 99)
Green beans
Broiled tomatoes
Mustard Sauce (see below)

Place roast on rack in shallow baking pan or broiler pan. Roast in 350°F. oven 1½ hours (about 15 minutes per pound), or until meat thermometer inserted in thickest part of meat registers 140°F. for medium rare, or 150°F. for medium well done. Remove meat to warm platter; let rest for 10 minutes.

Fill center of roast with pilaf. Arrange carrots, beans, and tomatoes around roast. Serve Mustard Sauce in a small bowl.

Yield: 8 to 10 servings (2 or 3 ribs per serving)

Nutrient analysis of 1 ounce of lamb (please note—nutrient analyses of various vegetables are listed with individual recipes): 1 medium-fat meat exchange; 75 Calories; 7 g protein; 5 g fat; 0 g carbohydrate; 70 mg sodium; 20 mg cholesterol.

Mustard Sauce

½ cup whipping cream
¼ cup prepared Chardonnay white wine mustard
2 tablespoons snipped parsley
1 tablespoon lemon juice

Blend cream and mustard in small saucepan. Stir in parsley and lemon juice. Heat through, stirring constantly, over low heat (do not boil). Serve with lamb or vegetables.

Yield: ¾ cup

Nutrient analysis of 1 tablespoon: 1 fat exchange; 36 Calories; 0 g protein; 4 g fat; 0 g carbohydrate; 64 mg sodium; 4 mg cholesterol.

*Cassoulet

1 pound dried northern beans
4- to 5-pound duckling (thawed if frozen)
Salt and freshly ground pepper
¾ pound lean boneless pork, cut into ½-inch cubes
¾ pound boneless lamb, cut into ½-inch cubes
3 to 4 garlic cloves, peeled and chopped
1 large onion, chopped
1 stalk celery, diced
2 bay leaves
¾ pound smoked ham, cut into ½-inch cubes
1 teaspoon dried thyme
2 teaspoons salt
28-ounce can tomatoes
2 cups dry white wine

Place beans in large saucepan and cover with water. Heat to boiling and boil for 2 minutes. Remove from heat, cover, and let stand for 1 hour. Add more water, if necessary, to cover beans, and simmer uncovered for 50 minutes, or until tender. (Do not boil or beans will burst.) Drain beans, reserving liquid.

Season duckling with salt and pepper. Roast on rack in 325°F. oven until tender, about 2 hours. Prick skin with fork while roasting to release fat. When duckling is cool enough to handle, cut into slices. Discard bones.

Heat 2 to 3 tablespoons of the drippings from the duckling in a large skillet. (Remainder of drippings can be discarded.) Add the cubes of pork and lamb and the garlic. Cook and stir until brown.

In a 4-quart casserole or crockpot, combine duckling slices, pork, lamb, garlic, onion, celery, bay leaves, ham, thyme, and salt. Add beans and mix carefully. Add tomatoes and wine and, if necessary, enough reserved bean liquid so that liquid comes to 1 inch below top of food. Cover tightly and bake in a 250°F. oven for 4 to 6 hours or in crockpot on low setting for 10 to 12 hours. Discard bay leaves before serving.

Note: This recipe is very high in cholesterol and should not be eaten by someone on a low-cholesterol diet.

Yield: 14 servings (1 cup each)

Nutrient analysis of 1 serving: 1 starch/bread exchange; 4½ lean meat exchanges; 1 vegetable exchange; 356 Calories; 37 g protein; 14 g fat; 22 g carbohydrate; 624 mg sodium; 702 mg cholesterol.

Skillet Pork Chops

2 tablespoons vegetable oil
4 4-ounce pork chops
1 pound tomatoes, peeled and sliced
1 large green pepper, seeded and cut into rings
1 large onion, sliced
1 stalk celery, chopped
2 teaspoons dried basil
1 teaspoon celery salt
Freshly ground pepper

Heat oil in large skillet. Add chops and brown on both sides. Top chops with vegetables and sprinkle with basil, celery salt, and pepper. Cover and cook over low heat until chops are tender, 45 to 60 minutes. If necessary, add small amount of water during cooking.

Yield: 4 servings

Nutrient analysis of 1 serving: 3 medium-fat meat exchanges; 1½ vegetable exchanges; 1 fat exchange; 316 Calories; 25 g protein; 20 g fat; 8 g carbohydrate; 277 mg sodium; 74 mg cholesterol.

Barbecued Spareribs

3 pounds lean spareribs
¼ cup vegetable oil
2 tablespoons parsley flakes
2 tablespoons dried oregano
2 teaspoons dried rosemary, crushed
¼ teaspoon salt
¼ teaspoon pepper
3 medium onions, sliced and separated into rings
2 cloves garlic, minced
Barbecue Sauce (page 199)

Rub ribs with oil and place in baking pan. Season with parsley flakes, oregano, rosemary, salt, and pepper. Sprinkle onion rings and garlic on ribs.

Roast in 375°F. oven until ribs are brown on both sides, about 1 hour. Drain fat from pan. Pour barbecue sauce on ribs.

Reduce oven temperature to 350°F. Bake for 1¾ hours; baste ribs frequently with sauce.

Yield: 4 servings (3 ounces each)

Nutrient analysis of 1 serving (meat only; count sauce separately): 3 medium-fat meat exchanges; 3 fat exchanges; 1 vegetable exchange; 381 Calories; 20 g protein; 30 g fat; 7 g carbohydrate; 155 mg sodium; 79 mg cholesterol.

**Chinese Peas with Pork and Water Chestnuts*

2 tablespoons vegetable oil
6 ounces lean pork loin slices (about 1/4 inch thick and 2 to 3 inches long)
1 cup chicken stock
1 pound snow peas (Chinese green peas)
1 cup sliced water chestnuts
1 tablespoon cornstarch
1 tablespoon water
2 tablespoons soy sauce

Heat wok or large skillet until 1 or 2 drops water skitter around when sprinkled in pan. Add oil; rotate to coat side of pan. Add pork and stir-fry until pork is no longer pink. Add stock, cover, and cook over medium heat for 3 minutes. Add peas and water chestnuts; stir-fry for 1 minute. Mix cornstarch, water, and soy sauce; stir into meat mixture. Cook and stir over medium heat until mixture thickens.

Yield: 6 servings

Nutrient analysis of 1 serving: 1 medium-fat meat exchange; 2 vegetable exchanges; 1/2 fat exchange; 147 Calories; 10 g protein; 8 g fat; 9 g carbohydrate; 520 mg sodium; 19 mg cholesterol.

**Pork Chops Dijon*

6 center-cut pork loin chops (4 ounces each)
1/2 cup all-purpose flour
1 egg
3/4 cup prepared Dijon mustard
1 cup bread crumbs

Spray baking pan, 13 x 9 x 2 inches, with vegetable spray. Coat chops with flour. Beat egg and mustard in flat bowl until blended. Dip chops in mustard mixture, then coat with bread crumbs. Arrange in baking pan. Bake in a 350°F. oven until chops are brown and tender, 1 hour.

Yield: 6 servings

Nutrient analysis of 1 serving: 1 starch/bread exchange; 3 medium-fat meat exchanges; 336 Calories; 26 g protein; 17 g fat; 19 g carbohydrate; 520 mg sodium; 119 mg cholesterol.

Pork Chops with Dill

4 4-ounce loin pork chops
1 medium onion, sliced
2 tablespoons snipped fresh dill
4 slices tomato

Arrange the pork chops in a shallow baking dish. Top each with onion slice. Sprinkle with some of the snipped fresh dill (or use dried dillweed). Add a slice of tomato to each chop and sprinkle with the remaining snipped dill. Top with another slice of onion. Bake in a 350°F. oven until chops are tender, about 1 hour. Serve with Dill Sauce (see below).

Dill Sauce

1 cup tomato slices
½ cup snipped fresh dill
6 ounces sliced mushrooms

Cook and stir all ingredients in saucepan until tomatoes are tender, about 6 minutes.

Yield: 4 servings

Nutrient analysis of 1 serving: 3 medium-fat meat exchanges; 1 vegetable exchange; 248 Calories; 27 g protein; 13 g fat; 4 g carbohydrate; 68 mg sodium; 74 mg cholesterol.

Paul's Alsatian Pork Roast

5-pound pork loin roast
¼ pound dried apricots
2 cups Gewürztraminer (German white wine)
6 potatoes, pared and quartered

Have butcher bone pork loin and cut pocket lengthwise in meat. Do not have meat tied at intervals.

Soak apricots in wine in ceramic or glass dish for at least 8 hours or overnight in refrigerator.

Drain apricots, reserving marinade, and insert in pocket of roast. Pour ¼ cup marinade into pocket; tie roast at 2-inch intervals.

Roast meat at 350°F. for 2 hours. Surround meat with potatoes, turning potatoes to coat with drippings. Roast meat and potatoes, basting occasionally with reserved marinade, until meat thermometer registers 170°F. and potatoes can be pierced with fork, about 1 hour more.

Yield: 6 servings

Nutrient analysis of 1 serving: 1 starch/bread exchange; 3 medium-fat meat exchanges; 1 fruit exchange; 341 Calories; 26 g protein; 16 g fat; 25 g carbohydrate; 161 mg sodium; 185 mg cholesterol.

Pork Cutlets

½ cup all-purpose flour
1 teaspoon dry mustard
1 teaspoon paprika
1½ pounds boneless pork loin cutlets
3 tablespoons vegetable oil
1 egg
2 tablespoons skim milk
¾ cup bread crumbs
1 tablespoon margarine
1 tablespoon flour (additional)
1 teaspoon dried dillweed
¾ cup chicken stock
½ cup plain low-fat yogurt
2 tablespoons spicy brown prepared mustard

Mix the ½ cup flour, dry mustard, and paprika together. Pound meat with mallet or edge of saucer until ¼ inch thick. Coat meat with flour mixture. Heat oil in large skillet. Beat egg and milk until blended. Dip meat into egg, then coat with crumbs. Cook meat in oil until brown and tender, 4 to 5 minutes per side. (Do not crowd meat in skillet; cook in 2 batches if necessary.) Remove meat to warm platter and keep warm.

Melt margarine in skillet. Blend in 1 tablespoon flour and dillweed. Cook over low heat, stirring constantly, until smooth. Stir in stock. Heat to boiling, stirring constantly. Reduce heat to low and stir in yogurt and prepared mustard. Heat through, but do not allow sauce to boil. Pass sauce with meat.

Variations: Use veal cutlets instead of pork; substitute ¾ cup dairy sour cream for the yogurt, and omit the prepared mustard.

Yield: 6 servings

Nutrient analysis of 1 serving: 1½ starch/bread exchanges; 3 medium-fat meat exchanges; 1 fat exchange; 381 Calories; 28 g protein; 21 g fat; 20 g carbohydrate; 327 mg sodium; 120 mg cholesterol.

*Fresh Ham Roast with Potatoes

6- to 8-pound fresh ham (rind removed)
1 cup prepared mustard
¼ cup margarine, melted
1 cup bread crumbs
8 medium potatoes, pared and quartered

Score top of meat in diagonal pattern. Place meat, fat side up, on rack in open shallow roasting pan. Insert meat thermometer so tip is in center of thickest part of meat and does not touch bone or rest in fat. Do not add water or cover. Roast meat in 325°F. oven (it is not necessary to preheat). Roast until meat thermometer registers 170°F. Allow 40 minutes per pound for roasting time of fresh ham.

Mix mustard, margarine, and bread crumbs. About 1½ hours before meat is done, spread mixture on meat. Add potatoes to pan, turning each to coat with drippings. Roasts are easier to carve if allowed to sit for 15 to 20 minutes after removal from oven.

Yield: 8 servings

Nutrient analysis of 1 serving: 2 starch/bread exchanges; 3 medium-fat meat exchanges; ½ fat exchange; 390 Calories; 30 g protein; 17 g fat; 28 g carbohydrate; 602 mg sodium; 75 mg cholesterol.

Ham, Broccoli, and Tomato Pie

1 cup broccoli flowerets
2 medium tomatoes, peeled and sliced
4 ounces sliced cooked ham, diced
1 cup shredded Swiss cheese
1 small onion, sliced thin
½ cup light cream
½ cup chicken stock
2 eggs, beaten
Whole Wheat Pastry for 9-inch one-crust pie (page 210)

Preheat oven to 450°F.

Layer broccoli, tomato slices, ham, cheese, and onion in 8-inch square baking pan. Mix cream, chicken stock, and eggs. Pour over ingredients in baking pan.

Roll out pastry 8 inches square. Fold in half and cut slits on folded edge. Place on ingredients, unfold, and seal to edges of pan. Bake at 450°F. for 10 minutes. Reduce oven temperature to 350°F. and bake until crust is golden brown, 25 to 30 minutes.

Yield: 8 servings

Nutrient analysis of 1 serving: 2 starch/bread exchanges; 1 medium-fat meat exchange; 2 fat exchanges; 332 Calories; 13 g protein; 19 g fat; 28 g carbohydrate; 322 mg sodium; 92 mg cholesterol.

**Ham and Cheese Quiche*

Unbaked 9-inch pastry shell, chilled
1 cup diced cooked ham
2 cups shredded Swiss cheese
3 eggs, beaten
⅔ cup chicken stock
½ cup cream

Preheat oven to 450°F.

Prick bottom and sides of pastry shell with fork. Bake at 450°F. for 5 minutes, then remove from oven and cool for 5 minutes. Layer ham and cheese in pastry shell. Mix eggs, chicken stock, and cream; pour into pastry shell. Bake 10 minutes at 450°F., then reduce oven temperature to 350°F. Continue to bake until knife inserted in center of quiche comes out clean, 20 to 25 minutes.

Yield: 6 main-dish or 12 appetizer servings

Nutrient analysis of 1 main-dish serving: 1 starch/bread exchange; 3 medium-fat meat exchanges; 3 fat exchanges; 440 Calories; 24 g protein; 31 g fat; 16 g carbohydrate; 745 mg sodium; 208 mg cholesterol.

Nutrient analysis of 1 appetizer serving: ½ starch/bread exchange; 1½ medium-fat meat exchanges; 1 fat exchange; 220 Calories; 12 g protein; 15 g fat; 8 g carbohydrate; 392 mg sodium; 104 mg cholesterol.

*Sausage and Lima Beans

2 pounds sweet Italian sausage
2 cups dry white wine or chicken stock
1 large onion, coarsely chopped
4 cloves garlic, coarsely chopped
2 tablespoons vegetable oil
3 large tomatoes, peeled and coarsely chopped
Dash freshly ground pepper
1 bay leaf
½ teaspoon dried sweet basil
1 teaspoon dry mustard
½ cup chicken stock (additional)
2 10-ounce packages frozen lima beans, thawed
⅓ cup snipped parsley

Place sausages in large, heavy skillet. Pour in 1½ cups wine and heat to boiling. Reduce heat and turn sausages. Cover only partially so steam can escape. Cook until sausages are brown on all sides and liquid has disappeared. Remove sausages and drain fat from skillet.

Cook and stir onion and garlic in oil in skillet until onion is tender. Stir in tomatoes, pepper, bay leaf, basil, and mustard. Cook about 3 minutes. Add chicken stock, sausages, and remaining ½ cup wine. Cook over medium heat for 3 minutes. Stir in lima beans and 3 tablespoons of the parsley. Heat to boiling. Reduce heat, cover, and simmer for 45 minutes, stirring occasionally. Sprinkle remaining parsley on top before serving.

Yield: 8 servings

Nutrient analysis of 1 serving: 1 starch/bread exchange; 3 medium-fat meat exchanges; 1 fat exchange; 324 Calories; 22 g protein; 20 g fat; 14 g carbohydrate; 1,188 mg sodium; 87 mg cholesterol.

POULTRY

*Chicken and Almonds

- 2 large chicken breasts, skinned, boned, and diced (about 1 pound of meat)
- ½ teaspoon salt
- ¼ teaspoon freshly ground pepper
- 2 teaspoons cornstarch
- 2 teaspoons soy sauce
- 1 egg white
- ½ cup vegetable oil
- 3 tablespoons slivered almonds
- 1 cup mushrooms, sliced thin
- ½ cup chicken stock
- 3 scallions, sliced thin (include green tops)

Place chicken in medium bowl. Add salt, pepper, cornstarch, soy sauce, egg white, and 1 tablespoon oil; mix thoroughly. Let stand for 30 minutes.

Heat wok or large fry pan. Add remaining oil and rotate pan to coat. Add almonds; stir-fry until golden. Remove with slotted spoon to paper towel. Add ⅓ of the chicken and stir-fry until tender (do not overcook). Remove from pan and drain on paper towel. Stir-fry remaining chicken, in 2 more batches, until tender. Remove from pan and drain on paper towel. Drain all but 1 tablespoon oil from pan; add mushrooms and stir-fry for 30 seconds. Add chicken stock and chicken; heat to boiling, stirring constantly. Remove to serving platter and sprinkle almonds and scallions on top.

Yield: 6 servings

Nutrient analysis of 1 serving: 3 medium-fat meat exchanges; 1 vegetable exchange; 1 fat exchange; 285 Calories; 24 g protein; 19 g fat; 5 g carbohydrate; 408 mg sodium; 51 mg cholesterol.

Sautéed Chicken Cutlets Dijonnaise

4 boneless chicken breast halves, split and pounded flat (4 ounces each)
¾ cup all-purpose flour
2 tablespoons unsalted margarine
2 tablespoons vegetable oil
½ cup dry vermouth
2 tablespoons prepared Dijon mustard
⅓ cup light cream
Salt and freshly ground pepper
2 tablespoons drained small capers

Coat both sides of cutlets with flour. Heat margarine and oil in large skillet until very hot. Cook cutlets, one at a time, in hot skillet until browned on both sides, about 5 to 6 minutes. Remove cutlets to warm platter and keep warm.

Pour vermouth into skillet; cook over low heat for 2 minutes, scraping loose any brown bits in pan. Stir in mustard and cream and cook 2 more minutes. (Do not boil.) Season with salt and pepper. Add cutlets to sauce, turning once to coat. Turn onto serving platter and sprinkle with capers.

Yield: 4 servings

Nutrient analysis of 1 serving: 1 starch/bread exchange; 4 lean meat exchanges; 306 Calories; 29 g protein; 14 g fat; 16 g carbohydrate; 227 mg sodium; 87 mg cholesterol.

**Chicken with Tomato*

6 ounces skinned and boned chicken breast
1 tablespoon cornstarch
2 tablespoons soy sauce
1 tablespoon dry sherry
2 tablespoons vegetable oil
1 medium onion, sliced thin
¼ cup chicken stock
¼ teaspoon salt
½ teaspoon sugar
2 medium tomatoes, peeled and cut into wedges

Cut chicken into ½-inch strips. Mix cornstarch, soy sauce, and sherry in medium bowl. Add chicken and toss to coat all pieces. Marinate chicken in mixture for 20 minutes, tossing occasionally.

Heat oil in wok or skillet. Add chicken and stir-fry 3 to 4 minutes. Add onion slices, and stir-fry 3 minutes more. Stir in chicken stock, salt, and sugar and heat to boiling. Gently stir in tomato wedges and heat through.

Yield: 4 servings

Nutrient analysis of 1 serving: ½ starch/bread exchange; 1½ lean meat exchanges; 123 Calories; 12 g protein; 5 g fat; 8 g carbohydrate; 833 mg sodium; 24 mg cholesterol.

**Grilled Chicken*

½ cup margarine
1 tablespoon lemon juice
1 tablespoon soy sauce
2 cloves garlic, crushed
¼ teaspoon dried thyme
1 teaspoon dried tarragon
⅛ teaspoon white pepper
2 2½-pound broiler-fryers, quartered
Freshly ground pepper
2 tablespoons coarse (kosher) salt
Snipped parsley

Set oven control at broil or 550°F.

Cream margarine, adding lemon juice a few drops at a time. Beat in soy sauce, garlic, thyme, tarragon, and pepper. Spread paste on both sides of chicken pieces.

Place chicken, skin side down, on broiler rack; season with pepper and 1 tablespoon coarse salt. Broil 4 inches from heat source for 15 minutes; baste chicken every 5 minutes with remaining paste, and then with drippings. Turn the chicken, and season with pepper and the remaining tablespoon of coarse salt. Broil 10 minutes longer, or until done. Chicken is done when thickest parts are fork-tender and drumstick meat feels soft when pressed between fingers.

Yield: 8 servings

Nutrient analysis of 1 serving: 3½ lean meat exchanges; 269 Calories; 25 g protein; 18 g fat; 0 g carbohydrate; 1,796 mg sodium; 75 mg cholesterol.

Lemon Chicken

2½-pound broiler-fryer chicken, cut up
¼ cup lemon juice
2 tablespoons vegetable oil
½ teaspoon dry mustard
¼ teaspoon dried rosemary
¼ teaspoon dried thyme
¼ teaspoon dried marjoram
¼ teaspoon sesame seeds
¼ teaspoon pepper

Preheat oven to 300°F.

Arrange chicken in lightly greased shallow pan. Mix all remaining ingredients. Brush part of mixture on chicken. Bake uncovered at 300°F. for 1 hour, brushing frequently with remaining mixture. Increase oven temperature to 500°F. and bake 15 minutes more.

Yield: 8 servings

Nutrient analysis of 1 serving: 3 lean meat exchanges; 196 Calories; 24 g protein; 10 g fat; 0 g carbohydrate; 57 mg sodium; 88 mg cholesterol.

Baked Lemon Chicken

2 chicken breasts, split (2 to 2½ pounds) or 2- to 2½-pound broiler-fryer, cut up
1 clove garlic, crushed
Juice of 1 large lemon
3 tablespoons vegetable oil
Snipped parsley
Cherry tomatoes or tomato slices

Place chicken in glass or ceramic bowl. Sprinkle with garlic and pour on lemon juice and oil. Turn chicken to coat both sides. Cover and refrigerate several hours or overnight, turning occasionally.

Preheat oven to 350°F.

Remove chicken from marinade. Place, skin side up, on rack in shallow roasting pan. Bake until tender and golden brown, 35 to 40 minutes. Remove to warm platter and garnish with parsley and tomatoes.

Note: Chicken can be broiled or grilled.

Yield: 4 servings

Nutrient analysis of 1 serving: 3 lean meat exchanges; 1 fat exchange; 230 Calories; 25 g protein; 15 g fat; 1 g carbohydrate; 60 mg sodium; 71 mg cholesterol.

**Onion-Smothered Chicken*

3-pound broiler-fryer, cut up
¼ cup skim milk
¼ cup whole wheat flour
3 tablespoons vegetable oil
3 medium onions, sliced
⅓ cup soy sauce
1 cup boiling water
2-inch piece fresh ginger, diced
Hot cooked rice

Preheat oven to 350°F.

Dip chicken into milk, then coat with flour. Heat 2 tablespoons oil in large skillet. Cook chicken in oil over medium heat until browned on both sides. Arrange chicken in baking pan, 13 x 9 x 2 inches.

Add remaining oil to skillet. Cook and stir onion until tender. Stir in soy sauce, water, and ginger and heat to boiling. Pour over chicken. Cover tightly and bake at 350°F. until fork-tender, about 45 minutes. Serve with rice.

Yield: 8 servings

Nutrient analysis of 1 serving: ½ starch/bread exchange; 4 lean meat exchanges; 248 Calories; 30 g protein; 11 g fat; 7 g carbohydrate; 768 mg sodium; 84 mg cholesterol.

*Chicken with Walnuts

3 tablespoons cornstarch
2 tablespoons dry sherry
8 ounces skinned and boned chicken breast, cut into 1-inch cubes
3 tablespoons vegetable oil
1 cup blanched walnut halves
1 tablespoon minced fresh ginger
½ cup diced bamboo shoots
4-ounce can mushrooms, drained (reserve liquid)
¼ cup chicken stock

Combine cornstarch and sherry in medium bowl. Add chicken and toss to coat cubes. Cover and refrigerate 20 minutes.

Heat wok or large skillet until 1 or 2 drops water sprinkled in pan skitter around. Add 1 tablespoon oil; rotate pan to coat sides. Add walnuts and stir-fry until browned. Remove walnuts with slotted spoon and set aside. Heat remaining 2 tablespoons of oil to pan. Add ginger to pan and stir-fry for 1 minute. Add chicken and stir-fry until chicken turns white. Stir in bamboo shoots, mushrooms, ¼ cup reserved mushroom liquid, and chicken stock. Cover and cook over medium heat about 3 minutes. Stir in walnuts and serve at once.

Yield: 4 servings

Nutrient analysis of 1 serving: 1 starch/bread exchange; 3 medium-fat meat exchanges; 2 fat exchanges; 392 Calories; 18 g protein; 30 g fat; 13 g carbohydrate; 940 mg sodium; 36 mg cholesterol.

*Chicken Marsala

2 tablespoons margarine
3 8-ounce chicken breasts, skinned, boned, and halved
10¾-ounce can condensed cream of chicken soup
⅓ cup Marsala wine
3 tablespoons snipped parsley

Melt margarine in large skillet. Cook chicken in margarine over medium-high heat, turning to brown both sides, about 15 minutes. Remove chicken to baking dish, 11¾ x 7½ x 1½ inches. Blend soup and wine and pour over chicken. Bake in a 325°F. oven until chicken is tender, about 30 minutes. Garnish with parsley.

Yield: 6 servings

Nutrient analysis of 1 serving: 3 lean meat exchanges; ½ fruit exchange; ½ fat exchange; 212 Calories; 20 g protein; 11 g fat; 5 g carbohydrate; 507 mg sodium; 75 mg cholesterol.

Williamsburg Chicken

- **4 boned chicken breasts (4 ounces each)**
- **Salt and freshly ground pepper to taste**
- **¼ cup all-purpose flour**
- **⅓ cup fine cracker crumbs**
- **2 tablespoons margarine**
- **2 tablespoons vegetable oil**
- **Grape Sauce (see below)**
- **4 thin slices cooked Virginia ham (½ ounce each)**

Season chicken with salt and pepper. Mix flour and cracker crumbs and coat chicken with mixture. Heat margarine and oil in a large skillet. Add chicken and cook over medium heat until golden brown, 5 to 10 minutes. Turn and cook until fork-tender and brown, about 5 minutes more. Set aside in a warm place.

Prepare Grape Sauce. To serve, place each chicken piece on slice of ham and pour sauce over all.

Grape Sauce

- **1 cup chicken stock**
- **½ cup orange juice**
- **¾ cup seedless red grapes**
- **¼ cup raisins**
- **¼ teaspoon sugar**
- **¼ teaspoon nutmeg**
- **⅛ teaspoon cinnamon**
- **1 tablespoon cornstarch**
- **1 tablespoon water**

Heat all ingredients except cornstarch and water to boiling. Mix cornstarch and water; stir into grape mixture. Cook over medium heat, stirring constantly, until mixture boils. Boil and stir for 1 minute.

Yield: 4 servings

Nutrient analysis of 1 serving: 4 lean meat exchanges; 1 fruit exchange; 300 Calories; 27 g protein; 14 g fat; 17 g carbohydrate; 288 mg sodium; 71 mg cholesterol.

Chicken with Peppers

2 pounds boneless chicken (thigh, leg, breast)
½ cup all-purpose flour
2 tablespoons margarine
2 tablespoons vegetable oil
½ cup dry white wine
1 teaspoon lemon juice
1 green pepper, seeded and cut into 1-inch narrow strips
1 small red pepper, seeded and cut into 1-inch narrow strips
1 lemon, sliced thin

Remove skin from chicken. Place between 2 pieces plastic wrap. Pound with mallet or side of saucer until ¼ inch thick. Take care not to tear meat. Coat with flour.

Heat margarine and oil in large skillet until margarine is melted. Cook chicken, a few pieces at a time, until golden brown, turning once. Drain and keep warm.

Return browned chicken to skillet; pour wine and lemon juice over chicken. Heat to boiling. Reduce heat, cover, and simmer until chicken is tender, about 5 minutes. Add peppers and lemon slices. Cover and simmer 5 minutes more.

Yield: 8 servings

Nutrient analysis of 1 serving: ½ starch/bread exchange; 3 lean meat exchanges; ½ fat exchange; 250 Calories; 26 g protein; 13 g fat; 7 g carbohydrate; 98 mg sodium; 71 mg cholesterol.

Chicken with Curried Rice and Almonds

1 cup uncooked long-grain rice
1 tablespoon curry powder
2 teaspoons dry mustard
2 tablespoons snipped chives
1 cup sliced almonds
2 cups chicken stock
3½-pound broiler-fryer, cut up

Preheat oven to 325°F.

Mix rice, curry powder, mustard, chives, and almonds in ungreased baking pan, 13 x 9 x 2 inches. Heat chicken stock to boiling, then stir into rice mixture. Arrange chicken pieces over rice. Cover tightly. Bake at 325°F. until chicken is tender and liquid is absorbed, about 1 hour.

Yield: 8 servings

Nutrient analysis of 1 serving: 1½ starch/bread exchanges; 3 medium-fat meat exchanges; 1 fat exchange; 368 Calories; 27 g protein; 20 g fat; 20 g carbohydrate; 297 mg sodium; 56 mg cholesterol.

*Family-Style Chicken Cordon Bleu

6 large boneless chicken breast halves (about 2½ pounds)
6 thin slices lean baked ham (½ ounce each)
6 slices Swiss cheese (½ ounce each)
2 tablespoons margarine
1 tablespoon vegetable oil
Parsley Rice (see below)

Flatten chicken breast halves to between ¼ and ½ inch thick. Cut ham and cheese slices in half. Place half slice each ham and cheese in center of chicken. (Reserve remaining ham and cheese.) Wrap chicken around ham and cheese. Roll up, jelly-roll fashion, and press to seal.

Heat margarine and oil in large skillet. Add chicken rolls and cook over medium heat until browned, about 10 minutes. Turn and brown other side, about 10 minutes. Prepare Parsley Rice (see below).

Preheat oven to 350°F. Spread rice on heatproof platter. Arrange rolls on rice. Top the rolls with the reserved half slices of ham and cheese. Place in oven and heat until cheese melts, about 10 minutes.

Parsley Rice

2 cups chicken stock
1 cup rice
1 cup snipped parsley

Heat chicken stock and rice to boiling in a large saucepan, stirring occasionally. Reduce heat, cover pan tightly, and simmer for 14 minutes (do not lift cover or stir). Remove from heat. Fluff rice with fork, cover, and let steam for 5 to 10 minutes. Remove cover, and stir in the snipped parsley.

Yield: 6 servings

Nutrient analysis of 1 serving: 1 starch/bread exchange; 4 lean meat exchanges; 2 fat exchanges; 360 Calories; 31 g protein; 21 g fat; 11 g carbohydrate; 520 mg sodium; 110 mg cholesterol.

*Pollo alla Milano

- **¼ cup plus 2 tablespoons seasoned bread crumbs**
- **2 tablespoons grated Parmesan cheese**
- **4 3-ounce boned and skinned chicken breast halves**
- **¼ cup chopped scallions (include green top)**
- **2 tablespoons margarine**
- **2 tablespoons flour**
- **1 cup skim milk**
- **2 tablespoons bran**
- **10-ounce package frozen chopped spinach, thawed and drained**
- **2 ounces thin-sliced boiled ham, cut up**

Preheat oven to 325°F. Spray 11¾ x 7½ x 1¾-inch baking dish with vegetable spray.

Mix bread crumbs and cheese together well. Coat chicken with crumb mixture. (Reserve the extra for topping.) Arrange crumbed chicken in baking dish.

Cook and stir scallions in margarine until tender. Stir in flour and cook over low heat until bubbly. Stir in milk. Heat to boiling, stirring constantly. Boil and stir for 1 minute, then stir in the bran, spinach, and ham. Pour ham mixture over chicken. Sprinkle remaining crumb mixture on top. Bake until bubbly, 30 to 40 minutes.

Yield: 4 servings

Nutrient analysis of 1 serving: 1 starch/bread exchange; 3½ lean meat exchanges; 1 vegetable exchange; 305 Calories; 28 g protein; 13 g fat; 19 g carbohydrate; 558 mg sodium; 86 mg cholesterol.

Poached Tarragon Chicken

- **3-pound broiler-fryer chicken**
- **½ cup chicken stock**
- **½ cup dry white wine**
- **2 sprigs fresh tarragon**
- **Freshly ground pepper**
- **¾ pound small new red potatoes**
- **2 large leeks, cut into 1-inch slices (include green tops)**
- **1 pound carrots, cut into narrow strips**
- **1 sprig fresh tarragon (additional)**
- **2 tablespoons margarine**

Soak top and bottom of clay pot in cold water for 10 minutes. Place whole chicken in pot. Pour stock and wine on chicken. Top with 2 sprigs tarragon. Season with pepper. Cover and bake in 350°F. oven until chicken is tender, about 45 minutes.

Heat ½ inch water to boiling in saucepan. Place steamer basket with unpared potatoes and leek slices in saucepan, and steam for 20 minutes. Add carrots and sprig of tarragon. Cover and steam 10 minutes more.

Remove chicken to large serving platter; surround with vegetables. Dot vegetables with margarine.

Yield: 6 servings

Nutrient analysis of 1 serving: 1 starch/bread exchange; 3 lean meat exchanges; 1 vegetable exchange; 1 fat exchange; 322 Calories; 28 g protein; 11 g fat; 23 g carbohydrate; 311 mg sodium; 75 mg cholesterol.

**Mediterranean Chicken*

- **1½ tablespoons margarine**
- **1½ pounds boneless chicken breast, cut into ½-inch cubes**
- **2-ounce can anchovies, drained and chopped**
- **½ cup chopped onion**
- **½ cup sliced mushrooms**
- **½ cup diced green pepper**
- **½ teaspoon salt**
- **¼ teaspoon cayenne pepper (optional)**
- **½ cup pitted black olives**
- **¼ cup dry white wine**
- **28-ounce can tomato sauce**
- **8-ounce package spaghetti**

Melt margarine in large skillet. Add chicken cubes. Cook and stir until light brown. Remove chicken from skillet and set aside. Add anchovies, onion, mushrooms, green pepper, salt, cayenne pepper, and olives to skillet. Cook, stirring occasionally, for 5 minutes. Stir in the wine, tomato sauce, and chicken cubes. Heat to boiling, reduce heat, and simmer, uncovered, for 30 minutes.

Cook spaghetti as directed on package. Drain. Serve chicken mixture on hot spaghetti.

Yield: 6 servings

Nutrient analysis of 1 serving: 2 starch/bread exchanges; 3 lean meat exchanges; 2 vegetable exchanges; 1 fat exchange; 414 Calories; 29 g protein; 14 g fat; 43 g carbohydrate; 1,141 mg sodium; 76 mg cholesterol.

*Lebanese Chicken and Rice

- 3 8-ounce boned and skinned chicken breasts
- 1 bay leaf
- ½ teaspoon dried coriander
- ½ pound lean ground lamb
- 2 ounces pine nuts, lightly toasted†
- 1 cup uncooked long grain rice
- 1 teaspoon salt
- Dash freshly ground pepper
- ¼ teaspoon allspice
- 2 tablespoons margarine
- 3 tablespoons snipped parsley
- Toasted almonds (optional)‡

Place chicken in large skillet. Add bay leaf and coriander and just enough water to cover chicken. Heat to boiling, reduce heat, and simmer until chicken is fork-tender, 10 to 15 minutes. Remove from heat and cool chicken in broth. Cut cooled chicken into 2-inch pieces. Reserve broth.

Cook and stir lamb in medium saucepan until light brown. Stir in pine nuts, rice, salt, pepper, allspice, margarine, and 2 cups reserved broth. Heat to boiling. Reduce heat, cover, and simmer until all liquid is absorbed, about 20 minutes. Stir in chicken and heat through. Season with salt and pepper. Garnish with parsley and, if desired, toasted almonds.

Yield: 6 servings

Nutrient analysis of 1 serving: 1½ starch/bread exchanges; 4 lean meat exchanges; 1 fat exchange; 397 Calories; 38 g protein; 17 g fat; 22 g carbohydrate; 452 mg sodium; 99 mg cholesterol.

†To toast nuts, spread nuts in shallow pan; bake in 350°F. oven until golden, 10 to 15 minutes.

‡Five almonds will add 2½ grams of fat and 27 calories per serving.

SAUCES

Horseradish Sauce

8-ounce carton plain low-fat yogurt
3 ounces prepared white horseradish, well drained
2 heaping tablespoons prepared spicy brown mustard

Mix all ingredients in small bowl. Cover and refrigerate until ready to use. Will keep for 1 to 2 days. Serve with cold roast beef or cold chicken.

Yield: 1 cup

Nutrient analysis of 2 tablespoons: 1 vegetable exchange; 26 Calories; 2 g protein; 1 g fat; 3 g carbohydrate; 87 mg sodium; 2 mg cholesterol.

Cranberry Relish

¾ cup orange juice
2 tablespoons sugar
1 12-ounce package cranberries†
2 tablespoons grated orange peel
1 orange, peeled, sectioned, pitted, and diced
1 apple, peeled, cored and diced

Measure orange juice and sugar into a 2-quart saucepan. Stir until sugar is dissolved. Heat to boiling. Add cranberries and heat to boiling. Boil, stirring occasionally, 5 to 7 minutes. Remove from heat and stir in orange peel, orange pieces, and apple. Pour into a 1-quart bowl and cool. Cover and refrigerate about 2 hours before serving. Serve with poultry. Will keep for several days.

Yield: 3 cups

Nutrient analysis of 2 tablespoons: free exchange; 14 Calories; 0 g protein; 0 g fat; 3 g carbohydrate; 0 mg sodium; 0 mg cholesterol.

†To wash cranberries, empty package into large colander. Sort out bruised or overripe berries and discard. Rinse berries in colander under cold running water, then drain.

Mexican Relish

2 cups diced firm tomato
1 cup minced onion
1 cup mixed sweet red and green peppers, finely chopped
1 tablespoon garlic or herb vinegar
¼ teaspoon grated lemon peel
2 teaspoons fresh lemon juice
⅛ teaspoon red pepper (optional)

Mix all ingredients thoroughly. Cover and refrigerate for 8 hours to blend flavors. Will keep several days in refrigerator. Serve with your favorite Tex-Mex dishes or with cold meats.

Yield: 4 cups

Nutrient analysis of ¼ cup: free exchange; 12 Calories; 0 g protein; 0 g fat; 3 g carbohydrate; 89 mg sodium; 0 mg cholesterol.

Sauce Peyzacola

2 to 3 cloves garlic, minced
2 tablespoons olive oil
16-ounce can whole tomatoes, drained (reserve ½ cup juice)
1 teaspoon dried basil or 1 tablespoon snipped fresh basil
¼ cup snipped parsley
Salt and freshly ground pepper to taste
2 tablespoons capers

Cook and stir garlic in oil in saucepan for 2 minutes. Cut tomatoes into quarters and add to garlic. Stir in reserved tomato juice, basil, and parsley. Season with salt and pepper. Heat to boiling. Reduce heat, and simmer 15 minutes. Stir in capers before serving.

Serve warm sauce on grilled steak, chicken, hamburgers, or veal chops. If desired, top with snipped parsley.

Yield: 1 cup

Nutrient analysis of ¼ cup: 1 vegetable exchange; 1½ fat exchanges; 86 Calories; 1 g protein; 7 g fat; 5 g carbohydrate; 242 mg sodium; 0 mg cholesterol.

Herb Margarine

2 tablespoons chopped fresh herbs (parsley, dill, or thyme) or 1 tablespoon parsley flakes, dillweed, or dried thyme
¼ cup unsalted margarine
¼ teaspoon hot pepper sauce

Melt margarine. Stir in pepper sauce and herbs. Serve on vegetables, broiled fish, or meat.

Yield: about ¼ cup

Nutrient analysis of 2 teaspoons: 2 fat exchanges; 94 Calories; 0 g protein; 11 g fat; 0 g carbohydrate; 1 mg sodium; 0 mg cholesterol.

Seasoned Margarine

½ cup unsalted margarine
¼ teaspoon hot pepper sauce

Mix margarine and pepper sauce until smooth. Serve on hot toasted bread, baked potatoes, or vegetables.

Yield: ½ cup

Nutrient analysis of 2 teaspoons: 2 fat exchanges; 94 Calories; 0 g protein; 11 g fat; 0 g carbohydrate; 1 mg sodium; 0 mg cholesterol.

Lemon Poultry Basting Sauce

¾ cup unsalted margarine
2 teaspoons paprika
1 teaspoon sugar
½ teaspoon pepper
¼ teaspoon dry mustard
Dash cayenne pepper
½ cup lemon juice
½ cup hot water
2 teaspoons grated onion

Melt margarine in saucepan. Stir in paprika, sugar, pepper, mustard, and cayenne pepper. Blend in lemon juice, hot water, and onion. Use to baste chicken or turkey during grilling or roasting.

Yield: about 1¾ cups

Nutrient analysis of 1 tablespoon: 1 fat exchange; 41 Calories; 0 g protein; 4 g fat; trace carbohydrate; 1 mg sodium; 0 mg cholesterol.

Meat-Basting Sauce

1 cup red wine
1 cup olive oil
¼ cup red wine vinegar
2 medium onions, chopped
2 cloves garlic, peeled
⅛ teaspoon rosemary leaves
⅛ teaspoon cayenne pepper

Shake all ingredients in tightly covered screw-top jar. Refrigerate for 24 hours to blend flavors. Remove garlic before using. Use for basting meat or poultry while roasting or broiling.

Yield: about 2½ cups

Nutrient analysis of 1 tablespoon: 1 fat exchange; 57 Calories; 0 g protein; 6 g fat; 1 g carbohydrate; 1 mg sodium; 0 mg cholesterol.

Low-Salt Tomato Paste

18-ounce can no-salt added tomato juice
¾ teaspoon sugar

Bring tomato juice to a boil in a small saucepan. Reduce heat, and simmer stirring occasionally until sauce is consistency of tomato paste, about 45 minutes. Stir in sugar. Will keep for several days in refrigerator.

Yield: ½ cup

Nutrient analysis of 1 tablespoon: free exchange; 15 Calories; 0 g protein; 0 g fat; 3 g carbohydrate; 8 mg sodium; 0 mg cholesterol.

Basic Marinade

3 parts vegetable oil
1 part acid (vinegar, lemon juice or dry wine)
Enhancements (garlic, herbs, spices, seeds)

Shake all ingredients in tightly covered screw-top jar. Will keep for up to 2 weeks in refrigerator. Use to marinate meats for grilling.

Yield: optional

Nutrient analysis of 1 tablespoon: 2 fat exchanges; 94 Calories; 0 g protein; 11 g fat; 0 g carbohydrate; 0 mg sodium; 0 mg cholesterol.

Chinese Mustard

½ cup dry mustard

Boiling water

Measure dry mustard into small bowl. Mix in enough boiling water to make thin smooth paste. Allow sauce to sit for 30 minutes at room temperature before using, to develop flavor.

Note: The Chinese make their mustard fresh before each meal because it loses flavor quickly. This mustard is good with beef and Chinese dishes. Beer can be substituted for the boiling water.

Yield: ½ cup

Nutrient analysis of 1 tablespoon: free exchange.

Low-Salt Dijon-Type Mustard

1½ cups tarragon vinegar
½ cup water
2 tablespoons sugar
¼ stick cinnamon
5 whole cloves
5 white peppercorns
5 black peppercorns
1 bay leaf
5 2-ounce cans dry English mustard
¼ to ⅓ cup olive oil

Simmer the vinegar, water, sugar, cinnamon stick, cloves, peppercorns, and bay leaf in a medium saucepan, uncovered, for 5 minutes. Strain and pour onto mustard in a medium bowl. Stir to mix well and cover bowl.

Let mustard stand in the bowl at room temperature, stirring every other day, for about 2 months. (If mustard becomes dry, stir in small amount boiling water or cream sherry.) Stir in olive oil. Pour into jar, cover, and store for up to 6 months in refrigerator. This Dijon-type mustard can be used in recipes throughout the book to lower the sodium content of recipes.

Yield: 3½ to 4 cups

Nutrient analysis of 2 teaspoons: free exchange; 11 Calories; 0 g protein; 1 g fat; 0 g carbohydrate; 0 mg sodium; 0 mg cholesterol.

Mock Hollandaise Sauce

¾ cup Low-Calorie Mayonnaise (page 94)
⅓ cup skim milk
¼ teaspoon salt
Dash white pepper
1 tablespoon grated lemon peel
1 tablespoon lemon juice

Blend mayonnaise, milk, salt, and pepper in a small saucepan. Cook over low heat, stirring constantly, until heated through, about 3 minutes. Stir in lemon peel and juice. Serve immediately with hot vegetables.

Yield: 1 cup

Nutrient analysis of 2 tablespoons: 1 fat exchange; 36 Calories; 1 g protein; 3 g fat; 1 g carbohydrate; 94 mg sodium; 12 mg cholesterol.

Hollandaise Sauce

¼ cup plus 2 tablespoons egg substitute
3 tablespoons lemon juice
½ cup margarine, melted

Measure egg substitute and lemon juice into blender container or food processor. Cover and process at high speed until smooth. Add margarine in a slow, steady stream while processing at low speed. Mix until smooth and creamy. Use immediately in recipes calling for hollandaise sauce or on vegetables.

Yield: about 1 cup

Nutrient analysis of ¼ cup: 5½ fat exchanges; 254 Calories; 3 g protein; 27 g fat; 1 g carbohydrate; 324 mg sodium; 0 mg cholesterol.

Nutrient analysis of 1 tablespoon: 1½ fat exchanges; 64 Calories; ½ g protein; 8 g fat; 0 g carbohydrate; 81 mg sodium; 0 mg cholesterol.

Béarnaise Sauce

1 tablespoon dry white wine
2 teaspoons tarragon vinegar
½ teaspoon lemon juice
½ teaspoon bottled meat glaze
2 egg yolks
¾ cup margarine (1½ sticks)
1 tablespoon snipped chives

Process wine, vinegar, lemon juice, meat glaze, and egg yolks in blender or food processor at high speed for 5 seconds.

Heat margarine over low flame until melted and bubbly. While processing at medium speed, add the hot margarine slowly to the egg yolk mixture. Continue to process until sauce is smooth. Mix in chives while at low speed. Refrigerate until ready to use. Serve at room temperature with steaks or to dress up a hamburger.

Yield: about 1 cup

Nutrient analysis of 1 tablespoon: 4 fat exchanges; 177 Calories; 1 g protein; 20 g fat; 0 g carbohydrate; 214 mg sodium; 68 mg cholesterol.

Barbecue Sauce

2 cloves garlic, minced
2 onions, chopped
¼ cup vegetable oil
1 tablespoon parsley flakes
28-ounce can tomato puree
2 tablespoons red wine vinegar
2 tablespoons brown sugar
1 teaspoon dry mustard
2 tablespoons Worcestershire sauce
⅛ teaspoon salt
½ teaspoon pepper
¼ teaspoon dried oregano
¼ teaspoon hot pepper sauce

Cook and stir garlic and onion in oil until onion is tender. Stir in remaining ingredients. Heat to boiling, stirring constantly. Reduce heat and simmer, uncovered, for 30 minutes. Will keep for 2 or 3 days in the refrigerator.

Yield: 4 cups

Nutrient analysis of ¼ cup: 1 vegetable exchange; 1 fat exchange; 57 Calories; 1 g protein; 4 g fat; 5 g carbohydrate; 47 mg sodium; 0 mg cholesterol.

DESSERTS

Summer Fruit Plate

For each serving, arrange attractively on plate:

¼ wedge pineapple†
4 strawberries
2 slices orange, halved
1 small wedge honeydew melon or cantaloupe
10 raspberries or blackberries
2 slices kiwi fruit
4 watermelon balls

Nutrient analysis of 1 serving: 3 fruit exchanges; 173 Calories; 3 g protein; 1 g fat; 42 g carbohydrate; 12 mg sodium; 0 mg cholesterol.

†Remove green top of pineapple if not perfect. Cut pineapple in half lengthwise, through green top, and then cut again, making 4 quarters. Cut core from pineapple quarters and cut fruit from shell with grapefruit knife. Turn shells upside down on paper towels to drain. Remove "eyes" from fruit. Place fruit back in shells; cut fruit lengthwise and then crosswise into bite-size pieces.

Fruit Platter Dessert

½ cantaloupe, rind removed and sliced
½ honeydew melon, rind removed and sliced
2 cups blueberries
2 cups strawberries or raspberries
2 kiwi fruits, pared and sliced

Arrange slices of cantaloupe and honeydew melon on large platter. Sprinkle blueberries and strawberries over slices. Top with kiwi fruit slices.

Yield: 6 servings

Nutrient analysis of 1 serving: 2 fruit exchanges; 105 Calories; 2 g protein; 1 g fat; 26 g carbohydrate; 18 mg sodium; 0 mg cholesterol.

Grapes and Pineapple in Sour Cream

2 cups seedless green grapes
8-ounce can pineapple chunks in unsweetened pineapple juice, drained
2 tablespoons brown sugar
1/3 cup dairy sour cream

Combine grapes and pineapple chunks. Mix sugar and sour cream; pour over fruits and toss. Chill.

Yield: 4 servings

Nutrient analysis of 1 serving: 2 fruit exchanges; 1/2 fat exchange; 142 Calories; 1 g protein; 3 g fat; 31 g carbohydrate; 13 mg sodium; 8 mg cholesterol.

Orange Snow

1 envelope (1/4 ounce) unflavored gelatin
2 tablespoons sugar
1/2 cup water
1 cup orange juice
3 medium oranges, sectioned, pitted, and cut into small pieces (about 3 cups)
1 tablespoon lime juice
2 egg whites

Mix gelatin and sugar in small saucepan. Stir in water and heat to boiling, stirring until sugar is dissolved. Remove from heat. Stir in orange juice, orange pieces, and lime juice. Refrigerate until thickened.

Beat egg whites until stiff peaks form. Beat gelatin until frothy. Fold gelatin mixture into egg whites. Pour into 5-cup mold and refrigerate until set. Unmold and, if desired, garnish with orange slices and whole strawberries.

Yield: 8 servings

Nutrient analysis of 1 serving: 1 fruit exchange; 65 Calories; 2 g protein; 1 g fat; 13 g carbohydrate; 83 mg sodium; 1 mg cholesterol.

Double Fruit Whip

- 1 envelope (¼ ounce) unflavored gelatin
- 1 cup canned unsweetened pineapple juice
- ½ teaspoon grated lemon peel
- 3 tablespoons honey
- 2 cups unsweetened applesauce
- Cinnamon or nutmeg

Sprinkle gelatin on pineapple juice to soften. Stir over low heat until gelatin is dissolved. Stir in lemon peel, honey, and applesauce. Refrigerate, stirring occasionally, until mixture mounds slightly when dropped from spoon.

Beat until fluffy. Divide among 8 dessert dishes. Refrigerate until firm. Sprinkle each with cinnamon.

Yield: 8 servings

Nutrient analysis of 1 serving: 1 fruit exchange; 69 Calories; 0 mg protein; 0 mg fat; 18 g carbohydrate; 4 mg sodium; 0 mg cholesterol.

Tapioca Cream

- 2 egg yolks, slightly beaten
- 2 cups milk
- 2 tablespoons sugar
- 2 tablespoons quick-cooking tapioca
- 1 teaspoon vanilla
- 2 egg whites
- ¼ cup sugar (additional)

Combine egg yolks, milk, 2 tablespoons sugar, and tapioca in saucepan. Cook over low heat, stirring constantly, until mixture boils. Cool slightly, and then chill. Stir in vanilla.

Beat egg whites until foamy. Beat in the ¼ cup sugar, 1 tablespoon at a time. Continue beating until stiff and glossy. Fold into tapioca mixture.

If desired, pudding can be poured over fresh or drained fruit in dessert dishes. Refrigerate until well-chilled, at least 1 to 2 hours, and serve with light cream.

Yield: 6 servings

Nutrient analysis of 1 serving: ½ starch/bread exchange; ½ skim milk exchange; 80 Calories; 5 g protein; 0 g fat; 11 g carbohydrate; 62 mg sodium; 88 mg cholesterol.

Fresh Melon Sherbet

1 envelope (¼ ounce) unflavored gelatin
¼ cup sugar
½ cup water
¼ cup lemon juice
1 cup water (additional)
4 cups cubed cantaloupe or honeydew melon

Mix gelatin and sugar in small saucepan. Stir in ½ cup water and heat to boiling, stirring until sugar is dissolved. Remove from heat, stir in lemon juice and cool.

Pour 1 cup water into blender or food processor container. Add melon cubes and process until smooth. Stir into gelatin mixture, then pour all into a loaf pan, 9 x 5 x 3 inches. Freeze until almost firm. Remove from freezer. Place mixture in a bowl and beat until mushy and thick. Return to loaf pan and freeze until firm.

Variation: Watermelon or casaba melon cubes can be substituted for the cantaloupe or honeydew. However, omit the 1 cup water when processing.

Yield: 12 servings

Nutrient analysis of 1 serving: ½ fruit exchange; 30 Calories; 1 g protein; 0 g fat; 7 g carbohydrate; 7 mg sodium; 0 mg cholesterol.

Strawberry Dessert

2 egg whites
10-ounce package frozen strawberries, partially thawed
2 tablespoons lemon juice
⅓ cup sugar
1 cup whipping cream

In a large bowl of an electric mixer, beat the egg whites, strawberries, lemon juice, and sugar until stiff, about 10 minutes. Beat the cream in a separate bowl until stiff. Fold the whipped cream into the strawberry mixture. Turn into a 13 x 9 x 2-inch pan. Freeze until firm. Cut into 15 squares.

Yield: 15 servings

Nutrient analysis of 1 serving: ¼ fruit exchange; 1 fat exchange; 62 Calories; 1 g protein; 6 g fat; 2 g carbohydrate; 12 mg sodium; 22 mg cholesterol.

Frozen Fruit Dessert

1½ cups graham cracker crumbs (18 square crackers)
3 tablespoons vegetable oil
½ cup nonfat dry milk powder
1 egg white
½ cup chilled orange juice
1 tablespoon lemon juice
¼ cup sugar
8¾-ounce can crushed pineapple in unsweetened pineapple juice, drained

Mix crumbs and oil. Reserve ⅓ cup of mixture for topping. Press remaining mixture into an 8- or 9-inch square pan.

Beat dry milk, egg white, and orange juice in small bowl of an electric mixer at high speed for 3 minutes. Add the lemon juice and beat 3 minutes more. Add sugar; beat at low speed for 30 seconds. Fold in the pineapple. Pour into prepared pan; sprinkle reserved crumb mixture over top. Freeze until firm.

Yield: 12 servings

Nutrient analysis of 1 serving: 1 fruit exchange; 1 fat exchange; 106 Calories; 2 g protein; 5 g fat; 15 g carbohydrate; 90 mg sodium; 1 mg cholesterol.

Lemon Soufflé

2 tablespoons margarine
3 tablespoons all-purpose flour
¾ cup skim milk
Grated peel and juice of 1 medium lemon
5 egg whites
4 egg yolks
¼ cup sugar

Preheat oven to 350°F.

Grease a 6-cup soufflé dish with margarine or butter. Make a 4-inch band of triple thickness aluminum foil or waxed paper 2 inches longer than circumference of dish. Grease 1 side of band. Tie band, greased side in, around top of dish so that it extends 2 inches above top of dish.

Melt the margarine in a saucepan over low heat. Stir in the flour. Cook over low heat until bubbly. Stir in milk. Heat to boiling, stirring constantly. Boil and stir for 1 minute. Remove from heat and stir in the lemon peel and juice.

Beat the egg whites in a large bowl until stiff peaks form. Set aside.

Beat the egg yolks and sugar in a medium bowl. Stir in 1 tablespoon of the hot milk mixture, then blend in remainder. Fold egg yolk mixture into egg whites.

Pour into prepared soufflé dish. Bake at 350°F. for 15 minutes. *Serve immediately.* Carefully remove band and divide soufflé into sections with 2 forks.

Yield: 6 servings

Nutrient analysis of 1 serving: 1 whole milk exchange; 132 Calories; 6 g protein; 8 g fat; 9 g carbohydrate; 108 mg sodium; 182 mg cholesterol.

Spicy Apple Tarts

Ingredients for 8- or 9-inch 1-crust pie (page 210)
2½ pounds unpared apples† **(6 or 7 large), cored and diced**
1 teaspoon grated lemon peel
Juice of 1 lemon
⅓ cup honey
1½ teaspoons cinnamon
¼ teaspoon cloves

To make tart shells, follow directions for standard pie pastry (page 210), but before adding water, add 2 tablespoons finely chopped filberts. Roll pastry into a 13-inch circle about ¼ inch thick. Cut circle into 4½-inch rounds. (If using individual pie pans or tart pans, cut pastry rounds 1 inch larger than inverted pans; fit into pans that have been lightly sprayed with a non-caloric vegetable spray.) Fit over backs of muffin cups or small custard cups, making pleats so pastry will fit closely. Prick with fork and place on baking sheet. Bake in a 475°F. oven for 8 to 10 minutes. Cool for several minutes before removing from cups.

Combine remaining ingredients in a large saucepan. Cook over medium heat approximately 10 to 15 minutes, stirring occasionally, until apples have softened but still retain their shape. Cool slightly. Spoon into tart shells and serve.

Yield: 8 servings

Nutrient analysis of 1 serving: 1 starch/bread exchange; 2 fruit exchanges; 2 fat exchanges; 258 Calories; 2 g protein; 10 g fat; 40 g carbohydrate; 3 mg sodium; 0 mg cholesterol.

†Granny Smith apple is a good cooking apple.

Spicy Melon Delight

1 medium honeydew melon
16-ounce can pineapple chunks in unsweetened pineapple juice, drained (reserve juice)
1 teaspoon powdered ginger
1 teaspoon cloves

Cut 1½-inch slice from top of melon and remove seeds. Refrigerate drained pineapple chunks. Heat reserved pineapple juice, ginger, and cloves just to simmer. Pour into the melon. Cover with aluminum foil and refrigerate for 2 hours.

Drain juice from melon. Cut melon into 6 wedges and top each with pineapple chunks.

Yield: 6 servings

Nutrient analysis of 1 serving: 2 fruit exchanges; 116 Calories; 1 g protein; 0 g fat; 28 g carbohydrate; 16 mg sodium; 0 mg cholesterol.

Orange-Pineapple Cream

1 cup cooked orzo
½ cup chilled, drained, crushed pineapple in unsweetened pineapple juice
½ cup chilled, drained, mandarin orange segments in light syrup, halved
½ cup Whipped Topping (page 207)
Mint leaves

Fold orzo, pineapple, and mandarin orange halves into topping. Divide among 4 sherbet dishes; garnish with mint leaves.

Yield: 4 servings (½ cup each)

Nutrient analysis of 1 serving: 1 starch/bread exchange; ½ fruit exchange; ½ fat exchange; 144 Calories; 5 g protein; 3 g fat; 24 g carbohydrate; 36 mg sodium; 10 mg cholesterol.

Banana Whip

1 cup cooked orzo
1 cup mashed ripe banana (about 2 small)
1 teaspoon lemon juice
1 cup Whipped Topping (see below)

Mix orzo, banana, and lemon juice. Fold into topping. Pour into 4 dessert dishes and refrigerate.

Yield: 4 servings (1/2 cup each)

Nutrient analysis of 1 serving: 1 starch/bread exchange; 1 fruit exchange; 1 fat exchange; 164 Calories; 5 g protein; 4 g fat; 29 g carbohydrate; 38 mg sodium; 10 mg cholesterol.

French Plums

16-ounce can plums in light syrup
3 tablespoons kirsch
2 tablespoons shredded lemon peel

Heat plums in their syrup, kirsch, and lemon peel just to boiling. Remove from heat and chill.

Yield: 6 servings (1/2 cup each)

Nutrient analysis of 1 serving: 1½ fruit exchanges; 85 Calories; 0 g protein; 0 g fat; 20 g carbohydrate; 17 mg sodium; 0 mg cholesterol.

Whipped Topping

6½-ounce can evaporated skim milk
2 tablespoons sugar
1 teaspoon vanilla

Pour evaporated skim milk into small mixing bowl. Place in freezer with the beaters until crystals form around edge of milk in bowl, about 15 to 20 minutes. Then, beat at high speed until stiff. Add sugar and vanilla; continue beating another 1 to 2 minutes.

Yield: about 1½ cups

Nutrient analysis of 1 tablespoon: free exchange.

Nutrient analysis of 1/4 cup: 1/4 whole milk exchange; 46 Calories; 2 g protein; 2 g fat; 4 g carbohydrate; 34 mg sodium; 10 mg cholesterol.

Apple Snow

1 pound apples (3 medium)
¼ cup water
1 tablespoon sugar
2 egg whites

Pare, core, and slice apples. Turn into a saucepan with the water and sugar. Cover and cook over low heat until apples are soft. Turn mixture into blender or food processor and process at high speed until smooth. Cool.

Beat egg whites until stiff. Fold in apple mixture and chill until firm.

Yield: 4 servings

Nutrient analysis of 1 serving: 1 fruit exchange; 75 Calories; 2 g protein; 0 g fat; 16 g carbohydrate; 25 mg sodium; 0 mg cholesterol.

Baked Apple Rice Pudding

⅓ cup egg substitute
2 cups pared and cored apples, finely chopped (2 medium)
1½ cups cooked white rice
½ cup pitted dates, snipped
¼ cup sugar
½ teaspoon cinnamon
2 tablespoons unsalted margarine, softened
1 teaspoon vanilla
2 egg whites
¼ teaspoon cinnamon

Preheat oven to 325°F.

Mix together the egg substitute, apples, rice, dates, sugar, cinnamon, margarine, and vanilla. Beat the egg whites until stiff peaks form; fold into rice mixture. Turn into a 1½-quart casserole or soufflé dish. Sprinkle cinnamon on top.

Place casserole in a pan of very hot water (1 inch deep). Bake at 325°F. about 70 minutes. Serve warm or chilled. If desired, garnish with fresh apple slices dipped in lemon juice.

Yield: 6 servings

Nutrient analysis of 1 serving: 1 starch/bread exchange; 1 fruit exchange; 1 fat exchange; 185 Calories; 4 g protein; 6 g fat; 31 g carbohydrate; 42 mg sodium; 0 mg cholesterol.

Fresh Fruit with Zabaglione

¾ cup egg substitute
2 tablespoons sugar
½ cup Marsala wine
2½ cups fresh fruit (blueberries, raspberries, sliced strawberries, peaches, plums, or nectarines)

Beat egg substitute and sugar in top of double boiler until light and fluffy. Continue beating while slowly adding wine. Place top of double boiler over simmering water. Cook, beating constantly, until thick and fluffy, about 20 minutes. Mixture will form soft peaks.

Spoon ½ cup fresh fruit into each of 5 sherbet dishes or tall wine glasses. Top each with ¼ cup sauce. If desired, top each with Whipped Topping (page 207).

Yield: 5 servings

Nutrient analysis of 1 serving: 1 medium-fat meat exchange; ¾ fruit exchange; 100 Calories; 4 g protein; 5 g fat; 10 g carbohydrate; 67 mg sodium; 0 mg cholesterol.

Frozen Chantilly Melba

10-ounce package frozen unsweetened raspberries, partially thawed, or 1 pint (1¼ cups) fresh raspberries
1 cup Whipped Topping (page 207)

Place raspberries in blender or food processor container. Cover and process at high speed until pureed, about 30 seconds. Fold raspberries into topping. Pour into refrigerator tray and freeze until firm.

Note: Other fresh fruit, such as strawberries or sliced peaches, can be substituted for the raspberries.

Yield: 4 servings (½ cup each)

Nutrient analysis of 1 serving: ½ fruit exchange; ¼ whole milk exchange; 70 Calories; 3 g protein; 3 g fat; 10 g carbohydrate; 35 mg sodium; 10 mg cholesterol.

Jamaican Jumble

1 medium banana
8½-ounce can crushed pineapple in unsweetened pineapple juice
2 cups sliced strawberries
1 ounce dark Jamaican rum

Slice banana into bowl. Stir in pineapple with juice, strawberries, and rum. Cover and chill.

Yield: 6 servings

Nutrient analysis of 1 serving: 1 fruit exchange; 57 Calories; 1 g protein; 0 g fat; 12 g carbohydrate; 1 mg sodium; 0 mg cholesterol.

Standard Pie Pastry

For 8- or 9-inch one-crust pie

¼ cup whole wheat flour
¾ cup all-purpose flour
⅓ cup plus 1 tablespoon unsalted margarine
2 to 3 tablespoons cold water

For 10-inch one-crust pie

⅓ cup whole wheat flour
1 cup all-purpose flour
½ cup unsalted margarine
3 to 4 tablespoons cold water

For 8- or 9-inch lattice-topped pie

½ cup whole wheat flour
1 cup all-purpose flour
½ cup plus 1 tablespoon unsalted margarine
3 to 4 tablespoons cold water

Measure flour into mixing bowl. Cut in margarine thoroughly. Sprinkle in water, 1 tablespoon at a time, mixing until all flour is moistened and dough almost cleans side of bowl (1 to 2 teaspoons water can be added if needed). Gather dough into ball; shape into flattened round on lightly floured cloth-covered board.

For One-Crust Pie: With floured stockinet-covered rolling pin, roll out dough 2 inches larger than inverted pie pan. Fold pastry into quarters; unfold and ease into pan. Trim overhanging edge of pastry 1 inch from rim of pan. Fold and roll pastry under, even with pan; flute. Fill and bake as directed in recipe.

For Baked Pie Shell: Prick bottom and sides thoroughly with fork. Bake at 475°F. for 8 to 10 minutes.

For Lattice-Topped Pie: Use ⅔ of dough; with floured stockinet-covered rolling pin roll out dough 2 inches larger than inverted pie pan. Fold pastry into quarters; unfold and ease into pie pan. Trim overhanging edge of pastry 1 inch from rim of pan. Turn desired filling into pastry-lined pie pan. Roll out remaining dough into circle about the size of inverted pie pan. Cut circle into strips about ½ inch wide. Place 5 to 7 strips (depending on size of pan) across filling in pie pan. Lay second half of strips across first strips. Fold trimmed edge of lower crust over ends of strips, building up a high edge. (A juicy fruit pie is more likely to bubble over when topped by lattice than when the juices are held in by a top crust; be sure to build up a high pastry edge.) Seal and flute. Cover edge with a 2- to 3-inch strip of aluminum foil to prevent excessive browning; remove foil for last 15 minutes of baking. Bake as directed in recipe.

Yield: 8 servings

Nutrient analysis of 1 serving:

	8- or 9-inch	10-inch	Lattice-topped
Exchanges	¾ starch/bread 2 fat	1 starch/bread 3 fat	1½ starch/bread 4 fat
Calories	137	200	287
Protein	2 g	2 g	2 g
Fat	10 g	14 g	20 g
Carbohydrate	11 g	15 g	19 g
Sodium	2 mg	2 mg	3 mg
Cholesterol	0 mg	0 mg	0 mg

Fruit Whip

1 envelope (¼ ounce) unflavored gelatin
1 cup canned unsweetened pineapple juice
½ teaspoon grated lemon peel
3 tablespoons honey
2 cups unsweetened applesauce
Cinnamon or nutmeg

Sprinkle gelatin on pineapple juice to soften. Stir over low heat until gelatin is dissolved. Stir in lemon peel, honey, and applesauce. Refrigerate, stirring occasionally, until mixture mounds slightly when dropped from spoon.

Beat until fluffy. Divide evenly among 8 dessert dishes. Refrigerate until firm. Sprinkle each with cinnamon.

Yield: 8 servings

Nutrient analysis of 1 serving: 1 fruit exchange; 64 Calories; 0 g protein; 0 g fat; 17 g carbohydrate; 0 mg sodium; 0 mg cholesterol.

Eggnog Fluff

2 eggs, separated
2 cups skim milk
3 tablespoons honey
½ teaspoon nutmeg
1 envelope (¼ ounce) unflavored gelatin
1 teaspoon vanilla
1 cup raspberries (optional)

Blend egg yolks and milk in small saucepan. Stir in honey, nutmeg, and gelatin. Cook over medium-low heat, stirring constantly, just until mixture boils. Remove from heat and stir in vanilla. Refrigerate until thickened but not set.

Beat egg whites until stiff peaks form. Beat gelatin mixture until smooth and fluffy. Fold gelatin mixture into egg whites. Divide evenly among 6 dessert dishes. Top each with 2 heaping tablespoons raspberries.

Yield: 6 servings plus berries (scant ½ cup each)

Nutrient analysis of 1 serving: ½ low-fat milk exchange; ¼ fruit exchange; 84 Calories; 5 g protein; 2 g fat; 12 g carbohydrate; 62 mg sodium; 88 mg cholesterol.

PART III

Recipes for Young Cooks

by Paul Margie

All the recipes in this section of the book were developed for and tested by young cooks. However, this does not mean they cannot be enjoyed by family members and friends of all ages. So, whether you are preparing a snack for yourself or cooking dinner for your family, we wish you "good eating"!

You will find that cooking is fun and easy. However, whether you are a beginner or experienced, be sure to review the information on the following pages before you start.

KITCHEN SAFETY RULES

1. Always dry your hands after washing them, to avoid having slippery fingers and to avoid an electrical shock.
2. Never pull on the cord of an electrical appliance to disconnect it. Pull on the *plug*. Never place a plugged-in appliance in water.
3. Learn how to use all appliances correctly. Have an adult stand by when you are using an electrical appliance.
4. Do's and don't's with appliances:

   Turn off the mixer before putting in or taking out the beaters.

   Turn off the blender or mixer before scraping the sides of the container or bowl.

   Open the oven door carefully—the hot air inside can burn you.

   The blades in a food processor are very sharp. Ask an adult for help. Always handle the blades with extreme care and unplug the processor before removing the top.

   Be careful not to touch the burners on the stove.

   Turn the handles of saucepans and skillets toward the middle or back of the stove so no one will accidentally bump into them.
5. Always use thick, dry potholders.
6. Ask someone older to drain foods that have been cooked in hot water and to remove hot items from the oven.
7. Sharp knives are dangerous. Always cut away from you. When chopping, dicing, or paring food, hold the food firmly on a cutting board.

Keep your fingers out of the way, and never hold food in your hand to cut it. Wash knives carefully. Never put them in a sink of sudsy water with other utensils because you won't be able to see them easily.

PREPARING A MEAL

1. Read the kitchen safety rules and review the cooking terms listed on pages 217–19.
2. Spend a few minutes getting ready. Check with an adult to make sure it is all right to use the kitchen. Read the recipe carefully. If you need assistance, ask an adult to help you. Make sure you have enough time to complete the entire recipe and that you have all the necessary ingredients. Wash your hands well, put on an apron, roll up your sleeves, and, if your hair is long, tie it back so it will not get in the food. Take out two cookie sheets (one for "clean," one for "dirty"), measuring cups, measuring spoons, and a scale if you need one.
3. Get out all the ingredients, utensils, bowls, and appliances you will need. Place all carefully measured recipe ingredients on one cookie ("clean") sheet. Then, as you add each ingredient, put the used container on the other ("dirty") cookie sheet.
4. Follow the recipe directions exactly and in the order the recipe specifies. For best results, use the pan size called for in the recipe. As you finish each step of the recipe, place any utensils you no longer need on the "dirty" cookie sheet.
5. Always clean up. All your used items should be on one cookie sheet, ready to be carried to the sink. Make sure everything is put away and all the counters are wiped. If you leave the kitchen clean, you will always be invited back.

INGREDIENTS AND HOW TO MEASURE THEM

All-purpose flour: Dip from cannister with measuring cup, then level with a spatula.

Baking powder, baking soda, cream of tartar, and spices: Dip and fill spoon, then level with a spatula.

Brown sugar: Spoon into dry measuring cup and pack down firmly, then level with spatula.

Cake flour: Spoon lightly into dry measuring cup, then level with spatula.

Egg and egg substitutes: Use medium or large eggs. Have someone show you how to separate the white from the yolk. To measure egg substitute, read directions carefully and follow package instructions regarding substitution and storage.

Granulated sugar: Dip from cannister with a measuring cup, then level with a spatula.

Lemon or orange peel: To grate, wash fruit and rub in short strokes across small holes of a grater onto waxed paper. Grate only the colored peel which contains the oil and flavor; the white peel is bitter. To measure, press grated peel into measuring spoon until level with top.

Liquids: Pour milk, water, and oil into a liquid measuring cup placed on a table or countertop. Check measurement at eye level. Measure corn syrup, honey, and molasses in the same way.

Margarine: For stick margarine, unwrap and cut, then soften to room temperature. For whipped margarine, dip measuring spoon in tub and level off with a knife.

Shredded cheese, soft bread crumbs, raisins, nuts: Pack lightly into dry measuring cup until level. For smaller amounts, dip and fill measuring spoon. Do not pack down these ingredients.

Yeast: Active, dry yeast usually comes in small packets. Always check expiration date on the packet before using, to be sure it is still fresh.

DICTIONARY OF COOKING TERMS

Terms for Preparing Ingredients

Beat: Make mixture smooth by vigorous over-and-over motion with a spoon, fork, whisk, rotary beater, or electric beater.

Blend: Thoroughly combine all ingredients until very smooth and uniform.

Chill: Cool in the refrigerator.

Chop: Cut into very small pieces with knife or sharp tool (hold one end of knife on board with one hand; pivot the rest of the blade up and down with the other).

Combine: Mix ingredients together.

Cool: Allow heated items to come to room temperature.

Cream: Mash until soft and smooth.

Crush: Pound into small pieces.

Cube: Cut into cubes ½ inch or larger.

Cut in: Mix fat into flour mixture with a pastry blender, fork, or two knives.

Defrost: Leave frozen food at room temperature or in refrigerator until it is no longer frozen.

Dot: Drop bits of margarine or cheese here and there over food.

Drain: Pour off all liquid.

Fold: Mix gently by lifting from the bottom to the top, then folding over with a spoon or spatula.

Flour: Dust greased pans with flour until they are well coated on the bottom and sides. Shake out extra flour.

Garnish: Decorate with pieces of colorful foods such as parsley, pimiento, or lemon.

Grate: Cut into tiny particles by using small holes of grater.
Grease: Cover the bottom and sides of baking pan with a small amount of margarine, shortening, or low-calorie nonstick vegetable spray. Hands may also be greased by spraying with vegetable spray.
Ingredient: A food item used in a recipe.
Knead: Work dough with hands by repeating a folding-back, pressing-forward, and turning motion.
Line: Cover inside of pan, sometimes with waxed paper. Muffin tins are often lined with paper cups.
Marinate: Let food stand in liquid to add flavor or to tenderize.
Mash: Flatten with the back of a fork or potato masher until soft and smooth.
Melt: Heat until liquid.
Mix: Stir ingredients together, usually with a spoon.
Mince: Chop or cut into tiny pieces.
Pare: Cut off outer covering with a knife or other sharp tool.
Peel: Strip off outer covering such as with bananas or oranges.
Precooked: Already cooked.
Quarter: Cut food into four equal parts.
Refrigerate: Store or chill in the refrigerator.
Roll out: Flatten and spread with a rolling pin.
Separate: Divide into parts.
Serving: Quantity of food needed for one person.
Shred: Cut into thin pieces by using large holes on a grater or shredder.
Snip: Cut into very small pieces with scissors.
Skin: Peel a strip off the outer layer of skin of a vegetable, fruit, chicken, or fish.
Slice: Cut into thin, flat pieces with a knife.
Soften: Leave food at room temperature so that it becomes soft.
Spread: Cover a surface smoothly with a thin layer of ingredient.
Sprinkle: Scatter one ingredient on top of another.
Stir: Combine ingredients with a circular or figure-eight motion until of uniform consistency.
Substitute: Use one food or ingredient in place of another.
Tender: Soft and suitable for eating.
Top: Place an ingredient on top of another.
Toss: Tumble ingredients lightly with a lifting motion.
Undiluted: As liquid comes from its container, with nothing added to it.
Utensil: Kitchen tool used for cooking.
Whip: Beat with a rotary egg beater or electric beater to add air.

Terms for Cooking Food

Bake: Cook in the oven.
Baste: Spoon a flavoring ingredient on a food during the cooking process.
Boil: Cook directly on the cooking unit until bubbles rise continuously and break the surface of the liquid.

Broil: Cook directly under heat source in the oven or broiler or over hot coals.

Brown: Cook until food changes color, usually in a small amount of fat over medium heat.

Cook and stir: Cook in a small amount of shortening, stirring occasionally, until tender and brown.

Preheat: Heat the oven to the temperature called for in the recipe before putting in the food.

Simmer: Cook in liquid just below the boiling point. Bubbles form slowly and collapse below the surface.

Toast: Brown in the oven or toaster.

BREAKFAST DISHES

Cottage Cheese Pancakes

6 eggs
1 cup creamed cottage cheese
1 cup low-fat buttermilk
¾ cup all-purpose flour
1 tablespoon sugar
½ teaspoon salt
¼ teaspoon baking soda
¼ teaspoon baking powder

Measure all ingredients into a mixing bowl.

Beat with rotary beater until smooth.

Heat griddle; grease if necessary. Heat is just right if bubbles skitter around when a few drops of water are sprinkled on it.

Pour batter from large spoon or soup ladle onto hot griddle. Turn each pancake as soon as it is puffed and full of bubbles. Cook other side until golden brown.

Yield: 6 servings (5 pancakes each)

Nutrient analysis of 5 pancakes: 1 starch/bread exchange; 1 medium-fat meat exchange; 167 Calories; 11 g protein; 7 g fat; 15 g carbohydrate; 323 mg sodium; 270 mg cholesterol.

Whole Wheat Crepes with Fruit

1 cup skim milk
½ cup all-purpose flour
1 cup whole wheat flour
1 egg
1 tablespoon margarine, melted
¼ teaspoon salt
1 cup creamed cottage cheese
Cinnamon
1½ cups blueberries or cut-up strawberries

Measure milk, flours, egg, margarine, and salt into blender container or food processor. Cover and process until smooth. Refrigerate at least 1 hour.

Brush a 6- to 7-inch crepe pan or skillet with vegetable oil. Place pan over medium heat until oil just begins to smoke. Pour ¼ cup batter into pan while rotating pan so bottom is coated evenly. Return pan to heat until underside of crepe is light brown. Turn crepe with spatula and cook other side for 30 seconds. Let finished crepes rest on a clean towel while cooking remaining batter.

After all the crepes are made, spread each one with 2 tablespoons cottage cheese and a sprinkle of cinnamon. Roll up crepe. Place on serving plate and top with berries.

Yield: 8 servings (2 crepes each)

Nutrient analysis of 1 serving: 1 starch/bread exchange; ½ medium-fat meat exchange; ½ fruit exchange; 142 Calories; 6 g protein; 3 g fat; 22 g carbohydrate; 103 mg sodium; 40 mg cholesterol.

Super French Toast

2 eggs
¼ cup orange juice
¼ teaspoon salt
½ cup cornflakes, crushed†
¼ cup wheat germ
¼ cup ground pecans
3 tablespoons margarine
8 slices whole wheat or French bread

Beat the eggs, orange juice, and salt in a flat bowl with a fork or whisk until blended. Mix the cornflakes, wheat germ, and nuts in a small pie pan or cake pan.

Heat the margarine in a large skillet. Dip bread slices into egg mixture and then into cornflake mixture, coating both sides. Place in skillet as many pieces as will fit comfortably in 1 layer (2 or 3 batches may be needed).

Cook until brown on both sides, turning slices carefully with wide spatula. Keep finished toast warm if cooking more batches.

Yield: 8 slices

Nutrient analysis of 1 slice: 1 starch/bread exchange; 1 medium-fat meat exchange; 1 fat exchange; 205 Calories; 9 g protein; 12 g fat; 18 g carbohydrate; 374 mg sodium; 66 mg cholesterol.

†To crush cornflakes, place in plastic bag, tie securely, and crush with hands.

*Waffles

2 eggs
1¾ cup skim milk
½ cup margarine, melted
1½ cups all-purpose flour
½ cup whole wheat flour
1 tablespoon plus 1 teaspoon baking powder
1 tablespoon sugar

Heat waffle iron. Measure all ingredients into mixing bowl. Beat with rotary beater until batter is smooth.

Pour batter from cup or pitcher onto center of hot waffle iron. Bake until steaming stops, about 5 minutes. Remove waffle carefully.

Yield: 3 10-inch waffles

Nutrient analysis of 1 plain waffle: 4 starch/bread exchanges; 1 high-fat meat exchange; ¾ low-fat milk exchange; 4 fat exchanges; 676 Calories; 17 g protein; 37 g fat; 68 g carbohydrate; 1,064 mg sodium; 175 mg cholesterol.

Variations:

Orange Waffles: Stir 1 tablespoon grated orange peel into batter. Serve waffles with Orange Margarine (½ cup softened margarine and ¼ teaspoon grated orange peel beaten together until fluffy).

Nut Waffles: Sprinkle 2 tablespoons coarsely chopped pecans on waffle before baking.

Be sure to add in extra calories and exchanges if you use a variation.

*Quick Breakfast Muffins

1 whole wheat English muffin
2 teaspoons margarine
¼ cup plus 2 tablespoons shredded part-skim-milk mozzarella cheese

Split muffin and toast in toaster. Spread each half with 1 teaspoon margarine. Sprinkle with 3 tablespoons cheese and place on baking sheet.

Set oven control at broil or 550°F. Broil muffin 4 inches from heat source until cheese is melted and bubbly, about 3 minutes.

Yield: 1 serving

Nutrient analysis of 1 serving: 2 starch/bread exchanges; 1½ lean meat exchanges; 2 fat exchanges; 327 Calories; 17 g protein; 17 g fat; 30 g carbohydrate; 519 mg sodium; 23 mg cholesterol.

*Breakfast Casserole

4 slices whole wheat bread
1 pound bulk pork sausage
1 cup shredded Cheddar cheese
6 eggs
2 cups skim milk
1 teaspoon salt
1 teaspoon dry mustard

Preheat oven to 350°F.

Cut bread into ½-inch cubes. Spread over the bottom of a buttered baking dish, 11¾ x 7½ x 1¾ inches.

Cook and stir sausage until brown. Drain off fat. Sprinkle sausage over bread cubes, then top with cheese.

Beat eggs, milk, salt, and mustard together. Pour over the layers in baking dish. (Can be baked right away or covered and refrigerated several hours or overnight.)

Bake uncovered at 350°F. for 35 to 40 minutes. Let stand for 10 minutes before serving. Cut into 8 equal pieces.

Yield: 8 servings

Nutrient analysis of 1 serving: ½ starch/bread exchange; 3 medium-fat meat exchanges; 2 fat exchanges; 366 Calories; 24 g protein; 26 g fat; 9 g carbohydrate; 807 mg sodium; 241 mg cholesterol.

Breakfast Cheese Grits

2 cups water
½ cup uncooked regular grits
3 eggs
1 tablespoon plus 1½ teaspoons margarine
1 cup shredded sharp Cheddar cheese

Preheat oven to 350°F. Heat water to boiling in saucepan. Stir in grits gradually. Cook, while stirring constantly, for 5 minutes.

Remove from heat and cool for 5 minutes. Beat in eggs, one at a time. Stir in margarine and cheese. Pour into a 1½- or 2-quart casserole.

Bake at 350°F. for 30 minutes.

Variation: For spicy grits, stir in 1 teaspoon dry mustard and 2 tablespoons onion flakes along with the cheese.

Yield: 4 servings (1 cup each)

Nutrient analysis of 1 serving: 1 starch/bread exchange; 2 medium-fat meat exchanges; 1 fat exchange; 282 Calories; 13 g protein; 18 g fat; 17 g carbohydrate; 277 mg sodium; 227 mg cholesterol.

Baked Eggs in Toast Cups

4 slices whole wheat or other variety bread
4 teaspoons margarine
4 eggs
Freshly ground pepper to taste

Preheat oven to 375°F.

Cut crusts from 4 thin slices whole wheat, rye, or white bread. Spread each slice with 1 teaspoon margarine. Press, buttered side down, into muffin cups.

Bake at 375°F. for 8 minutes.

Remove cups from oven. Break 1 egg into each toast cup. Season with pepper.

Return cups to oven and bake at 375°F. until eggs are set, about 5 minutes.

Variation: Sprinkle bread slices with sesame seeds, dillweed, or snipped parsley after spreading with margarine.

Yield: 4 servings

Nutrient analysis of 1 serving: ½ starch/bread exchange; 1 medium-fat meat exchange; 1 fat exchange; 161 Calories; 7 g protein; 11 g fat; 9 g carbohydrate; 253 mg sodium; 263 mg cholesterol.

Egg-in-a-Frame

1 slice whole wheat bread
2 teaspoons margarine
1 tablespoon margarine (additional)
1 egg

Spread both sides of bread with the 2 teaspoons margarine. Cut out center of bread slice with 2-inch biscuit cutter and save "hole."

Heat 1 tablespoon margarine in small skillet. Place bread slice and "hole" in skillet. Break an egg into center of bread slice.

Cook until egg is set and bread is brown on bottom. Turn and cook until brown on other side. Serve "hole" with framed egg.

Yield: 1 serving

Nutrient analysis of 1 serving: 1 starch/bread exchange; 1 medium-fat meat exchange; 2 fat exchanges; 235 Calories; 8 g protein; 17 g fat; 12 g carbohydrate; 376 mg sodium; 264 mg cholesterol.

Poached Egg

2 teaspoons white vinegar
1 egg
1 slice bread, toasted
1 teaspoon margarine
Freshly ground pepper to taste

In a small skillet, heat 1½ inches water to boiling. Reduce heat to simmer and add vinegar.

Break the egg into a cup or saucer. Hold cup or saucer close to surface of water and slip egg into water.

Cook to desired doneness, 3 to 5 minutes. Remove egg from water with slotted spoon. Place on toast and dot with margarine. Season with pepper.

Yield: 1 serving

Nutrient analysis of 1 serving: 1 starch/bread exchange; 1 medium-fat meat exchange; 1 fat exchange; 168 Calories; 8 g protein; 10 g fat; 12 g carbohydrate; 253 mg sodium; 264 mg cholesterol.

Scrambled Eggs

2 eggs
1 tablespoon water or milk
Dash pepper
2 teaspoons margarine

Break eggs into a small bowl. Add water and pepper. Stir with a fork or whisk, mixing thoroughly for an even color, or mixing lightly if streaks of yellow and white in the eggs are preferred.

Heat margarine in a small skillet over medium heat until just hot enough to sizzle a drop of water.

Pour egg mixture into skillet. As mixture begins to set at bottom and sides, gently lift cooked portions with spatula so that thin uncooked portion can flow to bottom. Repeat this several times. Do not stir.

Cook until eggs are thickened throughout but still moist, 3 to 5 minutes.

Variations: Add ½ teaspoon snipped chives, snipped parsley, or dry mustard for a nice flavor.

Yield: 1 serving

Nutrient analysis of 1 serving: 2 medium-fat meat exchanges; 2 fat exchanges; 259 Calories; 12 g protein; 18 g fat; 1 g carbohydrate; 240 mg sodium; 526 mg cholesterol.

Omelet

4 eggs
3 tablespoons water
2 tablespoons margarine

Beat eggs and water in a small mixing bowl until light and fluffy.

Heat margarine in a large skillet until just hot enough to sizzle a drop of water. As margarine melts, tilt pan to coat bottom.

Pour egg mixture into skillet. Cook over medium heat, lifting edge to allow uncooked portion to flow to bottom, until omelet is light brown on bottom. Do not stir.

Tip skillet and loosen omelet by slipping spatula or pancake turner underneath. Fold omelet in half, being careful not to break it. Slip onto heated platter.

Variations:

Cheese Omelet (My Favorite): Sprinkle ½ cup shredded Cheddar, Swiss, or part-skim-milk mozzarella cheese on half of omelet before folding it. (Add 1 medium-fat meat to exchanges.)

Jelly Omelet (My Brother's Favorite): Drop 1 tablespoon diet strawberry jam, in small amounts, onto half of omelet before folding it. (Add ½ fruit to exchanges.)

Zucchini Omelet (My Father's Favorite): Before beating eggs, cook and stir ½ small onion, sliced into rings, and ¼ cup thin-sliced unpared zucchini in 1 tablespoon vegetable oil until tender. Season with salt and pepper and set aside. Drop small spoonfuls of zucchini onto half of omelet before folding. (Add 1½ fat exchanges.)

Apple Omelet (Cousin Jamie's Favorite): Before beating eggs, cook and stir 1 small apple, cored, pared and sliced, in 2 teaspoons margarine until soft. Stir in ¼ teaspoon cinnamon and set aside. Drop small spoonfuls of apple mixture onto half of omelet before folding. (Add ½ fruit exchange.)

Yield: 2 servings

Nutrient analysis of 1 plain omelet: 2 medium-fat meat exchanges; 1 fat exchange; 192 Calories; 12 g protein; 16 g fat; 2 g carbohydrate; 230 mg sodium; 526 mg cholesterol.

Omelet Roll

1 egg per serving
1 teaspoon margarine per serving
Salt and pepper to taste

Prepare 1 omelet roll at a time.

For each, beat 1 egg in a small bowl.

Melt 1 teaspoon margarine in a 10-inch skillet; rotate pan to coat bottom with margarine. Pour egg into skillet; slowly rotate pan to spread mixture into thin circle. Cook over medium heat 2 to 3 minutes.

Loosen edge of egg; roll up, using small spatula and fork. Season with salt and pepper.

If preparing more than one, keep omelet rolls warm on an ungreased baking sheet in a 275°F. oven.

Variations: (Be sure to calculate in extra calories and food groups.)

Cheese Omelet Roll: Just before rolling egg, sprinkle 2 teaspoons shredded cheese and 1 tablespoon snipped chives on top.

Jelly Omelet Roll: Just before rolling egg, drop 1 teaspoon diet jelly or diet orange marmalade on top.

Yield: 1 serving (1 roll)

Nutrient analysis of 1 omelet roll: 1 medium-fat meat exchange; 1 fat exchange; 112 Calories; 6 g protein; 9 g fat; 1 g carbohydrate; 368 mg sodium; 263 mg cholesterol.

Breakfast Shake

¾ cup skim milk
1 egg
1 banana, cut up
½ teaspoon vanilla

Place all ingredients in blender container or food processor. Cover and process until smooth.

Pour into large glass.

Variations: Substitute 1 peach, peeled, pitted, and cut up, 1 cup strawberries, or 1 cup blueberries for the banana.

Yield: 1 serving

Nutrient analysis of 1 serving: 1 medium-fat meat exchange; 1 skim milk exchange; 2 fruit exchanges; 243 Calories; 15 g protein; 7 g fat; 30 g carbohydrate; 164 mg sodium; 283 mg cholesterol.

Blender Breakfast

1 cup skim milk
1 cup fresh or unsweetened canned or frozen fruit (½ banana, fresh berries, pitted cherries, cut-up peaches, nectarines, or other fruits)
2 tablespoons wheat germ
1 tablespoon bran
1 to 2 teaspoons vanilla
4 ice cubes

Measure all ingredients into blender container or food processor. Process until smooth.

Yield: 1 serving

Nutrient analysis of 1 serving: 1½ starch/bread exchanges; 1 low-fat milk exchange; 1 fruit exchange; 274 Calories; 17 g protein; 4 g fat; 47 g carbohydrate; 130 mg sodium; 8 mg cholesterol.

BREADS

Challah

1 package active dry yeast
¼ cup warm water (105 to 115°F.)
1 egg
¼ cup sugar
¼ teaspoon salt
¼ cup margarine, softened
2½ to 3 cups all-purpose flour

Dissolve yeast in the warm water in a large bowl.

Beat egg in a small bowl. Stir the egg, sugar, salt, margarine, and 2 cups of flour into the yeast mixture. Beat with a large spoon until smooth. Mix in enough of the remaining flour to make dough easy to handle. (The dough should leave side of bowl and not stick to hands.)

Turn dough onto a lightly floured board. Knead until smooth and elastic, 5 to 10 minutes. Place dough in a greased bowl; turn dough so greased side is up. Cover with clean tea towel and let rise in a warm place until double its original height, 1½ to 2 hours. Test dough by pressing fingertips ½ inch into dough. If an impression remains, the dough has risen enough.

Punch down dough with fist. Divide dough into 3 equal parts. On a lightly floured board, use hands to roll each part into a rope 14 inches long. Place ropes lengthwise and close together on a greased baking sheet. Braid ropes gently and loosely. (Do not stretch.) Pinch ends together and tuck under. Cover and let rise in a warm place until doubled, about 1 hour.

Preheat oven to 375°F. Bake challah for 30 to 35 minutes, or until braids sound hollow.

Note: For a shiny crust, beat 1 egg white and 1 tablespoon water in a small bowl and brush on braid 10 minutes before end of baking time.

Yield: 1 loaf (12 slices)

Nutrient analysis of 1 slice: 1¼ starch/bread exchanges; 1 fat exchange; 137 Calories; 3 g protein; 5 g fat; 20 g carbohydrate; 94 mg sodium; 22 mg cholesterol.

Blueberry Muffins

3 eggs
¼ cup vegetable oil
½ cup skim milk
1 cup all-purpose flour
½ cup whole wheat flour
2 tablespoons wheat germ
2 teaspoons baking powder
½ teaspoon salt
½ cup dry milk powder
¾ to 1 cup fresh blueberries (or use well-drained, defrosted frozen blueberries)

Preheat oven to 400°F. Grease 12 muffin cups or line with paper baking cups.

Beat eggs lightly in mixing bowl. Stir in vegetable oil and skim milk.

Mix in flours, wheat germ, baking powder, salt, and dry milk just until flour is moistened. (Batter will be lumpy.)

Fold in blueberries. Fill each muffin cup ⅔ full.

Bake at 400°F. for 20 to 25 minutes, or until muffins are golden brown.

Yield: 12 muffins

Nutrient analysis of 1 muffin: 1 starch/bread exchange; 1½ fat exchanges; 142 Calories; 5 g protein; 7 g fat; 16 g carbohydrate; 189 mg sodium; 66 mg cholesterol.

Bran Muffins

1 cup all-purpose flour
1 cup All-Bran cereal
¼ cup wheat germ
2½ teaspoons baking powder
½ teaspoon salt
1 egg
2 tablespoons margarine
¼ cup molasses
¾ cup skim milk

Preheat oven to 400°F. Grease 12 medium muffin cups.

Measure flour, bran cereal, wheat germ, baking powder, and salt into a medium bowl. Stir together and set aside.

Measure the egg, margarine, molasses, and milk into blender container or food processor. Cover and process until smooth.

Pour milk mixture onto flour mixture and mix just until flour is moistened. (Batter will be lumpy.) Pour an equal amount of batter into each muffin cup.

Bake at 400°F. for 20 to 25 minutes. Remove muffins immediately from cups.

Yield: 12 muffins

Nutrient analysis of 1 muffin: 1 starch/bread exchange; ½ fat exchange; 108 Calories; 4 g protein; 3 g fat; 17 g carbohydrate; 211 mg sodium; 22 mg cholesterol.

Fruit Bran Muffins

1½ cups All-Bran cereal
1 cup skim milk
1 egg
¼ cup vegetable oil
¼ cup sugar
1 cup all-purpose flour
2 teaspoons baking powder
½ teaspoon baking soda
½ teaspoon grated lemon peel
½ teaspoon cinnamon
⅓ cup diced, pared and cored apple
⅓ cup diced banana
⅓ cup snipped dried apricots

Preheat oven to 400°F. Grease 12 medium muffin cups or line with paper baking cups.

Combine All-Bran cereal and milk in mixing bowl and let stand for 5 minutes to soften.

Beat the egg and oil into the cereal mixture thoroughly. Blend in the sugar, flour, baking powder, baking soda, lemon peel, and cinnamon. Place 1 spoonful of batter in each muffin cup. In each of 4 muffin cups, top batter with a fourth of the apples (1 rounded tablespoon). Top the next 4 cups with a fourth of the banana, and top the remaining 4 cups with a fourth of the apricots. Fill cups ⅔ full with remaining batter.

Bake at 400°F. 20 to 25 minutes, or until golden brown.

Yield: 12 muffins

Nutrient analysis of 1 muffin: 1 starch/bread exchange; 1 fat exchange; 142 Calories; 3 g protein; 6 g fat; 19 g carbohydrate; 179 mg sodium; 22 mg cholesterol.

Popovers

2 eggs
1 cup skim milk
1 cup all-purpose flour
¼ teaspoon salt

Preheat oven to 450°F. Grease 10 custard cups, muffin cups, or popover cups thoroughly.

Measure all ingredients into blender container or food processor. Cover and process at high speed until smooth. Fill cups ½ full.

Bake for 10 minutes at 450°F.; reduce heat to 350°F. and bake 35 minutes more. *Do not open oven during baking.*

Note: Do not use egg substitute in this recipe. For higher popovers, heat greased muffin tins or popover cups before filling them.

Yield: 10 popovers

Nutrient analysis of 1 popover: ¾ starch/bread exchange; 66 Calories; 3 g protein; 1 g fat; 10 g carbohydrate; 74 mg sodium; 26 mg cholesterol.

Cheese Corn Bread

1 cup yellow cornmeal
1 cup all-purpose flour
2 tablespoons wheat germ
2 tablespoons sugar
1 tablespoon plus 1 teaspoon baking powder
½ teaspoon salt
1 egg
1 cup skim milk
¼ cup vegetable oil
⅓ cup shredded sharp Cheddar cheese

Preheat oven to 425°F. Grease baking pan, 8 x 8 x 2 inches.

Measure all ingredients into a mixing bowl. Mix thoroughly with large spoon, then beat vigorously until smooth, 1 to 2 minutes. Pour into prepared pan.

Bake at 425°F. for 20 to 25 minutes, or until golden brown. Serve hot.

Variations:

Corn Sticks: Grease and heat corn-stick pans. Fill pans ⅔ full. Bake at 425°F. for 15 minutes, or until golden brown.

Corn Muffins: Fill greased 12-opening muffin tin ⅔ full. Bake at 425°F. about 15 minutes, or until golden brown.

Yield: 12 servings

Nutrient analysis of 1 serving: 1½ starch/bread exchanges; 1½ fat exchanges; 159 Calories; 4 g protein; 7 g fat; 21 g carbohydrate; 324 mg sodium; 25 mg cholesterol.

Wheat Germ Casserole Bread

1½ cups whole wheat flour
1½ cups all-purpose flour
½ cup wheat germ
2 envelopes active dry yeast
2 teaspoons salt
1½ cups warm water (105 to 115°F.)
2 tablespoons margarine, softened
2 tablespoons molasses

Put ½ cup whole wheat flour, ½ cup all-purpose flour, the wheat germ, yeast, salt, water, margarine, and molasses into the large bowl of an electric mixer. Beat at low speed for 30 seconds, scraping bowl constantly. Add ¼ cup each of the remaining whole wheat flour and the all-purpose flour. Then beat at high speed, scraping bowl frequently.

Remove bowl from beater, and with wooden spoon mix in the remaining ¾ cup each of the whole wheat flour and all-purpose flour. Scrape batter from side of bowl. Cover bowl and let rise in a warm place until dough has doubled in size, about 45 minutes.

Preheat oven to 375°F. Grease a 1½-quart casserole.

Stir down dough by beating with a wooden spoon for about 30 seconds, then spread it in the prepared casserole.

Bake at 375°F. for 1 hour and 15 minutes, or until loaf sounds hollow when tapped. Remove loaf to wire rack and serve warm or cool.

Yield: 1 loaf (16 slices)

Nutrient analysis of 1 slice: 1½ starch/bread exchanges; ½ fat exchange; 129 Calories; 5 g protein; 3 g fat; 22 g carbohydrate; 263 mg sodium; 0 mg cholesterol.

Easy Whole Wheat Bread

1 package active dry yeast
3 cups warm water (105 to 115°F.)
1 tablespoon honey
1 teaspoon salt
5 cups whole wheat flour

Dissolve yeast in warm water in a large bowl.

Stir in the honey and salt. Let stand until yeast begins to act.

Preheat oven to 400°F. Grease loaf pan, 9 x 5 x 3 inches.

Mix flour into yeast mixture until smooth. Pour batter into loaf pan. Let stand in a warm place for 10 minutes.

Bake at 400°F. for 45 minutes, until loaf is dark golden brown and sounds hollow when tapped.

Yield: 1 loaf (16 slices)

Nutrient analysis of 1 slice: 2 starch/bread exchanges; 142 Calories; 6 g protein; 1 g fat; 31 g carbohydrate; 122 mg sodium; 0 mg cholesterol.

Drop Biscuits

1½ cups all-purpose flour
½ cup whole wheat flour
3 teaspoons baking powder
½ teaspoon salt
⅓ cup vegetable oil
1 cup milk

Preheat oven to 450°F. Grease baking sheet.

Measure flours, baking powder, and salt into mixing bowl. Stir with a fork. Add oil and milk, and stir until dough cleans side of bowl.

Drop rounded teaspoonfuls of dough onto prepared baking sheet.

Bake at 450°F. for 10 to 12 minutes, or until golden brown. Serve hot with margarine and, if desired, with jelly, honey, jam, or syrup.

Variation:

Cheese Biscuits: Place small cube of cheese (¼ ounce) in center of each biscuit before baking. Cover with small amount of dough. (Add ½ fat exchange and 25 calories.)

Yield: 2 dozen biscuits

Nutrient analysis of 1 biscuit: ½ starch/bread exchange; ½ fat exchange; 66 Calories; 1 g protein; 3 g fat; 8 g carbohydrate; 99 mg sodium; 1 mg cholesterol.

Corn Fritters

Oil for frying
1 cup all-purpose flour
1 teaspoon baking powder
½ teaspoon salt
⅛ teaspoon paprika
16-ounce can whole kernel corn, drained (reserve ½ cup liquid)
2 eggs, separated

Heat 3 to 4 inches of oil in deep-fat fryer or kettle to 365°F. *(Adult should be in the kitchen when you are cooking with hot oil. This is important.)*

Measure flour, baking powder, salt, and paprika into bowl and set aside.

Place ½ cup corn liquid, 1 cup of corn, and egg yolks in blender container or food processor. Cover and process at high speed for 1 minute. Add half the flour mixture and blend until smooth. (Stop blender and push ingredients from sides of container with rubber spatula.) Add remaining flour mixture and blend at medium speed until smooth. Add remaining corn and process for 10 seconds.

Beat egg whites in medium-size bowl with rotary beater until stiff peaks form. Fold corn mixture into egg whites.

Drop batter by tablespoonfuls into hot oil and fry until golden brown. Drain on absorbent paper. Serve hot and, if desired, with diet syrup.

Yield: 24 fritters

Nutrient analysis of 1 fritter: ½ starch/bread exchange; ½ fat exchange; 57 Calories; 1 g protein; 3 g fat; 7 g carbohydrate; 118 mg sodium; 22 mg cholesterol.

SALADS

Salad Bar

Tear washed and dried greens (lettuce, spinach, romaine, watercress, escarole) into bite-size pieces. Place in a large bowl. Allow ½ cup greens per serving.

Surround bowl of greens with smaller bowls containing:
- Finely shredded red cabbage
- Shredded carrot
- Thinly sliced celery
- Shredded cheese
- Bacon bits
- Croutons
- Sliced mushrooms
- Sliced cucumbers
- Sliced zucchini
- Chopped hard-cooked egg

Allow ¼ cup of each for each serving.

Place small bowls of several dressings on table. Allow about 2 tablespoons dressing per serving. Let guests make their own tossed salad.

Use the Food Exchange Lists (Chapter 2) to calculate the nutrient content of your salad.

Tossed Green Salad

½ clove garlic
3 or 4 washed lettuce leaves (iceberg, Boston, Bibb, leaf, or bronze)
1 teaspoon olive or vegetable oil
¼ teaspoon cider or wine vinegar
Freshly ground pepper

Rub small wooden salad bowl with cut side of garlic. Tear lettuce into bite-size pieces (there should be about 1 cup), and turn into a bowl. Drizzle with oil and toss until leaves glisten. Refrigerate until serving time.

Mix vinegar and pepper; drizzle onto lettuce and toss.

Yield: 1 serving

Nutrient analysis of 1 serving: 1 fat exchange; 41 Calories; 0 g protein; 5 g fat; 0 g carbohydrate; 0 mg sodium; 0 mg cholesterol.

Orange and Lettuce Salad

½ small head lettuce or 1 bunch leaf lettuce
½ cup shredded carrot
2 oranges, pared, pitted, sectioned, and cut up
½ green pepper, seeded and sliced thin
¼ cup orange juice
1 tablespoon vegetable oil

Wash lettuce and tear into bite-size pieces (there should be about 2 cups). Place in salad bowl.

Add the carrot, orange pieces, and green pepper to lettuce.

Mix orange juice and oil. Drizzle mixture onto salad and toss gently.

Yield: 5 servings

Nutrient analysis of 1 cup: 1½ vegetable exchanges; ½ fat exchange; 54 Calories; 1 g protein; 3 g fat; 7 g carbohydrate; 5 mg sodium; 0 mg cholesterol.

Waldorf Salad

2 cups diced, cored, unpared apple (2 medium apples)
1 cup diced celery
⅓ cup coarsely chopped walnuts or pecans
½ cup low-calorie mayonnaise
6 lettuce cups

Place apple, celery, nuts, and mayonnaise in a bowl and mix lightly.

Spoon salad into lettuce cups and, if desired, garnish with Maraschino cherries.

Yield: 6 servings

Nutrient analysis of 1 serving: ¾ fruit exchange; 1½ fat exchanges; 109 Calories; 2 g protein; 8 g fat; 10 g carbohydrate; 47 mg sodium; 11 mg cholesterol.

Sunny Citrus Mold

2 envelopes (¼ ounce each) unflavored gelatin
⅓ cup sugar
20-ounce can pineapple chunks in unsweetened pineapple juice, drained (reserve juice)
⅓ cup lemon juice
1 cup coarsely shredded carrot
1½ cups halved, pitted orange sections
Salad greens

Mix gelatin and sugar in saucepan.

Add enough water to reserved pineapple juice to make 2½ cups. Pour 1 cup of juice mixture onto gelatin in saucepan. Stir over low heat until gelatin is dissolved, about 5 minutes. Remove from heat and stir in lemon juice and remaining pineapple juice mixture. Chill until mixture mounds slightly when dropped from spoon.

Stir in carrot, orange sections, and pineapple chunks. Pour into a 5-cup mold and chill until firm.

Unmold onto serving plate and garnish with salad greens.

Yield: 5 servings (1 cup each)

Nutrient analysis of 1 serving: 2 fruit exchanges; 116 Calories; 4 g protein; 0 g fat; 26 g carbohydrate; 36 mg sodium; 0 mg cholesterol.

Apple-Cabbage Slaw

- **½ cup low-calorie mayonnaise**
- **1 tablespoon plus 1½ teaspoons sugar**
- **1 tablespoon plus 1½ teaspoons lemon juice**
- **1 tablespoon skim milk**
- **1 teaspoon celery seeds**
- **¼ teaspoon salt**
- **⅛ teaspoon freshly ground pepper**
- **8 cups shredded cabbage (1 large head)†**
- **1 cup seedless red or green grapes**
- **1 apple**

Mix mayonnaise, sugar, lemon juice, milk, celery seeds, salt, and pepper in a large bowl.

Add cabbage and mix. Cover and refrigerate 2 hours.

Halve grapes. Quarter apple. Remove core and cut apple into small pieces. Add grape halves and diced apple to cabbage and mix.

Note: This recipe can be cut in half.

Yield: 10 cups

Nutrient analysis of 1 cup: ¾ fruit exchange; ½ fat exchange; 52 Calories; 1 g protein; 2 g fat; 9 g carbohydrate; 77 mg sodium; 6 mg cholesterol.

†Remove outer bruised leaves of cabbage. Cut cabbage into quarters. Remove core; shred with knife or use shredder or food processor.

Grape Salad

- **½ small head lettuce or 1 bunch leaf lettuce**
- **½ pound seedless grapes, halved**
- **1 cup shredded carrot**
- **2 tablespoons lemon juice**
- **½ cup diced Cheddar cheese**
- **2 tablespoons vegetable oil**

Wash lettuce and tear into bite-size pieces (there should be about 2 cups). Place in salad bowl.

Add grape halves, carrot, and lemon juice; toss lightly.

Sprinkle cheese over all; drizzle oil onto salad and toss.

Yield: 6 servings

Nutrient analysis of 1 serving: 1 vegetable exchange; ½ fruit exchange; 1 fat exchange; 120 Calories; 3 g protein; 8 g fat; 11 g carbohydrate; 76 mg sodium; 10 mg cholesterol.

Carrot Salad

1 pound carrots, shredded
1 scallion, minced (include green top)
3 tablespoons lemon juice
¼ teaspoon mace
¼ teaspoon nutmeg
¼ cup raisins or currants
Dash salt and freshly ground pepper
Lettuce

Combine all ingredients except lettuce in a bowl. Toss.

Cover and refrigerate for at least 1 hour.

Serve on lettuce leaves.

Yield: 6 servings

Nutrient analysis of 1 serving: 1 vegetable exchange; ½ fruit exchange; 50 Calories; 1 g protein; 0 g fat; 12 g carbohydrate; 78 mg sodium; 0 mg cholesterol.

Apple and Pear Salad

2 medium apples, cored and sliced thin
2 medium pears, cored and cut up
1 cup diced celery
½ cup chopped walnuts
1 cup low-calorie mayonnaise
2 tablespoons skim milk
¼ teaspoon sugar

Combine apples, pears, celery, and nuts in a salad bowl.

Mix the mayonnaise, milk, and sugar. Pour over ingredients in bowl and mix.

Yield: 6 cups

Nutrient analysis of 1 cup: 1½ fruit exchanges; 2 fat exchanges; 191 Calories; 3 g protein; 12 g fat; 21 g carbohydrate; 58 mg sodium; 21 mg cholesterol.

*Honeydew Salad

1 medium honeydew melon
1½ cups low-fat cottage cheese
1 cup alfalfa sprouts
½ cup pared, seeded, and chopped cucumber
½ cup seedless green grape halves
¼ teaspoon salt
1 tablespoon snipped parsley
Leaf lettuce

Cut off ends of melon; wrap ends in plastic wrap and refrigerate for future use.

Cut remaining melon crosswise into 3 slices. Discard seeds. Cover slices and refrigerate.

Mix cottage cheese, sprouts, cucumber, grapes, salt, and parsley.

Cut melon slices to loosen fruit from rind by carefully running a knife between the fruit and the rind. Leave fruit sitting on top of rind. Score fruit crosswise (do not cut through) into bite-size pieces.

Place melon slice on lettuce leaf on plates and spoon cottage cheese mixture on top.

Yield: 3 servings

Nutrient analysis of 1 serving: 2 lean meat exchanges; 2 fruit exchanges; 220 Calories; 17 g protein; 6 g fat; 28 g carbohydrate; 640 mg sodium; 8 mg cholesterol.

VEGETABLES, RICE, AND POTATOES

Artichoke

4 artichokes
1 teaspoon salt
Juice of 1 lemon
Lemon-Margarine Sauce (see below)

Discard any discolored leaves and the small leaves at the base of each artichoke. Trim stem even with base of artichoke. Cutting straight across, slice 1 inch off top and discard top. Snip off points of the remaining leaves with scissors. Rinse artichokes under cold water.

Bring 6 quarts water to a boil in a large kettle. Add the salt, lemon juice, and artichokes. Heat to boiling, reduce heat and simmer, uncovered, until leaves pull out easily and bottom is tender when pierced with a knife, 30 to 40 minutes.

Remove chokes (fuzzy center) from centers with a teaspoon. Serve with Lemon-Margarine Sauce.†

† To lower fat intake, use only half of the Lemon-Margarine Sauce.

Lemon-Margarine Sauce

½ cup melted margarine
2 tablespoons lemon juice

Combine margarine and lemon juice and mix thoroughly.

Note: To serve artichokes cold, cover and refrigerate several hours. Serve with Italian Salad Dressing (page 92).

Yield: 4 servings

Nutrient analysis of 1 serving: 3 vegetable exchanges; 5 fat exchanges; 216 Calories; 8 g protein; 25 g fat; 13 g carbohydrate; 250 mg sodium; 0 mg cholesterol.

Acorn Squash with Citrus Filling

2 acorn squash (1 pound each)
Salt and freshly ground pepper to taste
3 tablespoons margarine
2 medium oranges, peeled, pitted, and sectioned
1 medium grapefruit, peeled, pitted, sectioned, and cut up

Cut each squash in half horizontally; discard seeds and fibers.

Place squash in ungreased baking dish, 13½ x 9 x 2 inches. Season cut sides with salt and pepper; dot with margarine. Pour water into dish to ¼-inch depth; cover with aluminum foil.

Bake in 400°F. oven until tender, about 30 minutes.

Mix orange sections and grapefruit pieces.

Remove foil from pan; fill squash halves with orange and grapefruit mixture.

Bake at 400°F. until filling is hot, about 15 minutes.

Yield: 4 servings

Nutrient analysis of 1 serving: 1 starch/bread exchange; 1 fruit exchange; 2 fat exchanges; 233 Calories; 4 g protein; 9 g fat; 34 g carbohydrate; 206 mg sodium; 0 mg cholesterol.

Stuffed Celery

6 celery stalks
2 ounces cream cheese, softened
2 tablespoons skim milk

Trim celery stalks and cut into 1- to 2-inch pieces.

Beat cheese and milk in small bowl until smooth and fluffy.

Fill celery pieces with cheese mixture, using a small spoon or spatula.

Variation: Shredded Cheddar cheese (2 ounces) can be substituted for the cream cheese (change exchange to ½ lean meat; calories to 55).

Yield: 6 servings

Nutrient analysis of 1 serving: 1 fat exchange; 40 Calories; 1 g protein; 4 g fat; 1 g carbohydrate; 57 mg sodium; 11 mg cholesterol.

Carrot Curls

Carrots

Scrape carrots. Cut carrots lengthwise with vegetable parer into paper-thin slices. Roll up each slice and fasten with wooden pick.

Place in bowl of ice water to crisp. Remove wooden picks before serving.

Yield: as desired

Nutrient analysis of ½ cup: 1 vegetable exchange; 25 Calories; 2 g protein; 0 g fat; 5 g carbohydrate; 20 mg sodium; 0 mg cholesterol.

Pineapple Carrots

2 cups sliced carrots
¼ cup unsweetened pineapple juice
¾ teaspoon cornstarch
¼ cup pineapple chunks in unsweetened pineapple juice, drained
1½ teaspoons margarine

Steam carrots as directed on page 99. Drain and set aside.

Blend pineapple juice and cornstarch in a 1-quart saucepan. Cook over medium heat, stirring constantly, until mixture thickens and boils.

Stir in carrots, pineapple chunks, and margarine and heat through.

Yield: 4 servings

Nutrient analysis of 1 serving (½ cup): ½ fruit exchange; ½ vegetable exchange; ½ fat exchange; 61 Calories; 1 g protein; 2 g fat; 10 g carbohydrate; 43 mg sodium; 0 mg cholesterol.

Corn on the Cob

3 large ears fresh corn
3 teaspoons margarine
Salt and pepper to taste

Remove husks and silk from corn.

In a large kettle, heat to boiling enough water to cover corn.

Add corn and heat to boiling again. Boil uncovered for 7 minutes.

Using tongs, remove corn to platter and brush with margarine. Serve with salt and pepper.

Yield: 3 servings

Nutrient analysis of 1 serving: 1½ starch/bread exchanges; 1 fat exchange; 150 Calories; 3 g protein; 5 g fat; 23 g carbohydrate; 275 mg sodium; 0 mg cholesterol.

Corn on the Cob for a Cookout

Corn
Margarine

Remove husks and silk from corn and reserve husks. Brush corn with margarine.

Dampen husks and wrap around corn. Wrap in aluminum foil.

Place on hot coals and cook for 20 to 30 minutes, or until tender.

Yield: as desired

Nutrient analysis of 1 ear: 1½ starch/bread exchanges; 1 fat exchange; 140 Calories; 3 g protein; 5 g fat; 21 g carbohydrate; 135 mg sodium; 0 mg cholesterol.

**Rice*

1 cup uncooked regular white rice
2 cups chicken or beef stock
1 tablespoon margarine
1 tablespoon snipped parsley

Measure all ingredients into saucepan. Heat to boiling, stirring occasionally.

Reduce heat, cover, and simmer until all liquid is absorbed, 20 to 25 minutes.

Fluff rice with fork. Serve immediately.

Yield: 4 servings (½ cup each)

Nutrient analysis of 1 serving: 2 starch/bread exchanges; 1 fat exchange; 165 Calories; 6 g protein; 4 g fat; 26 g carbohydrate; 516 mg sodium; 1 mg cholesterol.

Rice Pilaf

1 onion, finely chopped
2 stalks celery, diced (include leaves)
¼ cup minced green pepper
¼ cup margarine
1 cup chicken stock
1⅔ cups water
1 cup brown rice

Cook and stir onion, celery, and green pepper in margarine in saucepan until tender, about 5 minutes.

Stir in chicken stock, water, and rice and heat to boiling, stirring occasionally.

Reduce heat, cover, and cook over low heat until all liquid is absorbed, about 50 minutes.

Yield: 6 servings

Nutrient analysis of 1 serving: 2 starch/bread exchanges; 2 fat exchanges; 199 Calories; 4 g protein; 9 g fat; 26 g carbohydrate; 367 mg sodium; 0 mg cholesterol.

*Calico Rice

1 cup uncooked regular white rice
2½ cups water
1 teaspoon salt
½ cup finely chopped onion
¼ cup finely chopped green pepper
¼ cup shredded carrot
2 tablespoons snipped parsley
½ bay leaf
1 tablespoon margarine
Salt and pepper to taste

Measure all ingredients except salt and pepper into a large saucepan. Heat to boiling, stirring occasionally.

Reduce heat to simmer, cover pan tightly, and cook until rice is tender, 15 to 20 minutes. (Do not lift cover or stir.)

Remove pan from heat. Remove bay leaf and season rice with salt and pepper. Fluff rice lightly with fork. If desired, cover pan and let rice stand for 5 to 10 minutes.

Yield: 4 servings

Nutrient analysis of 1 serving: 2 starch/bread exchanges; ½ fat exchange; 148 Calories; 3 g protein; 3 g fat; 27 g carbohydrate; 752 mg sodium; 0 mg cholesterol.

Oven-Fried Potatoes

2 tablespoons vegetable oil
4 unpared medium potatoes

Preheat oven to 450°F. Pour vegetable oil onto baking sheet.

Wash and scrub potatoes. Cut into long thin slices, as for French fries.

Place potato slices on baking sheet and toss to coat with oil.

Bake at 450°F. for 20 minutes, until potatoes are crisp and light brown. Turn occasionally with a large spatula.

Yield: 4 servings

Nutrient analysis of 1 serving: 1 starch/bread exchange; 1½ fat exchanges; 138 Calories; 2 g protein; 7 g fat; 17 g carbohydrate; 3 mg sodium; 0 mg cholesterol.

MAIN DISHES

*Pizza

2 cups Thick Tomato Sauce (see below)
1 package active dry yeast
1 cup warm water (105 to 115°F.)
2 cups all-purpose flour
2 cups whole wheat flour
2 tablespoons unprocessed bran
1 teaspoon salt
½ cup vegetable oil
2 teaspoons dried oregano
¼ cup grated Parmesan cheese
1 cup shredded part-skim-milk mozzarella cheese

Prepare thick tomato sauce as directed and set aside.

Dissolve yeast in warm water.

Mix flours, bran, and salt in a large bowl. Make a "well" in center and pour in the oil and the yeast mixture. Mix with wooden spoon until smooth. If necessary, mix in more warm water, 1 tablespoon at a time, to make dough smooth.

With the hands, knead dough in bowl until dough is soft, pliable, and pulls away from side of bowl. Turn dough onto cloth-covered board and knead until pliable, 2 to 3 minutes. To test, press finger into dough; if dough pops back, dough is pliable enough. Place dough in bowl, cover, and let rise until it doubles in height, 1½ to 2 hours.

Punch down dough.

Preheat oven to 400°F. Spray baking sheet with vegetable spray.

Roll dough on cloth-covered board into a rectangle, 12 x 8 inches. Place on baking sheet; turn up edges to hold filling. Prick rectangle with fork. Spread 2 cups thick tomato sauce on dough. Sprinkle oregano, Parmesan cheese, and mozzarella cheese on top.

Bake until edges of crust are golden brown, about 30 minutes.

Thick Tomato Sauce

1 cup chopped onion
¼ cup vegetable oil
2 cups finely chopped, drained, canned Italian plum tomatoes
15-ounce can tomato puree
1 clove garlic, crushed
1 teaspoon dried oregano
Dash freshly ground pepper

Cook and stir onion in oil until tender.

Stir in remaining ingredients. Heat to boiling, stirring frequently.

Reduce heat, and simmer, uncovered, for 1 hour. Stir occasionally. (Sauce becomes smoother and thicker the longer it simmers.) If desired, sauce can be pureed in blender or food processor for smoother consistency.

Yield: Approximately 2 cups

Variations: Add your favorite topping to pizza, *but* be sure to add the calories and extra exchanges. Try:
1 cup sliced mushrooms 1 cup chopped green peppers 1 cup sliced pepperoni 1 cup thin-sliced onion rings

Yield: 8 pieces

Nutrient analysis of 1 piece: 3 starch/bread exchanges; 1 high-fat meat exchange; 2 vegetable exchanges; 2 fat exchanges; 506 Calories; 15 g protein; 26 g fat; 54 g carbohydrate; 781 mg sodium; 13 mg cholesterol.

Pizza Burgers

1½ pounds lean ground beef
½ cup unprocessed bran
¼ teaspoon pepper
1 teaspoon dry mustard
1 egg
⅔ cup skim milk
¼ cup chopped onion
⅓ cup diced green pepper
6 hamburger buns, split into halves
6-ounce can tomato paste
1 teaspoon garlic salt
½ to 1 teaspoon dried oregano
4 ounces part-skim-milk mozzarella cheese, cut into thin strips

Mix meat, bran, pepper, mustard, egg, milk, onion, and green pepper.

Divide into 12 portions; spread one portion over each bun half.

Set oven control at broil or 550°F. Broil burgers 3 inches from heat source until done as desired.

Mix tomato paste, garlic salt, and oregano. Spread on patties and top each with cheese strip.

Return to broiler and broil until cheese is melted.

Yield: 12 servings

Nutrient analysis of 1 serving: 1½ starch/bread exchanges; 2 medium-fat meat exchanges; 240 Calories; 19 g protein; 9 g fat; 22 g carbohydrate; 279 mg sodium; 66 mg cholesterol.

**Stuffed Green Peppers*

4 large green peppers
½ cup finely chopped onion
1 pound lean ground beef
1 teaspoon salt
2 tablespoons snipped parsley
1 tablespoon Worcestershire sauce
1 cup cooked rice
1¼ cups tomato sauce
1 egg
Freshly ground pepper

Soak clay pot in cold water for 10 minutes.

Remove stems, seeds, and membranes from peppers. Be careful not to cut through sides. Place peppers in boiling water in a large saucepan and boil for 5 minutes. Drain and set aside.

Cook and stir onion and meat in large skillet until meat is brown. Remove from heat and mix in salt, parsley, Worcestershire sauce, rice, ¼ cup of the tomato sauce, and egg. Season with pepper.

Fill each pepper with meat mixture and place upright in clay pot. Pour remaining tomato sauce on peppers.

Cover and bake at 425°F. for 40 minutes.

Yield: 4 servings

Nutrient analysis of 1 serving: 1 starch/bread exchange; 3 lean meat exchanges; 1 vegetable exchange; 293 Calories; 27 g protein; 11 g fat; 20 g carbohydrate; 722 mg sodium; 145 mg cholesterol.

Hamburgers

1 pound lean ground beef
1 small onion, minced (optional)
½ teaspoon freshly ground pepper
½ teaspoon dry mustard
¼ teaspoon salt
¼ cup iced water

Place all ingredients in mixing bowl. Mix thoroughly with hands.

Shape mixture into 4 patties, each about 3 inches in diameter and 1 inch thick.

To broil:

Set oven control at broil or 550°F. Broil patties on rack 3 inches from heat source, 3 to 4 minutes per side for rare, and 5 to 7 minutes per side for medium.

To pan-fry:

Heat 1 to 2 teaspoons vegetable oil in large skillet. Place patties in skillet and cook over medium heat, turning frequently, about 10 minutes.

To grill:

Place patties on grill 4 to 6 inches from hot coals. Cook about 12 minutes, or until done, turning once.

Yield: 4 servings

Nutrient analysis of 1 serving: 3 lean meat exchanges; 194 Calories; 24 g protein; 10 g fat; 2 g carbohydrate; 180 mg sodium; 79 mg cholesterol.

Topper for Hamburgers: Top each hot hamburger with thin slice of processed American cheese and thin slice of tomato. Spoon on ¼ cup hot mashed potatoes to which 1 tablespoon chopped onion has been added. Sprinkle with paprika.

Nutrient analysis of 1 serving of topping: 1 medium-fat meat exchange; 1 fat exchange; ½ bread exchange.

*Hamburger Surprise

2 pounds lean ground beef
1 egg
1 tablespoon capers
1 tablespoon Worcestershire sauce
1 teaspoon garlic salt
Dash freshly ground pepper
6 tablespoons crumbled blue cheese or shredded Cheddar cheese

Mix ground beef, egg, capers, Worcestershire sauce, garlic salt, and pepper thoroughly. Shape mixture into 6 patties, each about 3 inches in diameter and 1 inch thick.

Make an indentation in center of each patty and place 1 tablespoon cheese in each. Cover cheese completely with meat and seal well.

Set oven control at broil or 550°F. Broil patties 3 inches from heat source, 3 to 4 minutes per side for rare, and 5 to 7 minutes per side for medium.

Yield: 6 servings

Nutrient analysis of 1 serving: 4 medium-fat meat exchanges; 298 Calories; 34 g protein; 17 g fat; 1 g carbohydrate; 772 mg sodium; 159 mg cholesterol.

*Hamburger Stroganoff

1 pound lean ground beef
½ cup chopped onion
2 tablespoons vegetable oil
1 teaspoon dry mustard
½ teaspoon salt
¼ teaspoon pepper
⅛ teaspoon paprika
2 tablespoons unprocessed bran
10½-ounce can condensed cream of mushroom soup
1 cup dairy sour cream
Hot cooked noodles or rice

Cook and stir ground beef and onion in oil in large skillet until meat is browned and onion is tender. Drain fat from pan.

Stir in seasonings, bran, and soup. Cook, stirring frequently, over medium heat for 15 to 20 minutes.

Stir in sour cream and heat through. Do not boil. Serve over noodles.

Yield: 4 servings (1 cup each of sauce only)

Nutrient analysis of 1 serving: 1 starch/bread exchange; 3 medium-fat meat exchanges; 2 fat exchanges; 389 Calories; 27 g protein; 26 g fat; 12 g carbohydrate; 942 mg sodium; 103 mg cholesterol.

Meat Cakes

1½ pounds lean ground beef
½ pound bulk Italian sausage
½ cup minced onion
1 teaspoon Italian seasoning
1 teaspoon salt
2 teaspoons Worcestershire sauce
½ teaspoon dried sage
1 cup unsweetened applesauce
½ cup whole wheat bread crumbs
½ cup unprocessed bran

Preheat oven to 350°F.

Mix all ingredients together well.

Place ⅓ cup (2 ounces) mixture in each of 16 muffin cups.

Bake at 350°F. until done, about 1 hour. Remove from muffin tins. Serve hot or cold.

Note: These cakes are nice for a picnic.

Yield: 16 meat cakes

Nutrient analysis of 1 meat cake: ½ starch/bread exchange; 2 lean meat exchanges; 150 Calories; 12 g protein; 8 g fat; 8 g carbohydrate; 360 mg sodium; 41 mg cholesterol.

Meat Loaf

1 pound lean ground beef
4 ounces smoked ham, cut into ¼-inch cubes
3 tablespoons snipped parsley
1 egg, beaten
¾ cup (2 ounces) quick-cooking oats
1 cup tomato juice

Mix all ingredients together thoroughly.

Press mixture evenly into greased loaf pan, 7¾ x 3⅝ x 2¼ inches.

Bake 1 hour at 350°F.

Let stand for 5 minutes before slicing.

Yield: 8 slices

Nutrient analysis of 1 slice: ½ starch/bread exchange; 2 medium-fat meat exchanges; 166 Calories; 16 g protein; 8 g fat; 6 g carbohydrate; 296 mg sodium; 82 mg cholesterol.

**Mock Lasagna*

8-ounce package lasagna noodles, broken into 1-inch pieces
1 pound lean ground beef
2 teaspoons salt
¼ teaspoon pepper
¼ teaspoon garlic salt
8-ounce can tomato sauce
8-ounce carton creamed cottage cheese
1 cup dairy sour cream
1 cup plain yogurt
6 ounces shredded processed cheese

Cook noodles as directed on package. Drain and set aside.

Preheat oven to 350°F.

Cook and stir ground beef, salt, pepper, and garlic salt in large skillet until meat is browned. Drain off fat.

Stir in tomato sauce and simmer for 5 minutes.

Stir in noodles, cottage cheese, sour cream, yogurt, and ½ cup shredded cheese.

Pour into 2-quart casserole. Sprinkle remaining cheese on top.

Bake at 350°F. for 35 to 40 minutes.

Yield: 8 servings (1 cup each)

Nutrient analysis of 1 serving: 2 starch/bread exchanges; 3 medium-fat meat exchanges; 329 Calories; 22 g protein; 14 g fat; 27 g carbohydrate; 836 mg sodium; 73 mg cholesterol.

**Cheeseburger Pie*

Pastry for 8-inch one-crust pie (page 210)
½ cup sesame seeds
1½ cups shredded Cheddar cheese (about 6 ounces)
2 tablespoons flour
1 pound lean ground beef
¼ cup evaporated skim milk
½ cup catsup
⅓ cup bread crumbs
¼ cup chopped onion
½ teaspoon salt
2 tablespoons steak sauce
½ teaspoon dried oregano
¼ teaspoon freshly ground pepper

Preheat oven to 350°F.

Prepare pastry as directed. However, before cutting in shortening, add sesame seeds to flour and salt.

Mix cheese and flour. Sprinkle ¼ of mixture in pastry-lined pie pan.

Break up ground beef in bowl with fork. Mix in remaining ingredients. Pour mixture into pie pan and spread evenly.

Bake at 350°F. for 35 to 40 minutes, or until brown. Sprinkle remaining cheese mixture on top and bake 10 minutes more.

Remove from oven and let stand 10 minutes before cutting and serving.

Yield: 8 servings

Nutrient analysis of 1 serving: 2 starch/bread exchanges; 3 medium-fat meat exchanges; 3 fat exchanges; 453 Calories; 23 g protein; 29 g fat; 27 g carbohydrate; 803 mg sodium; 64 mg cholesterol.

**Chili con Carne*

1 pound lean ground beef
28-ounce can whole tomatoes in thick tomato puree
2 medium onions, chopped (about 1 cup)
1 clove garlic, crushed
1 tablespoon chili powder
1 teaspoon salt
1 teaspoon dried oregano
1 teaspoon Worcestershire sauce
20-ounce can kidney beans, drained

Cook and stir meat in medium saucepan until browned. Drain fat from pan. Add remaining ingredients, breaking up tomatoes with fork.

Heat to boiling. Reduce heat, cover, and simmer, stirring occasionally, for 1 to 2 hours.

Yield: 8 servings (1 cup)

Nutrient analysis of 1 serving: 1 starch/bread exchange; 2 medium-fat meat exchanges; 228 Calories; 17 g protein; 10 g fat; 17 g carbohydrate; 655 mg sodium; 40 mg cholesterol.

*Sloppy Joes

½ pound lean ground beef
1 small onion, chopped
½ small green pepper, seeded and chopped
2 medium tomatoes, peeled and cut up
1 cup tomato juice
¼ teaspoon paprika
½ teaspoon salt
Freshly ground pepper
4 sandwich whole grain buns

Cook and stir meat, onion, and green pepper in large skillet until meat is brown. Drain excess fat.

Stir in tomatoes, tomato juice, paprika, and salt. Season with pepper. Heat to boiling. Reduce heat, cover, and simmer for 15 to 20 minutes, stirring occasionally.

Cut buns horizontally into halves and toast in broiler. Serve meat mixture on bun halves.

Yield: 4 sandwiches

Nutrient analysis of 1 sandwich: 2 starch/bread exchanges; 1½ medium-fat meat exchanges; 1 vegetable exchange; 311 Calories; 19 g protein; 9 g fat; 36 g carbohydrate; 802 mg sodium; 40 mg cholesterol.

Fruit Bobs

12 1-inch cubes lean beef sirloin tip
3 tablespoons thawed frozen orange juice concentrate
½ small cantaloupe, pared and cut into 12 cubes
1 apple, quartered, cored, and cut into 12 wedges
Salt and pepper to taste

Sprinkle beef cubes in bowl with 2 tablespoons of the orange concentrate. Cover and refrigerate at least 1 hour, turning cubes occasionally.

Sprinkle cantaloupe cubes and apple wedges with remaining orange juice concentrate and let stand for 5 minutes.

Alternate beef cubes, cantaloupe cubes, and apple wedges on each of 4 skewers. Season with salt and pepper to taste.

Set oven control at broil or 550°F. Broil skewers 4 inches from heat source, 2 to 3 minutes. Turn skewers and broil 2 to 3 minutes more, or until done as desired.

Note: Bobs can be cooked on grill.

Yield: 4 servings

Nutrient analysis of 1 serving: 3 medium-fat meat exchanges; 2 fruit exchanges; 1 fat exchange; 352 Calories; 20 g protein; 22 g fat; 18 g carbohydrate; 121 mg sodium; 57 mg cholesterol.

Shish Kebabs

3 ounces lean beef or lamb cubes
1 small onion, quartered
4 cherry tomatoes
4 mushroom caps
½ green pepper, seeded and cut into four 1-inch pieces
1 tablespoon catsup
½ cup white vinegar
Dash pepper

Alternate half the meat cubes, onion, tomatoes, mushrooms, and green pepper on each of 2 skewers. Mix remaining ingredients in small bowl and brush mixture on kebabs.

Set oven control at broil or 550°F. Broil kebabs 4 inches from heat source, turning once, until done as desired.

Note: Kebabs can be grilled.

Yield: 1 serving

Nutrient analysis of 1 serving: 2½ lean meat exchanges; 3 vegetable exchanges; ½ fruit exchange; 235 Calories; 24 g protein; 5 g fat; 23 g carbohydrate; 261 mg sodium; 57 mg cholesterol.

Homestyle Pot Roast

1 tablespoon flour
½ teaspoon salt
½ teaspoon allspice
¼ teaspoon pepper
1 tablespoon plus 1 teaspoon vegetable oil
3 pounds lean beef chuck pot roast
2 cups water
2 small onions
2 cloves garlic, crushed

Mix flour, salt, allspice, and pepper. Rub mixture on meat.

Heat oil in large skillet or Dutch oven. Brown meat in oil over medium heat, about 15 minutes.

Reduce heat and add water, onions, and garlic. Cover and simmer for about 3 hours, or until meat is tender.

Note: Pared potatoes can be added during last hour of cooking. (Be sure to add the exchanges and calories for the potatoes.)

Yield: 12 servings (3 ounces)

Nutrient analysis of 1 serving: 3 medium-fat meat exchanges; 1 fat exchange; 297 Calories; 22 g protein; 22 g fat; 2 g carbohydrate; 121 mg sodium; 79 mg cholesterol.

Swiss Steak

- 3 tablespoons flour
- 1 teaspoon salt
- 1/4 teaspoon pepper
- 2 pounds beef round steak (1 inch thick)
- 2 tablespoons margarine
- 8-ounce can tomato puree
- 2 medium onions, sliced thin
- 1/2 cup chopped celery
- 1 clove garlic, crushed
- 1 tablespoon Worcestershire sauce

Mix flour, salt, and pepper. Sprinkle one side of meat with half the flour mixture and pound it with meat mallet or rim of heavy saucer. Turn meat and pound in remaining flour mixture. Cut meat into 8 serving-size pieces.

Melt margarine in large skillet. Brown meat on both sides over medium heat, about 15 minutes.

Add remaining ingredients and heat to boiling. Reduce heat, cover, and simmer about 2 hours, or until meat is tender.

Variation: Pared and quartered potatoes and carrot sticks can be added during the last 45 minutes of cooking. This makes a complete meal. (Be sure to add the exchanges and calories for the potatoes and carrots.)

Yield: 8 servings

Nutrient analysis of 1 serving: 1 starch/bread exchange; 3 medium-fat meat exchanges; 2 vegetable exchanges; 1 fat exchange; 395 Calories; 29 g protein; 19 g fat; 27 g carbohydrate; 374 mg sodium; 77 mg cholesterol.

Beef Cubes à l'Orange

1 pound lean beef cubes
½ cup Basic Marinade (page 196)
1 orange, sliced; each slice halved
Snipped parsley

Place beef cubes in glass baking dish; pour on marinade. Refrigerate 1 hour, turning cubes occasionally.

Drain beef cubes well. Place cubes and orange slices in broiler tray.

Set oven control at broil or 550°F. Broil 3 inches from heat source, turning occasionally, until browned and done as desired, 10 to 12 minutes.

Remove meat and orange slices to heated platter. Garnish with parsley.

Yield: 4 servings (3 ounces each)

Nutrient analysis of 1 serving: 3 medium-fat meat exchanges; 1½ fat exchanges; 299 Calories; 24 g protein; 22 g fat; 3 g carbohydrate; 51 mg sodium; 79 mg cholesterol.

**Lamb Patties*

4 slices lean bacon
4 lamb patties (4 ounces each)
½ cup steak sauce
2 to 3 teaspoons ground thyme
Freshly ground pepper

Wrap slice of bacon around edge of each patty and secure ends by pressing together.

Place patties in shallow baking dish. Top each with 1 tablespoon steak sauce and 1 teaspoon thyme and season with pepper.

Turn patties and repeat topping. Cover and refrigerate for at least 1 hour.

Set oven control at broil or 550°F. Broil patties on rack 3 inches from heat source for about 10 minutes per side, or until done as desired.

Yield: 4 servings

Nutrient analysis of 1 serving: 3 medium-fat meat exchanges; 1 fat exchange; 220 Calories; 23 g protein; 15 g fat; 1 g carbohydrate; 620 mg sodium; 90 mg cholesterol.

Veal Roll-Ups

6 boneless veal cutlets (about 3 ounces each)
6 thin slices part-skim-milk mozzarella cheese (½ ounce each)
6 thin slices cooked or boiled ham (½ ounce each)
2 tablespoons skim milk
1 egg
½ cup whole wheat flour
¼ cup wheat germ
¼ cup bread crumbs

Have butcher pound cutlets to ¼ inch thickness, or place them between pieces of waxed paper and flatten cutlets with wooden mallet or heavy saucer. (Have adult help with this.)

Place a slice cheese and ham on each piece of meat. Roll up carefully, beginning at narrow end. Secure the rolls with wooden picks.

Beat milk and egg in a flat bowl until blended. Measure flour into small pie pan. Stir wheat germ and bread crumbs together in another small pan or flat bowl. Coat rolls with flour, then dip into egg mixture and coat with wheat germ mixture. Place in greased baking dish, 9 x 9 x 2 inches. Cover with plastic wrap and refrigerate 1 hour.

Preheat oven to 350°F. Bake rolls for 35 minutes, or until tender and light brown. If desired, garnish with parsley.

Variation: To make Chicken Roll-Ups, substitute 2 or 3 chicken boneless, split breasts for the veal cutlets.

Yield: 6 servings

Nutrient analysis of 1 serving: 1 starch/bread exchange; 4 medium-fat meat exchanges; 385 Calories; 32 g protein; 19 g fat; 16 g carbohydrate; 374 mg sodium; 100 mg cholesterol.

**Baked Ham*

3- to 4-pound fully cooked, boneless ham
Whole cloves
2 tablespoons prepared mustard

Score top of ham lightly, cutting diamond shapes. Insert clove in each section.

Heat ham as directed on label.

Spread mustard on ham 30 minutes before ham is done.

Yield: 12 to 16 servings

Nutrient analysis of 1 serving (3 ounces): 3 medium-fat meat exchanges; ½ fat exchange; 248 Calories; 18 g protein; 19 g fat; 0 g carbohydrate; 656 mg sodium; 76 mg cholesterol.

**Chinese Pork Chops*

1 egg
3 tablespoons soy sauce
1 tablespoon water or dry sherry
¼ teaspoon dried ginger
½ teaspoon garlic powder
¼ cup plus 2 tablespoons bread crumbs
3 tablespoons wheat germ
6 lean pork loin chops (3 to 4 ounces each)

Beat egg, soy sauce, water, ginger, and garlic powder with a fork in a flat bowl or pie pan.

Mix bread crumbs and wheat germ in another pie pan.

Dip pork chops into egg mixture, then in bread crumb mixture, coating both sides. Place chops on greased jelly roll pan, 15 x 10 x 1 inches.

Bake in a 350°F. oven for 30 minutes. Turn chops carefully with wide spatula and bake 20 minutes more, or until tender.

Yield: 6 servings

Nutrient analysis of 1 serving: ½ starch/bread exchange; 3 medium-fat meat exchanges; 280 Calories; 29 g protein; 14 g fat; 8 g carbohydrate; 799 mg sodium; 118 mg cholesterol.

Italian Baked Chicken

½ cup bread crumbs
2 tablespoons Italian herb seasoning
¼ teaspoon salt
¼ teaspoon pepper
¼ teaspoon paprika
¼ cup grated Parmesan cheese
¼ cup skim milk
2½-pound broiler-fryer, cut up

Heat oven to 375°F. Grease baking dish, 11¾ x 7½ x 1¾ inches.

Measure bread crumbs, Italian seasoning, salt, pepper, paprika, and cheese into a plastic bag. Hold open end closed and shake to mix ingredients.

Measure milk into small flat bowl. Dip chicken pieces, 1 or 2 at a time, into milk, then place in plastic bag and shake until completely coated.

Place chicken in prepared baking dish, skin side up.

Bake at 375°F. until tender, 40 to 45 minutes. To serve cold, cool and refrigerate covered.

Yield: 6 servings

Nutrient analysis of 1 serving: ½ starch/bread exchange; 4 lean meat exchanges; 256 Calories; 29 g protein; 12 g fat; 7 g carbohydrate; 328 mg sodium; 128 mg cholesterol.

Summer Garden Chicken

- 1 teaspoon vegetable oil
- 3-ounce piece chicken (leg, thigh, breast)
- 1 small potato, pared and quartered
- 1 small tomato
- 1 small onion
- 2 fresh mushrooms
- 2 slices green pepper
- 2 tablespoons uncooked instant rice
- 1 tablespoon lemon juice
- ⅛ teaspoon paprika
- ⅛ teaspoon dry mustard
- ¼ teaspoon salt
- Dash freshly ground pepper

Preheat oven to 450°F.

Heat oil in small skillet. Brown chicken in oil over medium-high heat.

Put chicken on 8- or 9-inch square piece of double-thickness aluminum foil. Arrange vegetables on and around chicken. Sprinkle rice on top. Mix remaining ingredients and drizzle onto chicken and vegetables. Fold foil over and seal securely. Place package in shallow baking pan.

Bake, turning every 20 minutes, for 1 hour and 15 minutes, or until chicken and vegetables are tender.

Note: Chicken can be cooked on the grill.

Yield: 1 serving

Nutrient analysis of 1 serving: 2 starch/bread exchanges; 3 lean meat exchanges; ½ vegetable exchange; 351 Calories; 29 g protein; 11 g fat; 32 g carbohydrate; 560 mg sodium; 71 mg cholesterol.

Easy Grilled Chicken

- Four 3-ounce pieces chicken (leg, thigh, breast)
- ¼ cup chopped onion
- 4 teaspoons snipped parsley
- 4 teaspoons dried rosemary
- ½ teaspoon freshly ground pepper
- ½ teaspoon salt

Place each chicken piece on a 6-inch square of heavy-duty aluminum foil. Sprinkle each with 1 tablespoon onion, 1 teaspoon parsley, 1 teaspoon rosemary, ⅛ teaspoon pepper, and ⅛ teaspoon salt.

Fold foil over and seal each package securely.

Cook on grill, turning once, until chicken is tender, about 30 minutes.

Yield: 4 servings

Nutrient analysis of 1 serving: 2½ lean meat exchanges; 124 Calories; 19 g protein; 5 g fat; 0 g carbohydrate; 287 mg sodium; 53 mg cholesterol.

Turkey

Here are some tips if you buy a frozen turkey:

Refrigerator thawing: Leave original wrap on frozen turkey; place turkey on a tray. Refrigerate for 3 to 4 days, about 24 hours for each 5 pounds.

Cold-water thawing: Place frozen turkey in its original wrap in a sink filled with cold water. Change the water every 30 minutes. Allow about 1 hour of thawing time for each 2 pounds of turkey.

After thawing, remove the wrap, free the legs and tail, and then remove the giblets and neck piece from the cavity. Never defrost a frozen turkey by leaving out at room temperature until thawed.

Roast Turkey

Wash turkey and pat dry. If stuffing turkey, stuff just before roasting, not ahead of time. Fill wishbone area with stuffing first. Fasten neck skin to back with skewers. Fold wings across back with tips touching. Fill body cavity lightly. Do not pack, because stuffing expands while cooking. Tie drumsticks together with heavy string; then tie to tail or tuck drumsticks under band of skin of tail.

Preheat oven to 325°F. Place turkey on rack, breast side up, in open shallow roasting pan. Brush with oil, shortening, or margarine. Insert meat thermometer so tip is in thickest part of inside thigh muscle or thickest part of breast meat. Make sure it does not touch bone. Do not add water to pan and do not cover. Follow table for cooking time (see page 263). Meat thermometer will register 185°F. when turkey is done. If you do not use a thermometer, test for doneness about 30 minutes before timetable indicates: move a drumstick up and down—if done, the joint should move readily or break; or press drumstick meat between fingers; the meat should be very soft.

After serving the turkey, remove all stuffing from it. Cool stuffing, meat, and gravy and refrigerate separately. Use gravy and stuffing within 1 or 2 days; heat thoroughly before serving. Serve cooked turkey meat within 2 or 3 days after roasting. If frozen, it can be kept up to 1 month.

Foil-Wrapped Turkey

Prepare the turkey as directed for roast turkey. Place turkey, breast side up, in middle of large sheet of heavy-duty aluminum foil. (If turkey is large, use two widths of foil.)

Brush turkey with shortening, oil, or margarine. Place small pieces of aluminum foil over the ends of legs, tail, and wing tips to prevent puncturing. Bring long ends of foil up over breast of turkey and overlap 3 inches. Close open ends by folding foil so drippings will not run into pan. Wrap loosely; do not seal airtight.

Preheat oven to 450°F. Place foil-wrapped turkey, breast side up, in open shallow roasting pan. Follow timetable for approximate time. Open foil once or twice during cooking to judge doneness. When thigh joint and breast meat begin to soften, fold back foil completely to brown turkey and crisp skin. Insert meat thermometer at this time.

Timetable for Roast Turkey

Type of turkey	Ready-to-cook weight, pounds	Approximate cooking time, hours	Internal temperature, °F.
Stuffed	6–8	3–3½	
whole	8–12	3½–4½	
turkey	12–16	4–5	185
	16–20	4½–5½	
	20–24	5–6½	
Foil-	8–10	1¼–1¾	
wrapped	10–12	1¾–2¼	
turkey	12–16	2¼–3	185
(unstuffed)	16–20	3–3½	
	20–24	3½–4½	
Boneless	2½–4½	1¾–2½	
turkey	4½–6½	2½–3¼	170
	6½–7½	3¼–4	

Yield: if turkey weighs 12 pounds or less, allow ¾ to 1 pound per serving; if turkey weighs over 12 pounds, allow ½ to ¾ pound per serving.

Nutrient analysis of 1 serving (3 ounces): 3 lean meat exchanges; 165 Calories; 21 g protein; 9 g fat; 0 g carbohydrate; 70 mg sodium; 74 mg cholesterol.

*Dressing

8 cups dry bread cubes
1 cup diced celery
½ cup minced onion
2 teaspoons poultry seasoning
1 teaspoon dried thyme
1 teaspoon salt
½ cup margarine
½ cup chicken stock or water

Measure bread cubes, celery, onion, poultry seasoning, thyme, and salt into large bowl.

Heat margarine and stock to boiling. Pour onto bread cube mixture and mix lightly. Stuff turkey just before roasting.

Variations:

Corn Bread Stuffing: Substitute corn bread cubes for the bread cubes.

Meat Stuffing: Add 1 pound lean ground beef or bulk pork sausage, crumbled and browned, to bread cube mixture. If using pork sausage, drain fat from browned meat (½ cup adds 1 medium-fat meat exchange).

Fruit Stuffing: Decrease bread cubes to 7 cups and add 2 cups finely chopped pared and cored apple and ½ cup raisins to bread cube mixture (½ cup adds 1 fruit exchange).

Yield: about 8 cups (enough for 10-pound turkey or two 4- to 6-pound chickens)

Nutrient analysis of ½ cup: 2½ starch/bread exchanges; 1½ fat exchanges; 253 Calories; 7 g protein; 8 g fat; 37 g carbohydrate; 591 mg sodium; 3 mg cholesterol.

Boneless Turkey Roasts

Follow package directions.

If directions are not available, remove outer wrap from turkey roast. Do not remove the inside netting. If roast is not seasoned, rub surface lightly with salt and pepper. Follow directions for roast turkey. Baste or brush roast with margarine or pan drippings during roasting. Continue roasting until meat thermometer inserted in center of roast registers 170°F. Remove netting before slicing meat.

Carving Turkey or Chicken

Place legs to carver's right. Gently pull leg away from body and cut through joint between leg and body. Remove leg. Cut between drumstick and thigh; slice off meat. Make deep horizontal cut into breast just above wing. Insert fork in top of breast, then start halfway up breast and cut thin slices down to the cut.

William's Mother's Chicken

2½- to 3-pound broiler-fryer, cut up
½ cup margarine (1 stick)
1 teaspoon dried oregano
2 cloves garlic, crushed
Juice of 1 lemon (3 tablespoons)
Salt and freshly ground pepper to taste

Arrange chicken pieces skin side down in shallow baking pan, 11 x 7 x 1½ inches.

Melt margarine in small saucepan over low heat. Stir in oregano, garlic, and lemon juice. Stir over low heat for 3 minutes. Remove from heat and brush on chicken in pan.

Bake chicken, skin side down, in 325°F. oven for 15 minutes. Turn and bake 20 minutes longer. Baste chicken with lemon-margarine mixture every 10 minutes.

Set oven control at broil or 550°F. Broil chicken 6 inches from heat source until crisp and brown, 5 to 10 minutes. Season with salt and pepper.

Note: To grill, cook chicken pieces on hot grill for 15 minutes. Season with salt and pepper. Cook until tender and crisp, 20 to 30 minutes, basting frequently with lemon-margarine mixture and turning often.

Yield: 6 servings

Nutrient analysis of 1 serving: 4 lean meat exchanges; 1 fat exchange; 283 Calories; 30 g protein; 17 g fat; 0 g carbohydrate; 202 mg sodium; 112 mg cholesterol.

Citrus Chicken

¼ cup all-purpose flour
½ teaspoon salt
Dash freshly ground pepper
¼ cup margarine
2 tablespoons vegetable oil
2½- to 3-pound broiler-fryer, cut up
½ cup white vermouth or other white wine
2 oranges, peeled, pitted, and sectioned (reserve juice)
1 grapefruit, peeled, pitted, and sectioned (reserve juice)
1 green pepper, seeded and cut into thin slices

Mix flour, salt, and pepper.

Heat margarine and oil in large skillet.

Coat chicken with flour mixture. Brown chicken in skillet.

Pour in wine and reserved juices. Reduce heat and simmer uncovered, turning occasionally, until chicken is tender, about 40 minutes.

Add fruit sections and green pepper. Simmer until fruit is heated through, 3 to 5 minutes. If desired, serve with Curried Rice (page 188) or Yellow Rice Pilaf (page 115).

Yield: 6 servings

Nutrient analysis of 1 serving: 3½ medium-fat meat exchanges; 1 fruit exchange; 325 Calories; 26 g protein; 19 g fat; 14 g carbohydrate; 329 mg sodium; 75 mg cholesterol.

**Fish Sticks*

1 pound flounder fillets
1 egg
2 tablespoons water
½ cup all-purpose flour
¾ cup Italian bread crumbs
½ cup vegetable oil
Relish Sauce (page 267)

Cut fish into sticks, about 2 x 1 inches.

Beat egg and water with fork until blended. Coat fish sticks with flour. Dip into egg mixture, then coat with bread crumbs.

Heat oil in large skillet. Fry sticks in hot oil until golden brown on both sides. Remove to warm platter and serve with Relish Sauce (below).

Yield: 4 servings

Nutrient analysis of 1 serving fish sticks (sauce counted separately): 2 starch/bread exchanges; 4 lean meat exchanges; 2 fat exchanges; 450 Calories; 32 g protein; 23 g fat; 28 g carbohydrate; 852 mg sodium; 142 mg cholesterol.

Relish Sauce

¼ cup pickle relish
¼ cup low-calorie mayonnaise

Combine relish and mayonnaise and mix thoroughly.

Yield: ½ cup

Nutrient analysis of 1 tablespoon: ½ fat exchange; 31 Calories; 0 g protein; 3 g fat; 2 g carbohydrate; 155 mg sodium; 2 mg cholesterol.

**Flamboyant Flounder*

1 pound flounder fillets or other fish fillets
1 tablespoon grated onion
½ teaspoon salt
⅛ teaspoon pepper
1 medium tomato, peeled and chopped
1 medium green pepper, seeded and diced
1 tablespoon plus 1½ teaspoons margarine, melted
⅓ cup shredded Swiss cheese

Thaw fish if frozen. Remove any skin from fillets.

Grease a heatproof serving platter. Arrange fillets in a single layer on platter. Sprinkle with onion, salt, and pepper. Cover fillets with tomato and green pepper, then pour margarine over top.

Set oven control at broil or 550°F. Broil fillets about 4 inches from heat source until fish flakes easily with fork, 10 to 12 minutes.

Remove from heat and sprinkle cheese on top.

Return to broiler. Broil until cheese is melted, 2 to 3 minutes.

Yield: 4 servings

Nutrient analysis of 1 serving: 4 lean meat exchanges; 227 Calories; 29 g protein; 11 g fat; 2 g carbohydrate; 489 mg sodium; 83 mg cholesterol.

*Fish in Foil

1 pound fish fillets†
4 carrots, sliced
1 tablespoon chopped onion
2 stalks celery, cut into ½-inch pieces
1 lemon, cut into 8 slices
½ cup margarine
2 teaspoons dried chervil (optional)
Salt and freshly ground pepper to taste

Preheat oven to 400°F.

Cut fish into 4 pieces. Place fish in center of sheet of heavy-duty aluminum foil, 18 x 13 inches.

Cover fish with carrot slices, onion, celery, and lemon slices. Dot with margarine. Season with chervil, salt, and pepper. (If using fresh fish, sprinkle with 2 tablespoons water.)

Fold sides and ends of foil tightly around fish. Seal securely by pinching edges of foil together. Place on baking sheet.

Bake at 400°F. until fish flakes easily with fork, about 20 minutes.

Note: Package of fish and vegetables can be sealed with freezer tape and frozen. Remove tape before baking. Do not defrost. Place in oven at 400°F. and bake 30 minutes instead of 20.

Yield: 4 servings

Nutrient analysis of 1 serving: 3 medium-fat meat exchanges; 1 vegetable exchange; 254 Calories; 27 g protein; 12 g fat; 5 g carbohydrate; 463 mg sodium; 76 mg cholesterol.

†If frozen fish is used, *do not allow to thaw.* Place frozen fish on aluminum foil, quickly assemble remaining ingredients, and place in freezer immediately.

PASTA

Pasta Merry-Go-Round

Prepare several toppings:

Tomato Sauce (page 130)
Spaghetti Sauce (page 270)
Shredded part-skim-milk mozzarella cheese
Grated Parmesan cheese
Shredded zucchini
Shredded carrot
Cottage cheese
Raisins
Chopped nuts
Snipped parsley
Chopped apple

Cook 3 kinds of pasta (choose from shells, spinach linguine, macaroni, thin spaghetti, whole wheat pasta) as directed on packages. Plan ½ to 1 cup cooked pasta per serving.

Turn pastas onto hot large platter and surround platter with bowls of toppings. Guests choose pastas and toppings they desire.

Nutrient analysis of ½ cup plain pasta†: 1 starch/bread exchange; 70 Calories; 2 g protein; 0 g fat; 15 g carbohydrate; 1 mg sodium, 0 mg cholesterol.

†Check recipes for exchange and nutrient content of toppings.

Spaghetti Sauce

1 pound lean ground beef
2 medium onions, finely chopped
1 green pepper, seeded and finely chopped
3 cloves garlic, minced
28-ounce can whole tomatoes
6-ounce can tomato paste
2 8-ounce cans tomato sauce
2 tablespoons dried oregano
2 tablespoons Worcestershire sauce
Salt and pepper to taste

Cook and stir meat, onion, green pepper, and garlic in large saucepan until meat is browned and onion is tender.

Stir in whole tomatoes (with liquid), tomato paste, tomato sauce, oregano, and Worcestershire sauce. Heat to boiling, stirring occasionally. Reduce heat and simmer for 2 to 3 hours, stirring occasionally.

Skim any fat from sauce; season with salt and pepper. Serve on hot pasta or freeze for later use.

Yield: 8 cups

Nutrient analysis of ½ cup: 1 lean meat exchange; 2 vegetable exchanges; 91 Calories; 8 g protein; 3 g fat; 10 g carbohydrate; 119 mg sodium; 20 mg cholesterol.

**Manicotti*

15-ounce carton part-skim-milk ricotta cheese (Italian pot cheese)
¼ pound part-skim-milk mozzarella cheese, shredded
2 eggs
½ cup grated Parmesan cheese
1 tablespoon Italian herb seasoning
2 tablespoons wheat germ
¼ teaspoon dry mustard
¼ teaspoon salt
Dash freshly ground pepper
10 manicotti shells (90 size)
2 cups Spaghetti Sauce (see above)
¼ cup grated Parmesan cheese (additional)

Mix ricotta cheese, mozzarella cheese, eggs, ½ cup Parmesan cheese, Italian seasoning, wheat germ, mustard, salt, and pepper in bowl. Set aside.

Heat about 6 inches of water to boiling in a large kettle. Add manicotti shells, a few at a time, to boiling water. Stir carefully and heat to boiling. Cook for 6 minutes. (Do not overcook.) Have an adult help you remove kettle from range and pour off ¾ of the hot water. Add cold water to cool manicotti, then drain.

Fill manicotti with cheese mixture. Place in a single layer in a baking dish, 11¾ x 7½ x 1¾ inches.

Pour spaghetti sauce over manicotti. Cover tightly with aluminum foil.

Bake in a 350°F. oven for 30 minutes. Remove foil and sprinkle ¼ cup Parmesan cheese on top. Bake 10 minutes more.

Yield: 5 servings

Nutrient analysis of 1 serving (2 tubes): 2½ starch/bread exchanges; 4 medium-fat meat exchanges; 1 vegetable exchange; 500 Calories; 38 g protein; 21 g fat; 40 g carbohydrate: 652 mg sodium; 176 mg cholesterol.

**Baked Lasagna*

8-ounce package lasagna noodles
4 cups Spaghetti Sauce (page 270)
2 pounds part-skim-milk ricotta cheese (Italian pot cheese)
½ pound part-skim-milk mozzarella cheese, shredded
3 tablespoons grated Parmesan cheese

Cook lasagna noodles as directed on package. With an adult helping, drain noodles into large colander; then run cold water on them.

Preheat oven to 375°F.

Reserve about ½ cup of the spaghetti sauce for thin top layer. Spread several tablespoons of remaining spaghetti sauce over the bottom of a baking dish, 11¾ x 7½ x 1¾ inches.

Layer ⅓ each of the noodles, remaining spaghetti sauce, and ricotta and mozzarella cheeses in baking dish. Repeat 2 more times.

Spread reserved spaghetti sauce over all and sprinkle with Parmesan cheese. Cover tightly with aluminum foil.

Bake at 375°F. for 20 minutes. Remove foil and bake 5 minutes longer.

Yield: 8 servings

Nutrient analysis of 1 serving: 2½ starch/bread exchanges; 3½ medium-fat meat exchanges; 1 vegetable exchange; 475 Calories; 24 g protein; 19 g fat; 43 g carbohydrate; 444 mg sodium; 71 mg cholesterol.

Chris's Macaroni and Cheese

1½ cups uncooked macaroni
2 cups cubed processed American cheese
2 tablespoons minced onion
½ teaspoon salt
1¼ cups hot skim milk

Combine macaroni, cheese, onion, and salt in ungreased 1½-quart casserole. Stir in hot milk. Cover tightly. Bake in 350°F. oven until macaroni is tender, about 40 minutes.

Yield: 4 servings (1 cup each)

Nutrient analysis of 1 serving: 2½ starch/bread exchanges; 2 medium-fat meat exchanges; 1 fat exchange; 368 Calories; 20 g protein; 16 g fat; 36 g carbohydrate; 908 mg sodium; 53 mg cholesterol.

Ham and Macaroni Bake

8-ounce package elbow macaroni
¼ cup margarine
¼ cup all-purpose flour
2 tablespoons prepared mustard
¼ teaspoon salt
Dash pepper
2 cups skim milk
2 cups cubed cooked ham
2 medium apples, pared, cored and sliced thin (2 cups)
1 cup soft bread crumbs
2 tablespoons margarine, melted

Cook macaroni as directed on package. Drain and set aside.

Melt ¼ cup margarine in a large saucepan. Stir in flour, mustard, salt, and pepper. Cook and stir over low heat until mixture is smooth and bubbly. Remove from heat. Stir in milk. Heat to boiling, stirring constantly. Boil and stir for 1 minute.

Stir macaroni, ham, and apples into sauce. Pour into a 2-quart casserole.

Mix bread crumbs and melted margarine; sprinkle on casserole.

Bake in 350°F. oven for 30 to 35 minutes, until hot and bubbly.

Yield: 8 servings

Nutrient analysis of 1 serving: 2 starch/bread exchanges; 2 medium-fat meat exchanges; 2 fat exchanges; 382 Calories; 16 g protein; 20 g fat; 35 g carbohydrate; 620 mg sodium; 38 mg cholesterol.

BEVERAGES, SNACKS, AND SANDWICHES

Strawberry Milk Smoothee

1 cup skim milk
¾ cup sliced strawberries
1 teaspoon vanilla
1 teaspoon lemon juice
Nutmeg (optional)

Measure all ingredients into blender container. Cover and blend at high speed until smooth.

Pour into glasses and, if desired, sprinkle with nutmeg.

Yield: 2 servings

Nutrient analysis of 1 serving: ½ skim milk exchange; ½ fruit exchange; 60 Calories; 4 g protein; 0 g fat; 10 g carbohydrate; 60 mg sodium; 4 mg cholesterol.

Blender Banana

1 cup skim milk
1 teaspoon vanilla
1 small banana, peeled and cut up

Place all ingredients in blender container. Cover and blend at high speed until smooth, about 10 seconds.

Pour into 2 glasses or dessert dishes. Serve immediately or freeze for dessert.

Yield: 2 servings

Nutrient analysis of 1 serving: ½ skim milk exchange; 1 fruit exchange; 87 Calories; 5 g protein; 0 g fat; 18 g carbohydrate; 65 mg sodium; 5 mg cholesterol.

Peach Cooler

¾ cup skim milk
½ cup canned sugar-free sliced peaches
⅛ teaspoon vanilla
½ cup vanilla ice cream, slightly softened

Measure milk, peaches, and vanilla into blender container. Cover and blend until smooth. Add ice cream and blend for 3 to 5 seconds.

Pour into glasses and serve immediately.

Yield: 2 servings

Nutrient analysis of 1 serving: ½ starch/bread exchange; ½ whole milk exchange; 109 Calories; 4 g protein; 4 g fat; 16 g carbohydrate; 67 mg sodium; 11 mg cholesterol.

Pink Lassies

1 cup diet cranberry juice
¼ cup orange juice
1 cup vanilla ice cream, slightly softened

Measure all ingredients into blender container. Cover and blend until smooth.

Pour into glasses and serve with straws.

Yield: 2 servings

Nutrient analysis of 1 serving: 1 starch/bread exchange; ½ fruit exchange; ½ fat exchange; 150 Calories; 2 g protein; 7 g fat; 19 g carbohydrate; 41 mg sodium; 22 mg cholesterol.

Peanut Munch

1 cup roasted peanuts
1 cup sunflower seeds
1 cup raisins

Combine all ingredients and enjoy.

Yield: 3 cups

Nutrient analysis of ½ cup: 2 high-fat meat exchanges; 3 fruit exchanges; 3 fat exchanges; 438 Calories; 16 g protein; 29 g fat; 31 g carbohydrates; 297 mg sodium; 0 mg cholesterol.

Popcorn

3 tablespoons vegetable oil
½ cup popping corn

Pour vegetable oil into 4-quart popcorn popper.† Sprinkle ½ cup popping corn kernels onto oil. Place cover on popper and place handles in grooves. Plug in popper and let corn pop.

Note: If you do not have a self-buttering popper, place oil in large heavy saucepan. Add popping corn, cover and shake over medium heat until all kernels are popped.

Yield: 16 cups

Nutrient analysis of 1 cup: ⅓ starch/bread exchange; 1 fat exchange; 57 Calories; 1 g protein; 4 g fat; 5 g carbohydrate; 0 mg sodium; 0 mg cholesterol.

†You can eliminate the fat exchange by using an air-type popper.

*Corn Squares

1 cup all-purpose flour
1 cup yellow cornmeal
2 tablespoons unprocessed bran
1 tablespoon plus 1 teaspoon baking powder
1 teaspoon salt
1 cup skim milk
3 eggs
⅓ cup margarine, melted
¾ cup minced cooked ham
¾ cup shredded Cheddar cheese
2 tablespoons snipped parsley
¼ cup minced green pepper (optional)

Preheat oven to 400°F. Grease a 9-inch-square baking pan.

Mix flour, cornmeal, bran, baking powder, salt, milk, eggs, and margarine. Beat 1 minute.

Stir in ham, cheese, parsley, and green pepper. Pour into prepared pan. Bake at 400°F. until golden brown and wooden pick inserted in center comes out clean, 30 to 35 minutes.

Cool on rack for 10 minutes. Run knife around edges to loosen. Invert onto board and cut into 9 squares.

Yield: 9 servings

Nutrient analysis of 1 serving: 1½ starch/bread exchanges; 1 medium-fat meat exchange; 1 fat exchange; 242 Calories; 11 g protein; 11 g fat; 25 g carbohydrate; 630 mg sodium; 110 mg cholesterol.

Ever-Ready Snack

15-ounce box golden raisins
15-ounce box raisins
10-ounce box currants
7½-ounce jar sunflower seeds
16-ounce jar dry-roasted peanuts

Mix all ingredients in a large bowl.

Store at room temperature in airtight container. Will keep for 1 to 2 weeks.

Yield: 16 servings (4 ounces each)

Nutrient analysis of 1 serving: 2 medium-fat meat exchanges; 1 fat exchange; 2 fruit exchanges; 325 Calories; 15 g protein; 15 g fat: 33 g carbohydrate; 220 mg sodium; 0 mg cholesterol.

Nuts and Bolts Snack Bag

1 cup nonsugar-coated ready-to-eat cereal in shapes (Cheerios, Kix, Bran Chex, wheat squares)
1 cup peanuts
1 cup raisins
½ cup sunflower seeds
½ cup dried currants

Measure ingredients into bowl and stir.

Place ½ cup mix into each of 8 small plastic bags and seal.

Note: These snack bags are nice to take on a hike or for snacking while studying.

Yield: 8 servings

Nutrient analysis of 1 serving: 1 starch/bread exchange; 1½ high-fat meat exchanges; ¾ fruit exchange; 2 fat exchanges; 342 Calories; 12 g protein; 22 g fat, 26 g carbohydrate; 259 mg sodium; 0 mg cholesterol.

*Delicatessen Pickles

- **2 tablespoons mustard seed**
- **2 tablespoons whole allspice**
- **2 tablespoons black peppercorns**
- **2 tablespoons whole cloves**
- **2 tablespoons dill seed**
- **2 tablespoons coriander seed**
- **2 tablespoons whole mace**
- **2 bay leaves**
- **4 quarts water**
- **½ cup coarse salt**
- **8 unwaxed cucumbers (each about 5 inches long)**

Measure spices into jar. Cover and shake until mixed.

Heat water, salt, and 1 tablespoon plus 2 teaspoons spice mixture to boiling. Cover and boil for 10 minutes. Remove from heat and cool.

Place cucumbers in a 2-gallon crock or large bowl. Pour remaining spice mixture and the spiced salt water over cucumbers. (Liquid should reach 2 inches above cucumbers.) Place plate on top of crock and weight it down. Allow cucumbers to marinate 4 days at room temperature before refrigerating.

Yield: 8 pickles

Nutrient analysis of 1 pickle: free exchange (over 700 mg sodium).

*Hero Sandwich

- **6-inch piece French bread**
- **2 tablespoons low-calorie mayonnaise**
- **¼ teaspoon prepared white horseradish**
- **1 slice cooked lean roast beef**
- **1 slice boiled ham**
- **1 slice salami**
- **2 slices Swiss cheese or low-fat cheese**
- **4 thin slices onion**
- **4 thin slices tomato**
- **½ cup shredded lettuce**

Cut bread in half lengthwise. Mix mayonnaise and horseradish; spread on both sides of bread. Layer meats, cheese, onion slices, tomato slices, and lettuce on one slice of bread. Top with remaining bread slice; secure with wooden picks and cut across into halves.

Yield: 2 servings

Nutrient analysis of 1 serving: 3 starch/bread exchanges; 3 medium-fat meat exchanges; 425 Calories; 23 g protein; 18 g fat; 43 g carbohydrate; 818 mg sodium; 59 mg cholesterol.

Andrew's Deluxe Peanut Butter

¾ cup coarsely shredded carrot
¾ cup chunky peanut butter
2 tablespoons mayonnaise
¼ cup sunflower seeds
½ cup raisins

Measure all ingredients into bowl. Mix thoroughly. Store in covered container in refrigerator.

Yield: 2⅓ cups

Nutrient analysis of 2 tablespoons: ½ high-fat meat exchange; 1 fat exchange; ½ fruit exchange; 119 Calories; 4 g protein; 9 g fat; 6 g carbohydrate; 57 mg sodium; 1 mg cholesterol.

Tuna Salad Sandwiches

6½- or 7-ounce can tuna in water, drained
¼ cup chopped celery
⅓ cup finely chopped onion
¼ cup low-fat mayonnaise
Freshly ground pepper
6 slices bread

Empty tuna into bowl and flake with fork. Add celery, onion, and mayonnaise and season with dash of freshly ground pepper. Mix lightly with fork until ingredients are coated.

Spread ½ cup tuna mixture on each of 3 slices of bread. Top each with another bread slice.

Yield: 3 sandwiches

Nutrient analysis of 1 sandwich: 1½ starch/bread exchanges; 2 lean meat exchanges; 185 Calories; 14 g protein; 5 g fat; 23 g carbohydrate; 277 mg sodium; 24 mg cholesterol.

DESSERTS

Frozen Fruit Pops

1 orange, peeled, pitted, sectioned, and cut up
6 to 8 strawberries
2 cups orange juice

Divide orange pieces and strawberries among 6 small paper cups or popsicle molds. Pour orange juice over fruit. Place in freezer until partially frozen.

Insert popsicle stick in each cup and return to freezer.

Remove pops from cups by pushing up on bottom of cup until pop slides out.

Variation: Substitute 1 cup blueberries and 2 cups apple juice for the orange, strawberries, and orange juice.

Yield: 6 servings

Nutrient analysis of 1 serving: 1 fruit exchange; 50 Calories; 1 g protein; 0 g fat; 11 g carbohydrate; 1 mg sodium; 0 mg cholesterol.

Summer Frozen Fruit

3 peaches, peeled and sliced
1 cup strawberries, halved
1 cup blueberries
3 cups orange juice

Arrange fruits in baking pan, 8 x 8 x 2 inches. Pour in orange juice. Cover with aluminum foil and freeze. To serve, cut into 6 squares.

Yield: 6 servings

Nutrient analysis of 1 serving: 1½ fruit exchanges; 95 Calories; 1 g protein; 0 g fat; 23 g carbohydrate; 4 mg sodium; 0 mg cholesterol.

Super Summer Fruit Sundae

Strawberry Sauce (see below)
½ medium cantaloupe
3 peaches, peeled and sliced†
10 strawberries, hulled and cut into quarters
4 teaspoons whipped cream

Prepare strawberry sauce and set aside.

Remove seeds and fibers from cantaloupe. Cut half melon into 4 rings. Cut rind from rings.

Place each cantaloupe ring on a dessert plate. Fill centers with peach slices and pour strawberry sauce over fruit. Top each with quartered strawberries and 1 teaspoon whipped cream.

†To peel peaches, pour boiling water on peaches in bowl. Let stand for 3 minutes. Drain peaches and remove peel with knife.

Strawberry Sauce

10 or 12 hulled strawberries

Place strawberries in blender container or food processor. Blend at high speed until strawberries liquefy.

Yield: 4 servings

Nutrient analysis of 1 serving: 1 fruit exchange; 1 fat exchange; 84 Calories; 1 g protein; 5 g fat; 12 g carbohydrate; 10 mg sodium; 0 mg cholesterol.

Cantaloupe Sundae

1 medium cantaloupe
2 cups vanilla ice cream
1 pint strawberries, hulled and halved

Cut cantaloupe in half. Remove seeds and fibers with large spoon. Cut each half in half, to make 4 quarters.

Top each quarter with ½ cup ice cream and about ½ cup strawberries.

Yield: 4 servings

Nutrient analysis of serving: 1 starch/bread exchange; 1½ fruit exchanges; 1½ fat exchanges; 227 Calories; 4 g protein; 8 g fat; 37 g carbohydrate; 59 mg sodium; 21 mg cholesterol.

Strawberry Ice

½ cup sugar
1 cup boiling water
2 tablespoons lemon juice
1 pint strawberries, hulled and cut up

Measure sugar into bowl. Pour in boiling water and stir until sugar is dissolved. Cool.

Measure lemon juice into blender container or food processor; add strawberries. Blend at high speed for 2 to 3 minutes.

Stir strawberry puree into sugar water.

Pour into refrigerator tray or loaf pan, 8½ x 4¼ x 2 inches. Freeze.

Cut into 5 servings and serve in dessert dishes. If desired, top with whipped cream and a strawberry.

Yield: 5 servings

Nutrient analysis of 1 serving: 1 fruit exchange; 73 Calories; 1 g protein; 0 g fat; 17 g carbohydrate; 1 mg sodium; 0 mg cholesterol.

Your Own Fruit Plate

Arrange choice of suggested fruits attractively on large plate:

Red and green apple slices†
Red and green seedless grapes
Sliced canned or fresh peaches
Sliced oranges
Sliced pears
Sliced nectarines
Sliced plums
Melon slices
Sliced banana
Blueberries
Strawberries

For a complete meal, serve fruit plate with toasted cheese sandwiches.

Use your food exchange list to calculate the nutrient content of your fruit plate.

†Dip fruit slices into fruit juice or syrup to prevent darkening.

Hawaiian Dip

1 pineapple (approximately 4 cups of chunks)
8-ounce carton orange-flavored low-fat yogurt
1 pint strawberries

Remove top from pineapple. Cut thick slice from bottom and from top of pineapple and discard.

Cut remaining pineapple into 5 slices. Remove rind and core from each slice. Cut 3 slices into 1-inch chunks. Place in bowl, cover, and refrigerate.

Chop up remaining 2 slices and place in bowl. Stir in yogurt. Cover and refrigerate for 1 to 2 hours to blend flavors.

Wash strawberries but do not remove hulls. Drain thoroughly.

At serving time, insert wooden picks in pineapple chunks. Place bowl of yogurt-pineapple mixture in center of serving plate. Arrange pineapple chunks and strawberries around bowl. Guests spoon yogurt mixture onto dessert plates, then dip pineapple chunks and strawberries into mixture.

Yield: 8–10 servings

Nutrient analysis of ½ cup fruit and 1 ounce dip: 1 fruit exchange; 76 Calories; 2 g protein; 1 g fat; 17 g carbohydrate; 29 mg sodium; 1 mg cholesterol.

Watermelon Basket

10-pound long watermelon, chilled
1 cup watermelon balls
2 cups sliced strawberries
2 cups fresh blueberries or pineapple chunks
3 cups honeydew melon balls
2 cups cantaloupe balls
1 pound seedless grapes
1 cup cut-up apple
1 cup cut-up peach

Chill all fruits. Cut up apple and fresh peaches just before filling shell.

Cutting lengthwise, slice off top third of watermelon. Use larger part for basket. Remove watermelon from shell of this part with melon-ball cutter. Have an adult help you make an attractive edge on basket. Cover shell and refrigerate.

Just before serving, fill shell with fruits.

Yield: 13 cups

Nutrient analysis of 1 cup: 1½ fruit exchanges; 85 Calories; 1 g protein; 1 g fat; 21 g carbohydrate; 23 mg sodium; 0 mg cholesterol.

Pineapple Boats

1 pineapple with fresh green leaves
½ cup seedless grapes, halved
½ cup sliced strawberries
½ cup blueberries
½ cup cantaloupe balls
1 apple, diced
¼ cup orange juice

Cut pineapple in half lengthwise through green top; then cut each half again, to make 4 quarters.† Cut core from pineapple quarter and cut along curved edges with grapefruit knife to remove fruit from shells. Turn shells upside down on paper towels to drain.

Remove "eyes" from pineapple, then cut into bite-size pieces.

Combine pineapple, grapes, strawberries, blueberries, cantaloupe balls, and apple in bowl. Pour orange juice on fruit and toss.

Spoon fruit onto shells.

Yield: 4 servings

Nutrient analysis of 1 serving: 2 fruit exchanges; 115 Calories; 1 g protein; 1 g fat; 29 g carbohydrate; 10 mg sodium; 0 mg cholesterol.

†An adult should help you cut fresh pineapple.

Fruit Kebabs

12 pineapple chunks†
12 cantaloupe balls
12 honeydew melon balls
12 strawberries
6 thin cantaloupe wedges

Place 1 pineapple chunk, 1 cantaloupe ball, 1 honeydew melon ball, and 1 strawberry on each of 12 skewers. Insert 2 skewers in each melon wedge.

Yield: 6 servings

Nutrient analysis of 1 serving: 1 fruit exchange; 51 Calories; 1 g protein; 0 g fat; 12 g carbohydrate; 18 mg sodium; 0 mg cholesterol.

†An adult should help you cut fresh pineapple. Twist off top of pineapple. Cut pineapple in half, then into quarters. Hold pineapple quarter firmly and slice fruit from rind. (A grapefruit knife can be used for removing rind.) Cut off pineapple core and remove any "eyes." For chunks, slice quarter lengthwise, then crosswise.

Baked Apple

1 baking apple
1 teaspoon raisins
½ teaspoon margarine
Dash cinnamon

Preheat oven to 350°F. Core apple and pare upper ⅓ to prevent skin from splitting. Place apple upright in small baking dish.

Fill center of apple with raisins and margarine. Sprinkle with cinnamon. Pour water to ¼ inch depth into dish.

Bake at 350°F. for 30 to 45 minutes, or until apple is tender when pierced with fork. Serve hot or cool.

Note: Use an apple corer to remove core, or cut carefully around core with knife. Ask an adult for help.

Yield: 1 serving

Nutrient analysis of 1 serving: 1½ fruit exchanges; ½ fat exchange; 105 Calories; 0 g protein; 2 g fat; 23 g carbohydrate; 25 mg sodium; 0 mg cholesterol.

Fruit Cocktail Fritters

Oil for frying
½ cup skim milk
2 eggs
1½ cups all-purpose flour
1½ teaspoons baking powder
½ teaspoon salt
1 tablespoon sugar
1 cup fruit cocktail, well drained

Pour 3 to 4 inches of oil into a deep fat fryer or kettle. Heat to 375°F. *(An adult should be in the kitchen when you are cooking with hot oil. This is important.)*

Measure milk, eggs, flour, baking powder, salt, and sugar into blender container or food processor. Cover and blend until mixture is smooth. Stir in fruit.

Drop batter by tablespoonfuls (4 or 5 per batch) into hot fat. Turn fritters as they rise to surface. Fry until golden brown, 2 to 3 minutes per side. Remove from hot oil and drain on absorbent paper.

Serve hot, with margarine or diet syrup if desired.

Yield: 32 fritters

Nutrient analysis of 1 fritter: ⅓ starch/bread exchange; ½ fat exchange; 47 Calories; 1 g protein; 3 g fat; 5 g carbohydrate; 57 mg sodium; 16 mg cholesterol.

Apple Pie

Pastry for 8-inch lattice topped pie (page 210)
1/3 cup sugar
3 tablespoons flour
1/4 teaspoon nutmeg
1/4 teaspoon cinnamon
5 cups thin-sliced pared tart apples (about 5 medium)
1 tablespoon margarine

Preheat oven to 425°F. Prepare pastry and set aside.

Stir together sugar, flour, nutmeg, and cinnamon and mix lightly with apples. Pour into pastry-lined pie pan. Dot with margarine.

Cover with lattice top pastry. Seal and flute. Cover edge with 2- to 3-inch strip of aluminum foil to prevent excessive browning. Remove foil for last 15 minutes of baking.

Bake at 425°F. for 40 minutes or until crust is brown and juice begins to bubble through lattice. Serve warm.

Yield: 8 servings

Nutrient analysis of 1 serving: 1 1/4 starch/bread exchanges; 1 fruit exchange; 3 fat exchanges; 285 Calories; 4 g protein; 16 g fat; 35 g carbohydrate; 179 mg sodium; 0 mg cholesterol.

Cinnamon-Blueberry Sauce

2 tablespoons sugar
1 teaspoon cornstarch
1 cup blueberries
2 tablespoons water
1 tablespoon lemon juice
1/2 teaspoon cinnamon

Mix sugar and cornstarch in small saucepan. Stir in remaining ingredients. Cook over medium heat, stirring constantly, until mixture thickens and boils. Reduce heat and simmer for 5 minutes, stirring occasionally.

Serve warm on ice cream, pancakes, or waffles.

Yield: 1 1/4 cups

Nutrient analysis of 1/4 cup: 1/2 fruit exchange; 32 Calories; 1 g protein; 2 g fat; 8 g carbohydrate; 2 mg sodium; 0 mg cholesterol.

New-Fashion Oatmeal Cookies

1 cup all-purpose flour
½ cup whole wheat flour
1 cup rolled oats
1 teaspoon baking powder
½ teaspoon salt
¼ teaspoon baking soda
⅛ teaspoon ground ginger
½ teaspoon grated orange or lemon peel
½ cup coarsely chopped nuts (walnuts or pecans)
2 tablespoons sesame seeds
¾ cup raisins
4 to 6 medium-sized ripe bananas
⅓ cup margarine, softened
½ cup molasses
1 egg
¼ cup powdered milk
½ cup sugar

Preheat oven to 400°F. Grease baking sheet.

Measure flours, oats, baking powder, salt, baking soda, ginger, orange peel, nuts, sesame seeds, and raisins into a bowl and set aside.

Mash bananas by slicing them into a large bowl. Beat with an electric mixer at low speed, scraping bowl constantly. Increase speed to medium and beat until mixture is smooth. Measure mashed banana to be sure it is 1½ cups; return banana to bowl. Add remaining ingredients; beat until smooth, scraping bowl occasionally.

Mix in flour mixture with a spoon. Drop dough by teaspoonfuls onto prepared baking sheet.

Bake at 400°F. about 10 minutes, or until golden brown. Cool on wire rack.

Yield: 48 cookies

Nutrient analysis of 3 cookies: 2 starch/bread exchanges; 1 fat exchange; 198 Calories; 3 g protein; 6 g fat; 33 g carbohydrate; 136 mg sodium; 15 mg cholesterol.

Nutty Orange Oatmeal Cookies

⅓ cup unsalted margarine, softened
⅓ cup plain low-fat yogurt
¼ cup brown sugar (packed)
1 teaspoon vanilla
1½ cups all-purpose flour
1 cup rolled oats
¼ teaspoon baking soda
2 tablespoons finely chopped walnuts
¼ teaspoon grated orange peel

Preheat oven to 325°F.

Blend margarine, yogurt, sugar, and vanilla. Mix in remaining ingredients. Shape dough by rounded teaspoonfuls into 1-inch balls. Place about 2 inches apart on ungreased baking sheet; flatten slightly with fork.

Bake at 325°F. for 12 to 15 minutes. Remove from baking sheet immediately.

Variation:

Nutty Orange Oatmeal Balls: Place 1-inch balls 1 inch apart on baking sheet. (Do not flatten.) Bake at 325°F. 15 to 20 minutes.

Yield: 54 cookies

Nutrient analysis of 3 cookies: 1 starch/bread exchange; ½ fat exchange; 102 Calories; 3 g protein; 3 g fat; 12 g carbohydrate; 15 mg sodium; 0 mg cholesterol.

Grandma B's Oatmeal Cookies

- ¼ cup unsalted margarine, softened
- ¼ cup sugar
- ¼ cup molasses
- ¼ cup egg substitute
- 6-ounce can frozen orange juice concentrate, thawed
- ½ cup rolled oats
- ¼ cup raisins
- ¼ cup chopped walnuts
- 2 cups all-purpose flour
- 1 teaspoon baking soda
- ½ teaspoon ground ginger
- ½ teaspoon cinnamon
- ¼ teaspoon salt
- ¼ teaspoon cloves
- ¼ teaspoon nutmeg

Preheat oven to 325°F. Spray baking pan, 13 x 9 x 2 inches, with vegetable spray.

Cream margarine and sugar until fluffy. Stir in molasses, egg substitute, and orange juice concentrate. Mix in remaining ingredients. Spread in pan.

Bake at 325°F. for 25 to 30 minutes. Cool. Cut into bars, about 2 x 1½ inches.

Yield: 32 bars

Nutrient analysis of 1 bar: 1 starch/bread exchange; 72 Calories; 2 g protein; 3 g fat; 11 g carbohydrate; 45 mg sodium; 0 mg cholesterol.

Dessert Crepes with Fruit

1½ cups all-purpose flour
1 tablespoon sugar
½ teaspoon baking powder
2 cups skim milk
⅓ cup egg substitute
½ teaspoon vanilla
2 tablespoons unsalted margarine, melted
Choice of fresh fruits (blueberries, raspberries, sliced strawberries, peaches)

Measure all ingredients except fruit into bowl; beat with rotary beater until smooth.

Lightly grease 7- or 8-inch skillet with margarine; heat over medium heat until margarine is bubbly. For each crepe, pour scant ¼ cup batter into skillet; immediately rotate skillet until batter covers bottom. Cook until light brown. Loosen around edge with wide spatula; turn and cook other side until light brown. Stack crepes, placing waxed paper or paper towel between them. Keep crepes covered to prevent them from drying out.

Place ¼ cup fruit on each crepe and roll up. Roll crepes so most attractive side is on outside.

Yield: 16 crepes

Nutrient analysis of 2 crepes: 1 starch/bread exchange; ¾ fruit exchange; 1 fat exchange; 166 Calories; 5 g protein; 5 g fat; 25 g carbohydrate; 75 mg sodium; 1 mg cholesterol.

White Mountain Sherbet

2 cups unsweetened applesauce
3 tablespoons sugar
3 egg whites
¼ cup frozen lemonade concentrate, thawed
¼ teaspoon grated lemon rind

Combine all ingredients in large bowl of electric mixer.

Beat at high speed until mixture is stiff, about 10 minutes.

Pour into 13 x 9 x 2 inch pan. Freeze until firm.

Cut into 15 squares.

Yield: 15 servings

Nutrient analysis of 1 serving: ½ fruit exchange; 27 Calories; 1 g protein; 0 g fat; 6 g carbohydrate; 10 mg sodium; 0 mg cholesterol.

Prune Bars

- **¼ cup unsalted margarine, softened**
- **½ cup sugar**
- **1 cup all-purpose flour**
- **¾ cup whole wheat flour**
- **1 teaspoon baking soda**
- **½ teaspoon salt**
- **½ teaspoon cinnamon**
- **¼ teaspoon nutmeg**
- **¼ teaspoon ground cloves**
- **½ cup unsweetened prune juice**
- **½ cup water**
- **1 cup chopped cooked prunes**
- **½ cup egg substitute**

Preheat oven to 350°F. Spray baking pan, 13 x 9 x 2 inches, with vegetable spray.

Cream margarine and sugar thoroughly. Mix in flours, soda, salt, cinnamon, nutmeg, and cloves alternately with prune juice and water. Stir in prunes.

Beat egg substitute with rotary beater 2 minutes. Fold into batter. Spread in pan.

Bake at 350°F. for 35 to 40 minutes, until wooden pick inserted in center comes out clean. Cool for 30 minutes. Cut into bars, 2½ x 1½ inches.

Yield: 36 bars

Nutrient analysis of 1 bar: ¾ starch/bread exchange; 63 Calories; 1 g protein; 2 g fat; 11 g carbohydrate; 56 mg sodium; 0 mg cholesterol.

Strawberry Dessert

- **1 pint strawberries (2 cups)**
- **2 tablespoons lemon juice**
- **¼ cup sugar**
- **2 egg whites**
- **1 cup whipping cream**

Place strawberries, lemon juice, and sugar in blender container. Cover and blend at high speed until strawberries are crushed, about 30 seconds.

Pour strawberry mixture into large bowl of electric mixer. Add egg whites; beat at high speed until stiff, about 10 minutes.

Beat cream separately until stiff; fold into strawberry mixture. Turn into 13 x 9 x 2 inch pan. Freeze until firm.

Cut into 12 servings.

Yield: 12 servings

Nutrient analysis of 1 serving: ½ fruit exchange; 1½ fat exchanges; 91 Calories; 1 g protein; 7 g fat; 6 g carbohydrate; 16 mg sodium; 27 mg cholesterol.

Fortune Cookies

3 egg whites
½ cup sugar
⅛ teaspoon salt
¼ teaspoon vanilla
1 cup all-purpose flour
1 teaspoon instant tea
2 tablespoons water
½ cup margarine, melted
Fortunes on slips of paper

Mix egg whites, sugar, and salt thoroughly with spoon. Mix in remaining ingredients, except fortunes. Cover bowl with plastic wrap and chill for 30 minutes.

Preheat oven to 350°F. Grease baking sheet. Have clean white cotton gloves ready to use when folding and shaping the hot cookies. If gloves are not available, use two pieces of paper towelling folded to several thicknesses to protect fingers from the hot cookies. Also, have some clean muffin tins ready to hold baked cookies while they cool.

Shape and bake 2 cookies at a time. For each cookie, drop 1 teaspoon batter onto baking sheet. Spread the batter with back of spoon to make a 3-inch circle.

Bake at 350°F. for 3 to 5 minutes, or until edges turn light brown.

Work very quickly. Remove one cookie with wide spatula to counter top. Place a fortune paper across center of cookie. Using gloves or paper towelling, fold edge of cookie over to make a semicircle. Hold cookie on the ends and place the middle of folded edge over top of muffin pan; bend ends down. Place folded cookie carefully in a muffin cup to cool. Repeat process.

Yield: 36 cookies

Nutrient analysis of 2 cookies: ½ starch/bread exchange; 1 fat exchange; 80 Calories; 2 g protein; 6 g fat; 6 g carbohydrate; 84 mg sodium; 0 mg cholesterol.

PART IV

Understanding Diabetes

by P. J. Palumbo, M.D., F.A.C.P.

5

INSULIN-DEPENDENT DIABETES MELLITUS

The term *insulin-dependent diabetes mellitus* describes the condition in which the beta cells of the pancreas fail to produce any insulin. The first symptoms are usually constant, increased urination and increased thirst. The increased excretion of urine causes a loss of sugar from the body, which in turn leads to loss of calories and usually loss of weight, even when the appetite is hearty and the food intake is adequate.

Insulin-dependent diabetes is more likely to become apparent during the fall and winter (particularly in children), which increases the danger of its being confused with flu. In fact, the patient indeed may have flu, and this will serve to unmask the underlying diabetes. Since flu is usually an illness of the upper respiratory tract, the presence of nausea and vomiting should alert one to the possibility of diabetes.

Hereditary factors may play a role in the development of insulin-dependent diabetes mellitus. Research has shown that the frequency of diabetes is increased in the siblings of diabetics and in identical twins.

HOW IS DIABETES DIAGNOSED?

The diagnosis of diabetes is made by measuring the blood glucose (sugar) level. Blood glucose levels of 140 mg per 100 ml or higher are arbitrarily defined as representing diabetes. In the insulin-dependent patient, there usually is little question about the diagnosis because the blood glucose level will be markedly elevated, usually to greater than 200 mg per 100 ml, and the urine will contain sugar. Normal persons have no sugar in the urine. The urine test is almost as good as the blood test for the diagnosis of insulin-dependent diabetes. In any patient with the symptoms described above and who has a positive test for sugar in the urine, the blood sugar level is likely to be greater than 200 mg per 100 ml.

Patients with insulin-dependent diabetes do not need specialized testing, since they usually have the most reliable sign of diabetes—fasting hyperglycemia—that is, a blood sugar level greater than 140 mg per 100 ml after an overnight fast. Detecting fasting hyperglycemia requires only one blood test, made at least 12 hours after the last meal the night before. (The test should be repeated on another day to make certain that the first one was not in error.) A glucose tolerance test is not necessary.

With high blood sugar levels and the absence of insulin production, fat breakdown occurs at an increased rate in the insulin-dependent diabetic and leads to production of ketoacids (ketoacidosis) that exceeds the body's capacity to utilize them. These ketoacids therefore are flushed out in the urine, leading to further water loss. A positive test for sugar and ketoacids in the urine is strong evidence of marked increase in the blood sugar level. When ketoacidosis is present along with high blood sugar levels, regardless of the time of day, it is not necessary to perform the two fasting blood sugar determinations for the diagnosis.

GOALS OF TREATMENT

The immediate goal of therapy is to restore the blood sugar level to normal or near normal. The long-term goal is the prevention of acute and chronic complications.

Rapid changes in blood sugar levels may have a deleterious effect on various organs of the body. The aim of the treatment program is to prevent a blood sugar level greater than 200 mg per 100 ml for more than 15 to 30 minutes. The current preference is to maintain the blood sugar level between 80 and 120 mg per 100 ml before meals and not more than 150 mg per 100 ml after meals.

One approach to controlling the blood sugar level uses "self blood glucose monitoring." This is done by the patient and involves pricking the finger to obtain a drop of capillary blood, placing the blood on a strip of paper, and comparing the color change to a standard scale or placing the strip in an instrument known as a reflectance meter for a more precise measurement. The physician advises the patient on how to adjust the insulin dosage on the basis of these blood sugar determinations.

Testing urine for sugar is used less frequently. Tests for ketoacids in the urine are still used in conjunction with self blood glucose monitoring to determine whether a particular blood sugar level is associated with ketoacid production, in which case an aggressive program of treatment may be needed to prevent serious problems.

The sugar content of hemoglobin in the blood (glycosylated hemoglobin level) is another measure of control. When the blood sugar level increases, the glycosylated hemoglobin level also increases. This measurement provides a more prolonged gauge of diabetes control than does the single blood sugar determination. Currently, the test is carried out at intervals of two to three months and provides information about diabetes control for the one to three months prior to the determination. In the future, it may be possible to measure the glycosylated hemoglobin on capillary blood specimens just as is being done now for glucose. The goal of therapy is to maintain the glycosylated hemoglobin level in the normal range, usually between 4 and 7 percent, depending on the laboratory in which the test is being done.

DIETARY MANAGEMENT

Diet control and insulin therapy are begun as soon as the diagnosis of insulin-dependent diabetes is made. The diet plan is based on the patient's weight and caloric need.

For those who are overweight, a calorie-restricted diet of 1,000 to 1,400 Calories may be prescribed. If you are at or near ideal weight, 12 to 15 Calories per pound of ideal weight generally represents an adequate caloric intake. For those who are near ideal weight, continued weight loss or unusual weight gain indicates the need for a visit to the physician or dietitian to restructure the caloric intake.

The frequency and timing of meals are coordinated with the insulin therapy. The absorption of insulin can vary from day to day in the same individual, depending on the blood sugar level and the site of injection (for example, leg versus abdomen). Having more than three meals a day may help maintain the blood sugar level at a satisfactory value. A midmorning snack may be necessary for older patients with insulin-dependent diabetes or for children who use fast-acting insulin prior to breakfast. Frequently, a midafternoon meal may be needed because of the time at which insulin has its maximum effect on the blood sugar. In addition, most diabetics on insulin need a bedtime snack.

Recent research indicates that mixed meals (mixtures of carbohydrate, fat, and protein) provide for slower absorption of carbohydrate and therefore lead to smoother control of the blood sugar level. In addition, an intake of complex carbohydrate and fiber helps avoid too rapid absorption and quick upswings in the blood sugar level. This is discussed more fully on pages 5–9.

MANAGEMENT WITH INSULIN

As the name implies, insulin-dependent diabetics require insulin for treatment. Several varieties of insulin are available. Some preparations contain insulin from animal species such as cows or pigs and others contain human insulin, synthesized in bacteria by recombinant DNA techniques. The currently available preparations are quick-acting, intermediate-acting, and long-acting. Quick-acting insulin has an effect for 3 to 6 hours; intermediate-acting lasts for 18 to 24 hours; and long-acting lasts for 24 to 36 hours. There are some other insulins, such as semilente insulin, that act for 6 to 12 hours.

Most insulin-dependent diabetics will require at least two insulin injections a day—usually one before breakfast and one before supper—with approximately two thirds of the insulin being given before breakfast and one third given before supper. However, this varies from person to person, and the individual treatment program must be determined by a physician. Sometimes it may be necessary to take the same amount of insulin before breakfast and before supper, or to combine quick-acting and intermediate-acting insulins in the same syringe before breakfast and supper. This information will be provided by your physician when the insulin dosage is being adjusted to provide the best control of your blood sugar.

For more intensified treatment programs, it may be necessary to take a dose of quick-acting insulin before every meal and a dose of long-acting insulin at suppertime or before breakfast. The daily dosages of quick-acting and long-acting insulin are determined by self blood glucose monitoring.

Insulin infusion pumps are currently being used by some diabetics. These pumps provide a continuous infusion of insulin. They require close supervision by a physician to adjust the doses of insulin between meals and at meal time.

Oral hypoglycemic agents are not appropriate treatment for insulin-dependent diabetics.

COMPLICATIONS OF INSULIN TREATMENT

The most common complication of insulin treatment is low blood sugar (hypoglycemia), more popularly known as "an insulin reaction." The usual symptoms are increased sweating, irritability, palpitations, blurring of vision, hunger, and headache.

Hypoglycemia can result from the administration of too much insulin, from inadequate food intake, from a delay in meals, or from excessive exercise. When hypoglycemia occurs, it must be treated promptly by consuming a simple carbohydrate such as sugar in water or orange juice or a special sugar preparation which can be swallowed easily (see the table on page 297 for suggestions). Low-calorie diet drinks or low-calorie diet foods will not correct hypoglycemia. It is important for you to ask your physician how to recognize the warning signs of hypoglycemia and how to treat it promptly. When hypoglycemia is more severe, causing confusion or inability to respond, it may be necessary to administer sugar by vein or to administer the hormone glucagon which stimulates the production of sugar within the body.

Treatment of hypoglycemia should never be delayed. Prompt recognition and treatment of severe hypoglycemia by family members or friends are essential to avoid a catastrophe. A diabetic can lapse into coma and die if hypoglycemia is not treated promptly.

Hypoglycemia is a special hazard to the diabetic driver. Therefore, it is important to have food available in the car and to be sure that meals are not skipped during a long trip. If the slightest suspicion arises that an insulin reaction may be coming on, food should be ingested promptly. Fortunately, insulin reactions are not a major problem for most diabetics who take insulin, but the diabetic driver needs to be alert to this potential problem when he or she gets behind the wheel of a car.

Some Fast-Acting Carbohydrates

Carbohydrate	Amount
Soda pop, regular	½ cup (4 ounces)
Orange juice, grapefruit juice, or apple juice	½ cup
Vanilla ice cream	⅓ cup (2½ ounces)
Sherbet	¼ cup (2 ounces)
Corn syrup, maple syrup, or honey	2 teaspoons
Honey (flat pack)	1 prepared packet
Sugar	3 teaspoons (1 packet = 1¼ teaspoons)
Sugar cubes	2 (½-inch square)
Sweetened gelatin (Jell-O) dessert	6 tablespoons
Raisins	2 tablespoons (half of a small box)
Lifesavers	6 pieces
Jelly beans	8 pieces
Dextrosol®	4 pieces
Monogel®	1 package (10 grams)

Another complication of treatment is the development of antibodies to the insulin injection. These antibodies are more likely to develop when insulin from an animal (particularly bovine insulin) is used. High antibody levels prevent the injected insulin from producing its effect on the blood sugar level. Your physician can advise you regarding appropriate treatment for such high antibody levels. With use of the currently available highly purified insulin preparations, and particularly the highly purified human insulin preparations, such excess antibodies are a rare occurrence.

Skin reaction to injected insulin is another possible complication. Most of these reactions appear in the area of the injection and occur within the first six weeks after therapy is started. Such localized reactions usually clear up spontaneously and require no specific treatment. Occasionally, injection of Benadryl® along with the insulin may help. However, just continuing the insulin injection eventually serves to decrease localized skin reactions in most people.

Another skin reaction is the loss of subcutaneous fat or the accumulation of excess fat in response to the insulin injected. These changes in skin fat usually show up in the area of the injection. An accumulation of excess fat is more likely to occur in men, whereas the loss of fat is more likely to occur in women. With the more highly purified insulin preparations, and particularly the human insulin preparations, such reactions occur less frequently.

Insulin allergy is very rare. When it does occur, it may cause generalized hives, swelling of the lips, or difficulty in breathing. If you had an allergy or eczema in infancy or childhood, you may be susceptible to insulin allergy. Starting and stopping insulin may produce an allergic response in susceptible individuals. If you suspect an allergic reaction, you should see your physician.

EFFECTS OF OTHER MEDICATIONS

You need to be alert to possible interactions when you take drugs for other conditions. Some medications, such as cortisone, can affect insulin action and it may be necessary to adjust the insulin dosage when certain medications are used.

Others, such as the beta-adrenergic blocking agents which are often used in heart disease, may make it difficult for the patient to recognize the reaction or for the body to produce enough sugar to overcome the reaction. Always check with your doctor before starting a new drug.

PREGNANCY

When an insulin-dependent diabetic becomes pregnant, it is especially important to maintain strict control of the blood sugar level and to prevent ketoacidosis which is very hazardous to the growing fetus. It is essential that blood sugar levels be normal or near-normal from the very start of pregnancy in order to prevent malformations or immaturity in the organ systems that develop in the fetus within the first 12 weeks of life. Good diabetes control later in pregnancy promotes healthy growth of the fetus in the uterus and a healthy child at birth. High blood sugar levels in the mother produce excessive sensitivity to blood sugar levels in the beta cells of the fetus. This sensitivity is associated with hypoglycemia in the newborn, which can produce brain damage and could lead to death. (For this reason, the infant of a diabetic mother should be monitored carefully for the development of hypoglycemia.)

Keeping the blood sugar level nearly normal in the diabetic mother also will prevent an excessive accumulation of fluid and fat in the infant, which can make delivery more difficult, and it will avoid maternal complications such as toxemia, high blood pressure, and excess amniotic fluid.

Occasionally, diabetes occurs only during pregnancy. This form of diabetes carries the same risk of complications as does insulin-dependent diabetes. Pregnant women who develop gestational diabetes run a relatively high risk of developing diabetes later on in life. The treatment for gestational diabetes is a well-balanced diet with adequate calories for growth of the fetus and for prevention of ketoacidosis. Insulin treatment may be necessary if the fasting blood sugar level is more than 105 mg per 100 ml and if the sugar level two hours after a meal is more than 120 mg per 100 ml.

INFECTIONS

A high blood sugar level (greater than 300 mg per 100 ml) impairs the activity of the white blood cells and other defense mechanisms that the body utilizes to fight infection. Therefore, when diabetes is poorly regulated, infections of the skin, urinary tract, vagina, and penis are more likely to develop. The infections of the vagina and penis are usually fungal. Skin infections and infections of the urinary tract usually are caused by bacteria. The drugs used for the treatment of both kinds of infections are more effective when the blood sugar is controlled.

DIABETIC KETOACIDOSIS

The major acute complication of insulin-dependent diabetes is diabetic ketoacidosis. This condition is a result of inadequate insulin dosage. The symptoms usually develop over a period of a few days. First, a high blood sugar level develops, followed by excessive production of keto-acids. Next, disturbances occur in water metabolism, electrolytes, and the acidity of the blood. As ketoacidosis develops, there is increased thirst with frequent urination. Ketoacidosis causes nausea, vomiting, increased breathing or overbreathing, and a state of weakness, fatigue, and lethargy. If these symptoms go unrecognized, the diabetic may lapse into coma and can die. This condition requires hospitalization and prompt intravenous administration of fluids and insulin.

Today, the death rate from ketoacidosis is low because it is quickly recognized—by the diabetic, by family members, and by physicians. A physician should be contacted immediately if you suspect this condition is developing.

LONG-TERM COMPLICATIONS

Complications can occur in any diabetic, but they are more likely to develop when the diabetes is poorly controlled.

One of the long-term complications is microangiopathy, a term used to describe diseases of small blood vessels, particularly those in the eyes and kidneys. The small vessels of the eye become damaged and the new vessels that may form are of poor quality, leading to bleeding within the chamber of the eye. The bleeding may be excessive and may lead to increased pressure or glaucoma and eventually to blindness. With early recognition and treatment using laser photocoagulation, it may be possible to control the blood vessel changes related to diabetes. Therefore, it is important to have frequent eye examinations. The small blood vessels of the kidney may also be affected, causing high blood pressure and, in advanced cases, kidney failure.

Damage to the nerves in the legs can also occur. This damage appears to be related to loss of the covering of the nerve or to decreased blood supply to the nerve. This leads to changes in the nerve's function, and pain may occur in the feet and legs. Impairment of the blood supply to the nerve also causes weakness in the leg. Rarely, there may be damage to the nerves controlling the muscles of the eye. When this happens, pain and weakness in the eye may occur.

Fortunately, the symptoms caused by these changes in the nerves will gradually go away. Usually, no specific treatment is necessary, although use of a drug to relieve pain or a tranquilizer may be necessary for short periods to control severe symptoms.

Diabetics need to be alert to damage to the nerves in the feet because when there is a loss of sensation, an injury to the feet may not be noticed. Foot care is an important part of the treatment of diabetes. Unrecognized small injuries can lead to ulceration and infection and, ultimately, to loss of the foot or leg. Therefore, it is very important to inspect your feet frequently and to be certain that all footwear fits properly. Avoid any rubbing in the shoe because this might cause ulceration. Inspect anything you put on your feet to be certain that there is no hidden foreign body.

Occasionally there may be damage to the nerves that control the heart rate or to the nerves that control the blood vessels. When these nerves are damaged, the heart rate increases and there may be a decrease in blood pressure, producing dizziness when you stand up. In diabetic men, there may be damage to the nerve that controls penile erections, and impotency will result.

Another major complication of diabetes is macroangiopathy—disease of the large blood vessels. Macroangiopathy can involve the arteries to the heart, the legs, and the brain. Arteriosclerosis (hardening of the arteries) occurs, and the arteries become narrow, which in turn impairs circulation and decreases the amount of blood reaching the organ systems. The result can be a heart attack, gangrene, or a stroke. Special dietary modifications may be necessary for patients with this condition.

OTHER RISK FACTORS

If you have diabetes, it is important that any other factors that might possibly increase the risk of blood vessel disease be corrected. For example, smoking is detrimental, and diabetics should not smoke. High blood pressure should be controlled by weight loss in the obese, low salt intake, and, if necessary, medication. High blood cholesterol and triglyceride levels should be corrected. However, the high triglyceride levels may result from poor regulation of diabetes. So, make sure your diabetes is well controlled. If cholesterol and triglyceride levels remain high, more specific treatment may be needed. Those who are overweight or obese need to reduce body weight because weight reduction alone often will result in correction of high blood pressure and cholesterol and triglyceride levels.

POSSIBLE FUTURE TREATMENT PROGRAMS

The search for more effective treatment—to restore beta cell function or to mimic it more closely—continues.

Success with pancreas transplantation has been limited. Such treatment is still under investigation. Sufficient numbers of human beta cells have been isolated from the pancreas, but so far attempts at implantation of these beta cells into other humans have not been successful.

A computer program to mimic the activity of the beta cells of the pancreas in recognizing the blood sugar level and in providing insulin in an appropriate amount in response to that level is being developed. Ultimately, this program will be housed in a device small enough to be implanted in the human body. This device, referred to as "the artificial pancreas," will act as an artificial beta cell.

Another possibility is based on techniques of genetic engineering. The idea is to reprogram the defective beta cells to produce insulin again or to program different cells of the body to do the work of the beta cells. The production of insulin in bacteria makes this potential form of diabetes treatment a viable theory.

RELATIONSHIP BETWEEN PHYSICIAN AND DIABETIC PATIENT

It is important to have a physician—if possible, one who specializes in diabetes—readily available when you have difficulties or are ill. It is important to be able to talk with your physician freely about any problems that may arise. If you have difficulty finding such a physician, contact your local American Diabetes Association Affiliate for a list of diabetes specialists in your locality.

6

NON-INSULIN-DEPENDENT DIABETES MELLITUS

"Non-insulin-dependent diabetes mellitus" is the term used to describe the condition in which some insulin is being produced by the body but not enough to control the blood sugar level. This may result from defective production of insulin or from resistance of the body's cells to the action of insulin.

Often weight reduction and weight control are all that are needed to control this type of diabetes. Approximately 10 to 20 percent of patients will have to take certain drugs by mouth and 20 to 30 percent will require insulin treatment for the control of blood sugar levels.

GOALS OF TREATMENT

The long-term goal is prevention of the complications, which are the same as those with insulin-dependent diabetes (see pages 299–300). The immediate goal of treatment is to achieve normal or near-normal blood sugar levels. Most doctors currently prefer to maintain a blood sugar level between 80 and 120 mg per 100 ml before meals and not more than 150 mg per 100 ml after meals. The glycosylated hemoglobin level, which indicates diabetes control over a period of two to three months, should be within the normal range (usually 4 to 7 percent, although it may vary from laboratory to laboratory).

DIETARY MANAGEMENT

Since the majority of non-insulin-dependent diabetics are overweight, diet control is the major component of the treatment. The dietary principles are the same as those for the insulin-dependent diabetic. At least 50 percent of the caloric intake should be from carbohydrates, 10 to 20 percent from protein, and 25 to 30 percent from fat. Complex carbohydrates and carbohydrates high in fiber are preferred, and simple carbohydrates, like refined sugar, in very limited quantities, can be eaten in mixed meals to meet your caloric needs.

For the obese, a balanced intake of 1,000 to 1,400 calories per day should produce weight reduction. For non-insulin-dependent diabetics who are lean or at ideal weight, the daily calorie needs are outlined on page 4. Late night or midafternoon snacks are only necessary if insulin therapy is used.

INSULIN MANAGEMENT

Insulin is the best treatment for diabetes when diet alone does not control the blood sugar level. Most non-insulin-dependent diabetics require only one insulin injection per day; however, occasionally, more than one injection may be necessary for optimal control. For a discussion of insulin treatment, see pages 295–98. The non-insulin-dependent diabetic on insulin therapy is susceptible to the same complications as the insulin-dependent diabetic. Be alert to the fact that hypoglycemic reactions are not well tolerated by older individuals and may affect mental functions or mimic a stroke.

ORAL MEDICATIONS

For the non-insulin-dependent diabetic whose blood sugar level does not respond to diet control alone, an oral hypoglycemic agent can be used. Currently, two types of oral hypoglycemic agents are available: the sulfonylurea drugs (related to the sulfa drugs) and the biguanide drugs. Only the sulfonylurea agents are available in the United States. The sulfonylurea drugs increase the production of insulin by the beta cell and render the body's cells more receptive to the insulin produced. The biguanides decrease sugar absorption and production and may have an effect on the utilization of sugar by the cells. In countries where both types of agents are available, the sulfonylureas and biguanides may be used together to correct high blood sugar levels.

Unfortunately, oral drugs have a high rate of failure. One of the reasons suggested for failure is poor adherence to diet. Therefore, it is important to adhere closely to the diet prescribed for you. It also appears that some patients become resistant to the effects of these drugs over time and require a change to insulin treatment.

Hypoglycemic reactions can occur in non-insulin-dependent diabetics taking a sulfonylurea-type drug. The recognition and treatment of this kind of reaction is discussed in the preceding chapter. If such hypoglycemic reactions occur, you should be seen by a physician.

EXERCISE

A program of regular exercise combined with an appropriate diet is an important part of treatment. Exercise results in better utilization of sugar, decreases insulin need, and promotes good body tone, physical fitness, and improved circulation to the organ systems of the body.

Walking two to four miles a day is an excellent form of exercise for older, lean individuals. If you are overweight, however, walking and other exercises that affect the large joints can cause damage to these joints. You should try swimming and physical fitness programs until you reach your ideal weight. More information regarding exercise programs is given in the final chapter.

EFFECTS OF OTHER MEDICATIONS

It is important to identify all drugs that you are taking, both over-the-counter and prescribed, and to discuss them with your physician. This will help pinpoint potential drug interactions that may cause problems.

CONSIDERATIONS ABOUT TRAVEL

If you are being treated by diet alone, no special precautions are necessary while traveling, other than to follow your dietary plan. Those taking an oral hypoglycemic agent need no special precautions other than to continue taking the drug according to the suggestions described on page 303.

Treatment with an oral agent should not pose any particular hazard in driving an automobile. However, the sulfonylureas can sometimes cause hypoglycemic reactions. Therefore, to be on the safe side, follow the same precautions outlined for patients taking insulin.

SICK DAYS

When any diabetic becomes ill, testing of the urine for sugar and ketoacids is necessary. During an acute illness, you may require insulin treatment. The blood and urine sugar levels and the urine ketoacid level should be checked frequently when you are ill.

Anyone on insulin who becomes ill should follow the guidelines outlined on pages 47–49.

INFECTION

A high blood sugar level may impair the body's defenses against infection. The comments in the preceding chapter apply to all diabetics.

COMA

Diabetic ketoacidosis is unusual in the non-insulin-dependent patient. When it does occur, recognition and management are the same as in the insulin-dependent patient. A more likely complication is hyperosmolar nonketotic coma. This occurs in a poorly regulated diabetic who becomes dehydrated—for example, during an illness with fever. The blood sugar level may increase to 1,000 mg per 100 ml or higher, and even though there is enough insulin circulating to prevent the breakdown of body fat to ketoacids, there is not enough to control the blood sugar level. The combination of an extremely high blood sugar level and dehydration leads to lethargy and coma. The condition is treated by giving the patient water (by mouth if possible or by intravenous injection of fluids if the patient is unable to drink). Small doses of insulin will help to correct the blood sugar level. The patient should recover without incident. If it is suspected that this condition is developing, a physician should be consulted immediately. If the problem is not corrected, the patient may die.

LONG-TERM COMPLICATIONS

The long-term complications of diabetes are discussed in the preceding chapter. For the non-insulin-dependent diabetic, the most frequent complications are the development of macroangiopathy, or large blood vessel disease, involving the arteries of the heart, the legs, and the brain, and the development of nerve damage described on page 300. Blood vessel changes in the eye or in the kidney occur less frequently in the non-insulin-dependent diabetic. When they do occur, they follow the same course as in the insulin-dependent diabetic.

Your physician should be contacted when there are difficulties in controlling diabetes or when an illness occurs. It is important to discuss any problems that arise or cause concern. A good working relationship between the diabetic and his or her physician is important in helping to cope with this disorder and its treatment.

7

DIABETES MELLITUS IN CHILDREN AND ADOLESCENTS

Diabetes mellitus in children and adolescents (under 18 years of age) can affect physical growth and psychological development. Management of diabetes in this age group requires a continuing cooperative effort among those concerned with the diabetic child—the medical team, the parents, and members of the community (the school nurse, teachers, the director of athletics, and the school counselor). However, the final responsibility still remains with the person who has diabetes. Parents need to make sure that their diabetic children know everything that they, the parents, know about diabetes. Even very young diabetics need to know the warning signs and treatment for hypoglycemia and ketoacidosis. Children should be encouraged to take increasing responsibility for themselves just as soon as they are able. Most are quite capable and most, particularly adolescents, do not want their parents hovering about, trying to control all aspects of their lives.

When diabetes develops in a person under 18 years old, it almost always is insulin-dependent diabetes. Good control of the diabetes is necessary to maintain normal metabolism and health. All insulin-dependent diabetics should read and understand the information in Chapter 5 of this section, as well as information given in the chapter on exercise. The importance of blood sugar monitoring, regular exercise, and careful attention to adjustment of insulin dosage should be stressed to the young diabetic.

Before puberty, the body is extremely sensitive to insulin, and usually only very small doses are required to maintain normal or nearly normal blood sugar levels and normal protein and fat metabolism. During puberty and the accompanying growth spurt, the insulin needs increase. Poor regulation of insulin-dependent diabetes, especially during the period of rapid growth, may result in ketoacidosis.

"WHY ME?"

Each diabetic, young and old, faces diabetes with the usual reaction: "Why me?" The impact of having diabetes is immense. Feelings of isolation, of being different, of being singled out by having diabetes are fertile ground for long-term emotional and behavioral problems. To be reminded daily, by the need to pay attention to details of diet and medication, that you are diabetic with constraints on your freedom can adversely affect the developing personality of the young diabetic.

Even with a strongly supportive family, the diabetic child or adolescent often continues to feel rejected, unloved, and the victim of unjust circumstances. Anger leads to detrimental "acting-out" behavior. It is as if these children are testing to see whether the limits imposed by diabetes are real.

The rebellious attitude of normal adolescents often is compounded in the diabetic, who may do things that can have dangerous long-term consequences.

Some refuse to carry out the testing procedures needed to monitor the diabetes control. Some skip insulin doses or gradually decrease the size of the insulin dose. Some refuse to vary the injection sites and administer the insulin in a small area which soon becomes insensitive. Many cheat on their diets. Some may even provide fake test results so that they appear to be conforming to their diet. Unfortunately, all of these kinds of behavior lead to poor regulation of the diabetes and can lead to ketoacidosis, coma, and death.

Some diabetics use their condition to obtain the love and attention that they wrongly feel they have lost because of their disease. However, with strong support from parents, other family members, the physician, and community resources, young diabetics can learn to handle their disease and focus attention on the positive aspects of life.

It is important for every diabetic to assume responsibility for his or her own health. Those who do can take pride in their ability to deal with a very serious problem. Having learned to deal with this problem, they are well prepared to deal with almost any problem in life. Many find that joining support groups of other diabetics who are experiencing the same feelings and problems is a great help. The local chapter of the Juvenile Diabetes Association and of the American Diabetes Association can provide information on local youth programs.

SCHOOL

It is important that diabetics participate in all school activities, including athletics. In most cases, there are no limitations on activities other than those related to diet and insulin treatment. Ask the school nurse to help arrange midmorning and midafternoon feedings that will not call attention to the student and to provide information to the faculty regarding behavioral changes that signal poor regulation of the diabetes—either high blood sugar level or low blood sugar level.

Participation in athletic activities should be encouraged. Some very fine athletes are diabetics and have proved that the diabetic can be resourceful enough to be successful in competitive sports. Always be alert to the possibility of hypoglycemic reactions during the exercise program, particularly vigorous team sports, and keep a quick-acting carbohydrate handy. If the school staff is properly informed, errors in judgment can be minimized and appropriate treatment can be provided when necessary.

Students can select meals from the school cafeteria or can bring lunch from home. However, it is important to be part of student activities, and every effort should be made to make it possible for the young diabetic to eat the same meals as other students. They need to learn how to select appropriate foods for meals, snacks after school, and at parties. The goal is to minimize the differences between the diabetic and other children while making it clear that he or she is responsible for avoiding irregularities in diabetes control.

8

THE ROLE OF EXERCISE

Regardless of the type of diabetes or type of treatment program, exercise is an important component in therapy. Exercise is helpful in controlling the blood sugar level throughout the day. In fact, many non-insulin-dependent diabetics who follow a regular exercise program and control their weight find that medications are no longer necessary. Exercise provides a sense of physical well-being, with muscle conditioning and improved circulation to the organ systems of the body. These beneficial effects improve the quality of life and may actually prolong it.

In developing an exercise program, you should consider the following factors: age, weight, current physical condition, possible physical impediments, individual interests, and the timing of the exercise and its effect on your blood sugar level.

Age plays a significant role in the choice of exercise and in the ability to carry out specific exercises. For example, a younger person is better able to perform more vigorous exercise; older persons tend to be more sedentary. In fact, exercise testing to assess physical condition, ability to perform an exercise, and the adverse effect that the exercise may have on the heart should be an important part of the overall physical assessment of the older diabetic.

All exercise should incorporate a warm-up period of several minutes and a cooling-down period of several minutes. This will allow for more favorable transitions between the nonactive and the active states.

Unless there are physical handicaps, walking and swimming are good exercises for any age group. More vigorous exercises such as bicycling, contact sports, or tennis require a certain level of physical fitness. However, before participating fully in any vigorous sports, isometric exercises, or exercises that develop muscles, remember it is necessary to increase your physical conditioning gradually.

PHYSICAL CONDITION

Weight is an important consideration in developing an exercise program. Exercises such as walking may precipitate or aggravate joint problems in the knees and feet in obese or overweight individuals. Isometric or bodybuilding exercises and swimming are probably more appropriate since these activities minimize the effect of excess weight on the joints.

The status of the heart, eyes, and feet is an important consideration in planning an exercise program. Severe heart disease (inability to move without pain or shortness of breath) restricts the amount and type of exercise that can be undertaken. Arthritis or other joint problems make certain forms of exercise undesirable because the involved joint may be used in the exercise. The wrong exercise may aggravate arthritis. The diabetic who has severe blood vessel disease in the eye must avoid vigorous exercise to prevent bleeding into the eye.

The diabetic who has foot ulcers, has had a stroke, or has damage to the peripheral nerves (neuropathy) should utilize forms of exercise that do not produce pressure on areas of the body susceptible to ulceration. Swimming or physical fitness programs with bodybuilding and muscle conditioning are better choices for those with foot problems or neuropathy.

TIMING OF EXERCISE

Exercise generally decreases the blood sugar level. This differs among people because each person exercises at a different level of intensity and utilizes insulin and food differently. Therefore, consideration needs to be given to the intensity and the timing of exercise and their effect on the blood sugar level.

If at all possible, exercise should be done at a time that is most effective in controlling the blood sugar level. For example, exercising in the afternoon (between 3 and 5 P.M.), when the blood sugar level is high, may bring the blood sugar level down. Whenever you exercise, be alert to the possibility of hypoglycemic reactions (insulin reactions).

You may need to eat promptly before or after exercise or even during exercise if hypoglycemia occurs or is a recurrent problem with exercise. In some instances, exercise actually can decrease the insulin requirement, and it may become necessary to decrease the insulin dose on the day of exercise. Consult your physician regarding how to adjust the insulin dosage or meals in conjunction with the exercise program.

SELECTION OF APPROPRIATE EXERCISE

The type of exercise you choose to do depends on your interests and ability. If you are unable or not inclined to do vigorous exercise, try walking, swimming, or pedaling an exercise cycle for 20 to 30 minutes. Walking two to four miles a day is excellent exercise if you are not overweight. You can walk anywhere—on the golf course or to and from work. If inclement weather rules out an outdoor walk, walk indoors in an enclosed area such as a shopping mall.

Vigorous exercise uses more calories and leads to better conditioning and physical fitness. Running, contact sports, and tennis are examples of vigorous exercise. However, these exercises are not possible for everybody, and the advice of a physician is important. The goal is to use up at least 100 to 200 calories during each exercise period. The chart on page 313 outlines the approximate calorie expenditure for various activities. Remember, to be effective, the exercise must be done on a regular basis.

Ideally, your exercise program should increase your heart rate. This promotes calorie expenditure and improves circulation and muscle conditioning. Have your physician explain how to measure heart rate and what to look for in evaluating the effects of exercise. Start out gradually and work up to a minimum of 90 aerobic minutes (see below) a week in three to five weekly sessions. Each exercise session should last approximately 20 to 30 minutes. Always warm up before starting and include a cool-down period at the end of each session. Remember, do not overdo.

AEROBIC EXERCISE

The word *aerobic* means "with oxygen." It refers to any sustained exercise that increases the heart rate. A good aerobic activity is one in which the large muscle masses of the body are used. Jogging, cycling, swimming, aerobic dancing, and cross-country skiing are good examples of aerobic activities. These activities burn calories, tone muscles, and, if performed correctly, strengthen the heart and blood vessels. There are three essential criteria for aerobic conditioning:

1. Frequency: the activity must be done at least three times a week, preferably on alternate days.
2. Intensity: the heart rate must reach the target zone—70 to 80 percent of the maximum attainable heart rate.
3. Duration: the exercise must be maintained at the target heart rate for at least 20 minutes.

The target heart rate is determined by the maximum attainable heart rate, and this is related to age. The advice of a physician should be obtained in setting the target heart rate and learning how to measure the rate. Exercising at less than 70 percent of one's maximum heart rate will not provide a great enough workload for aerobic conditioning. Exercising at more than 85 percent will lead to fatigue and injury. Therefore, you must pace yourself by checking the heart rate periodically during aerobic exercise:

1. About two minutes after aerobic activities are begun.
2. Midway through the activity.
3. After the activity is completed.

If the heart rate is higher than the target rate, the pace of the activity should be slowed. If the rate is lower than the target rate and no symptoms of overexertion are present, the pace can be increased slightly.

SPECIAL PRECAUTIONS FOR INSULIN-DEPENDENT DIABETICS

Pick an exercise that you enjoy and then find out how it affects your blood sugar level by use of careful self-monitoring. Your physician's advice should be obtained about any adjustments in the timing of the insulin doses and food intake.

A good time to exercise is one or two hours before meals. Exercise should not be done immediately after a dose of insulin is taken or when an insulin dose is at its peak level of effectiveness. The blood sugar level should be checked prior to exercise and a snack should be eaten according to the recommendations on pages 314–15. Exercise should be avoided during an illness, when ketoacids are in the urine, or after a large meal. Avoid consuming alcohol immediately before or after an exercise session. Try to avoid temperature extremes, and always drink enough water to replace fluid lost by perspiring.

No matter what kind of exercise is planned, always eat before engaging in any *extra* exercise that is not part of your normal routine. Never skip an insulin dose unless directed by your physician, and try to use a site for insulin injections not affected by the exercise. Select shoes and clothing that will not increase the body temperature and use shoes that minimize strain and trauma to the joints and muscles.

Allow 10 to 15 minutes for a warm-up period and 10 to 15 minutes for a cool-down period. When exercising, try to breathe out (exhale) during the effort cycle. If pain is felt in the chest, teeth, jaw, or arm or if an irregular heart rate occurs, stop the activity immediately and report these symptoms to your doctor. If possible, avoid exercising alone, and carry extra glucose tablets or a form of simple sugar for use in case a hypoglycemic reaction occurs.

All-day activities, such as skiing or backpacking, will require careful planning regarding insulin doses and eating schedules. Be overprepared: Carry extra food and easy-to-carry carbohydrates such as glucose tablets or gel for use in case of a hypoglycemic reaction. The potential for hypoglycemia can last for several hours after the exercise has been completed.

GUIDELINES FOR NON-INSULIN-DEPENDENT DIABETICS

For non-insulin-dependent diabetics, regular physical activity combined with weight loss may be all that is necessary to control blood sugar levels. Those taking medications often find that their dosages can be cut down or even eliminated once an exercise program has become part of their regular routine. Select an enjoyable activity and work out a regular exercise schedule that fits easily into your life-style. Before a new exercise program more strenuous than walking is begun, discuss it with your physician.

Start out gradually and work up to the desired level of activity. Always warm up before an exercise session and cool down after it. Do not overdo! Have your physician explain how to measure heart rate and what the signs of an adverse effect of exercise are. Once again, if pain occurs in the chest, teeth, jaw, or arm, or an irregular heartbeat occurs, stop the activity immediately. Report these symptoms to your doctor.

Approximate Calories Expended in Various Activities

Activity	**Calories per hour**
Moderate:	
Bicycling (5½ mph)	210
Exercise cycle (5 mph)	210
Walking (2½ mph)	210
Canoeing (2½ mph)	230
Golf (with a power cart)	240
Bowling	270
Rowing (2½ mph)	300
Swimming (¼ mph)	300
Walking (3¾ mph)	300
Badminton	350
Horseback riding (trotting)	350
Square dancing	350
Volleyball	350
Ice-skating or roller-skating	350
Vigorous:	
Tennis, doubles	360
Tennis, singles	420
Aerobic dancing	420
Water-skiing	480
Hill-climbing (100 feet/hour)	490
Paddleball	600
Skiing, downhill	600
Jogging (5 mph)	600
Squash or handball, practice	600
Running (5½ mph)	650
Cycling (13 mph)	660
Scull rowing (race)	840
Running (10 mph)	900

Recommended Snacks Before Exercise

Type of exercise	Example	If blood sugar (mg/100 ml) is	Increase food intake by	Suggested foods
Moderate intensity of short duration	Walking 1 mile or leisure cycling for less than ½ hour	80 or above	Not necessary	
		Less than 80	10–15 grams of carbohydrate	1 fruit or bread exchange
Moderate intensity	Tennis, swimming, jogging, leisure cycling, gardening, golfing, vacuum-cleaning for 1 hour	80–180	10–15 grams of carbohydrate per hour of exercise	1 fruit or bread exchange
		Less than 80	25–30 grams of carbohydrate prior to exercise; 10–15 grams per hour of exercise	½ meat sandwich with 1 milk or fruit exchange
		180–300	Not necessary to increase food	
		300 or above	Do not exercise until blood sugar is under better control*	

Strenuous	Football, hockey, racquetball, or basketball, strenuous cycling or swimming, shoveling heavy snow for 1 hour	80–180	25–30 grams of carbohydrate, depending on intensity and duration	½ meat sandwich with 1 milk or fruit exchange
		Less than 80	50 grams of carbohydrate; monitor blood sugar carefully	1 meat sandwich (2 slices of bread) with 1 milk and 1 fruit exchange
		180–300	15 grams of carbohydrate per hour of exercise	1 fruit or bread exchange
		300 or above	Do not exercise until blood sugar is under better control*	

*When the blood sugar level is 300 mg per 100 ml or greater, exercise may cause the blood sugar level to increase further.

GLOSSARY

Acidosis—Too much acid in the body. For a person with diabetes, this usually is ketoacidosis. *See also* Ketoacidosis.

Amino acids—The building blocks of proteins, the main material of the body's cells. Insulin is a protein made of 51 amino acids joined together.

Antidiabetic agent—A substance that helps a person with diabetes to control the level of glucose (sugar) in the blood so that the body works as it should. *See also* Insulin; Oral hypoglycemic agents.

Arteriosclerosis—The walls of the arteries get thick and hard. In one type of arteriosclerosis, fat builds up inside the walls and slows the blood flow (*see* Atherosclerosis). This often occurs in people who have had diabetes for a long time.

Artery—A large blood vessel that carries blood from the heart to other parts of the body. Arteries are thicker and have walls that are stronger and more elastic than the walls of veins. *See also* Blood vessels.

Artificial endocrine pancreas—A man-made device that constantly measures glucose (sugar) in the blood and, in response, releases the exact amount of insulin that the body needs at that time. This is a large bedside machine that also goes by the name "artificial beta cell."

Aspartame—A man-made sweetener that can be used in place of sugar because it provides very few calories.

Atherosclerosis—Fat builds up in the walls of the large- and medium-sized arteries. This fat may slow down or stop the flow of blood. This disease can occur in people who have had diabetes for a long time.

Beta Cell—A type of cell in the pancreas in areas called the islets of Langerhans. Beta cells make and release insulin, a hormone that controls the level of glucose (sugar) in the blood.

Biguanides—A group of oral hypoglycemic agents that lower the glucose (sugar) level in the blood (see also oral hypoglycemic agent).

Blood glucose—The main sugar that the body makes from the three elements of food—proteins, fats, and carbohydrates—but mostly from carbohydrates. Glucose is the major source of energy for living cells and is carried to each cell through the bloodstream. However, the cells cannot use glucose without the help of insulin.

Blood glucose monitoring—A way of testing how much glucose (sugar)

*Adapted from *The Diabetes Dictionary,* The National Diabetes Information Clearinghouse, National Institute of Arthritis, Diabetes, and Digestive and Kidney Diseases, National Institutes of Health, Bethesda, Maryland, 1984.

is in the blood. A drop of blood from the tip of a finger or an earlobe is placed on the end of a special strip of paper. The paper strip has a chemical on it that makes it change color according to how much glucose is in the blood. Whether the level of glucose is low, high, or normal can be determined in one of two ways. The first is visually, by comparing the end of the paper strip to a color chart that is printed on the side of the test strip holder. Types of test strips for self blood glucose testing are Chemstrip, bG, Dextrostix, Visidex, and Glucostix. In the second way, instead of comparing the strips to a color chart, some people use a machine (reflectance meter). They insert the strips into the meter and read the correct level of glucose in the blood. The types of meters are: Accuchek, Dextrometer, Glucocheck, Glucometer, Glucoscan, and Stattek.

Blood pressure—The force of the blood on the walls of the arteries. Two levels of blood pressure are measured: the higher or *systolic* pressure which occurs each time the heart pushes blood into the vessels, and the lower or *diastolic* pressure which occurs when the heart rests. In a blood pressure reading of 120/80 mm Hg, for example, 120 mm Hg is the systolic pressure and 80 mm Hg is the diastolic pressure. A reading of 120/80 mm Hg is in the normal range. Blood pressure that is too high can cause health problems such as heart attacks and strokes.

Blood vessels—Tubes that act like a system of roads or canals to carry blood to and from all parts of the body. The three main types of blood vessels are arteries, veins, and capillaries. The heart pumps the blood through these vessels. The blood can carry oxygen and nutrients to the cells and take away waste that the cells do not need.

Brittle diabetes—A term used when a person's blood glucose (sugar) level often swings very quickly from high to low and from low to high. This also is called "labile diabetes" or "unstable diabetes."

Calorie—Energy that comes from food. Some foods provide more calories than others: fats provide many calories; most vegetables provide few. People with diabetes are advised to follow meal plans with suggested amounts of calories for each meal or snack. *See also* Meal plan; Exchange lists.

Carbohydrate—One of the three main classes of foods. Carbohydrates are mainly sugars and starches which the body breaks down into glucose (a simple sugar that the body can use to feed its cells). The body also uses carbohydrates to make a substance called glycogen that is stored in the liver and muscles for future use. If the body does not have enough insulin or cannot use the insulin it has, then the body will not be able to use carbohydrates for energy the way it should, and the condition is called diabetes. *See also* Fat; Protein.

Cholesterol—A fat-like substance found in blood, muscle, liver, brain, and other tissues in people and animals. The body makes and needs some cholesterol. Too much cholesterol, however, may cause fat to build up in the artery walls, producing a disease that slows or stops the flow of blood. Butter and egg yolks are foods that have a lot of cholesterol.

Coma—A sleep-like state (not conscious) that can be due to too high or too low a level of glucose (sugar) in the blood. *See also* Diabetic coma.

Coronary heart disease—Damage to the muscles of the heart from inadequate blood flow through the vessels that feed the heart muscle because these vessels are blocked with fat or have become thick and hard. People with diabetes are at a higher risk of coronary disease.

Diabetic coma—A severe emergency in which a person is not conscious because the blood glucose (sugar) is too high and the body has too many ketoacids. The person usually has a flushed face, dry skin and mouth, rapid and labored breathing, a fruity breath odor, a rapid, weak pulse, and low blood pressure. *See also* Ketoacidosis.

Diabetic retinopathy—A disease of the small blood vessels of the retina of the eye. When it starts, the tiny blood vessels in the retina become larger, and they leak a little fluid into the center of the retina. The person's sight is blurred from this—called "background retinopathy." About 80 percent of the people with this leaking never have serious vision problems, and the disease never goes beyond this first stage. However, at the next stage, the harm to sight can be more serious. Many new, tiny blood vessels grow out and across the eye. This is called "neovascularization." The vessels may break and bleed into the clear gel that fills the center of the eye, and this blocks vision. Scar tissue also may form near the retina, pulling it away from the back of the eye. This stage is called "proliferative retinopathy" and it can lead to loss of vision and even blindness.

Diabetologist—A doctor who treats people who have diabetes mellitus.

Dietitian—An expert in nutrition who helps people to plan the kinds and amounts of foods to eat for special health needs. A registered dietitian (R.D.) has special qualifications.

Edema—A swelling or puffiness of some part of the body such as the ankles. This swelling is caused by water or other body fluids collecting in the cells.

Endocrinologist—A doctor who treats people who have problems with endocrine glands—for example, the pancreas.

Epidemiology—The study of a disease that deals with how many people have it, where they are, how many new cases are found, and how to control it.

Exchange lists—A grouping of foods to help people on special diets stay on the diet. Each group lists foods in a serving size. The lists put foods in six groups: (1) starch/bread; (2) meat; (3) vegetables; (4) fruits; (5) milk; and (6) fats. Within a food group, each serving provides about the same amount of carbohydrate, protein, fat, and calories. A person can exchange a food serving in a group for any other food serving in that same group.

Fasting blood glucose test—A method for finding out how much glucose (sugar) is in the blood. The test can show if a person has diabetes. A blood sample is taken in a lab or a doctor's office (usually in the morning before breakfast because 8 hours have elapsed since the last meal). If the blood glucose level is 70 to 110 mg/dl (depending on the type of blood that is tested), it is in the normal range. If the level is over 140 mg/dl, it usually means that the person has diabetes (except for newborns and some pregnant women).

Fat—One of the three main classes of foods and a source of energy in the body. Fats help the body to use some vitamins and keep the skin healthy. It is also the major form in which the body stores energy. In food, there are three types of fats: saturated, unsaturated, and polyunsaturated.

Saturated fats are solid at room temperature and come chiefly from animal food products. Some examples are butter, lard, and meat fat. They tend to raise the level of cholesterol, a fat-like substance in the blood.

Unsaturated (or monounsaturated) fats are neutral in that they neither raise nor lower blood cholesterol. Olive oil and peanut oil are examples of unsaturated fats.

Polyunsaturated fats are liquid at room temperature and come from vegetable oils such as corn, cottonseed, sunflower, safflower, and soybean. These fats tend to lower the level of cholesterol in the blood. *See also* Carbohydrate; Protein.

Fatty acids—A basic unit of fats. When insulin levels are too low or there is not enough glucose (sugar) to use for energy, the body burns fatty acids for energy. The waste products of this process are ketoacids which cause the acid level in the blood to become too high (ketoacidosis), a serious problem. *See also* Ketoacidosis.

Fructose—A type of sugar found in many fruits and vegetables and in honey. Fructose is used to sweeten some diet foods.

Gangrene—The death of body tissues. It is most often caused by a loss of blood flow, especially in the legs and feet.

Glucose—A simple sugar found in the blood. It is the body's main source of energy; also known as dextrose. *See also* Blood glucose.

Glycosuria—Having glucose (sugar) in the urine.

Glycosylated hemoglobin test—A blood test that measures a person's average blood glucose (sugar) level for the two to three months before the test.

Gram—A unit of weight in the metric system. There are 28 grams in 1 ounce. In some diet plans for people with diabetes, the suggested amounts of food are given in grams.

Human insulin (artificial)—A man-made insulin that is very much like the insulin made by the body. The artificial human insulin is made in a lab by using special strains of a bacterium called *E. coli*. The

Food and Drug Administration has approved the sale of human insulin.

Hyperglycemia—Too high a level of glucose (sugar) in the blood; a sign that diabetes is out of control. Many things can cause hyperglycemia. It occurs when the body does not have enough insulin or cannot use the insulin it does have. Signs of hyperglycemia are: a great thirst and hunger, a dry mouth, and a need to urinate often. For people with insulin-dependent diabetes, this may lead to diabetic ketoacidosis.

Hyperinsulinism—Too high a level of insulin in the blood. This occurs when the body makes too much insulin on its own or when a person takes too much insulin. Too much insulin in the body may cause the blood glucose (sugar) level to go too low. People with this problem feel shaky, nervous, weak, confused, sweaty, and have a headache and hunger. *See also* Hypoglycemia.

Hyperlipidemia—Too high a level of fats (lipids) in the blood. This occurs when diabetes is out of control.

Hypertension—Blood pressure that is above the normal range.

Hypoglycemia—Too low a level of glucose (sugar) in the blood. This occurs when a person with diabetes has injected too much insulin, eaten too little food, or exercised without extra food. A person with hypoglycemia may feel nervous, shaky, weak, or sweaty and have a headache, blurred vision, and hunger. Taking small amounts of sugar, juice, or food with sugar will usually help the person feel better within 10 to 15 minutes.

Insulin—A hormone that helps the body use glucose (sugar) for energy. The beta cells of the pancreas (in areas called the islets of Langerhans) make the insulin. When the body cannot make enough insulin on its own, a person with diabetes must inject insulin.

Insulin allergy—When a person's body has an allergic or bad reaction to taking insulin made from pork or beef or from bacteria because it is not exactly the same as human insulin or because it has impurities.

The allergy can take one of two forms. Sometimes an area of the skin becomes very red and itchy right around the place where the insulin is injected. This is called "local allergy."

In another form, a person's whole body can have a bad reaction. This is called "systemic allergy." The person can have hives or red patches all over the body or may feel changes in the heart rate and in the rate of breathing. A doctor may treat this allergy by prescribing purified insulins or by desensitization.

Insulin pump—A man-made device that pumps insulin into the body all the time at a low (basal) rate. A plastic tube with a small needle inserted under the skin is attached to the body. The pump keeps the level of insulin steady between meals. At mealtimes, the person uses either a switch or a dial on the pump to inject a larger dose (bolus) of insulin just before eating. The pump runs on batteries. It is used by people with insulin-dependent diabetes.

Insulin reaction—Too low a level of glucose (sugar) in the blood (hypoglycemia). This occurs when a person with diabetes has injected too much insulin, eaten too little food, or exercised without extra food. The person may feel hungry, nauseated, weak, nervous, shaky, confused, and sweaty. Taking small amounts of sugar, juice, or food with sugar will usually help the person feel better within 10 to 15 minutes.

Islet cell transplantation—Moving the beta cells from the pancreas of one living being to another. The beta cells make the insulin that the body needs to use glucose (sugar) for energy. Someday, transplanting beta cells may help people with diabetes, but it is still in the research stage at present.

Islets of Langerhans—Special groups of cells in the pancreas. They make and secrete hormones that help the body to break down and use food. Named after Paul Langerhans, the German who discovered them in 1869, these cells are in clusters in the pancreas. There are five types of cells in an islet: beta cells, which make insulin; alpha cells, which make glucagon; delta cells, which make somatostatin; and PP cells and D_1 cells, about which little is known.

Ketoacidosis (DKA)—Diabetic ketoacidosis (DKA) happens when the blood does not have enough insulin (because the person is ill, did not take a large enough dose of insulin, or got too little exercise). When the insulin level is too low, the body starts using stored fat for energy, and then ketoacids (ketone bodies) build up in the blood. The ketoacidosis starts slowly and becomes more and more severe. Emergency treatment may be needed. The signs include nausea and vomiting (which can lead to serious loss of water from the body), stomach pain, and deep and rapid breathing. If the person is not given fluids and insulin right away, the ketoacidosis can lead to coma and even death.

Ketone bodies—Chemicals that the body makes when there is not enough insulin in the blood and it must break down fat for its energy. Ketone bodies can poison and even kill body cells. When the body does not have the help of insulin, the ketones build up in the blood and then "spill" over into the urine so that the body can get rid of them. The body can also rid itself of one type of ketone called acetone through the lungs. This gives the breath a fruity odor. Buildup of ketones in the body for a long time leads to serious illness and coma. *See also* Ketoacidosis.

Ketonuria—Having ketone bodies in the urine; a warning sign of diabetic ketoacidosis.

Ketosis—A condition of having ketone bodies build up in body tissues and fluids. The signs of ketosis are nausea, vomiting, and stomach pain. Ketosis can lead to ketoacidosis.

Lipid—A term for fat. The body stores fat as energy for future use, just like a reserve fuel tank in a car. When the body needs energy, it can break down the lipids into fatty acids and burn them like glucose (sugar).

Macrovascular disease—A disease of the large blood vessels that occurs when someone has had diabetes for a long time. Fat and blood clots build up in the large blood vessels and stick to the vessel walls.

Meal plan—A guide for controlling the amount of calories, carbohydrates, proteins, and fats a person eats. People with diabetes can use plans like the exchange lists or the point system to help them plan their meals so that they can keep their diabetes under control.

Metabolism—The term for how the cells chemically change food so that it can be used to keep the body alive. It is a two-part process. One part, called *catabolism,* is when the body uses food for energy. The other, called *anabolism,* is when the body uses food to build or mend cells.

Microvascular disease—A disease of the smallest blood vessels that sometimes occurs when someone has had diabetes for a long time. The walls of the vessels become so thick and weak that they bleed, leak protein, and slow the flow of blood. Then some cells—for example, the ones in the eye—may not get enough blood and they may be damaged, leading to impairment of vision.

Nonketotic coma—A type of coma caused by having too little insulin in the system. A nonketotic crisis means: (1) very high levels of glucose (sugar) in the blood; (2) absence of ketoacidosis; (3) great loss of body fluid; and (4) a sleepy, confused, or comatose state. Nonketotic coma often results from some other problem, such as a severe infection or kidney failure.

Nutrition—The process by which the body draws nutrients from food and uses them to make or mend its cells.

Nutritionist—A person who is trained to count the calories and nutrients needed for normal growth and daily activity and to help plan meals and long-term eating habits.

Obesity—When a person has 20 percent or more extra body fat than he or she should for age, height, sex, and bone structure. Fat works against the action of insulin. Extra body fat is thought to be a risk factor for diabetes.

Oral hypoglycemic agents—Pills or capsules that people take to lower the level of glucose (sugar) in the blood. They work for some people whose pancreas still makes some insulin. The pills can help the body in several ways, such as causing the cells in the pancreas to release more insulin.

Six types of these pills are for sale in the United States. They are called "sulfonylureas." Each type of pill is sold under two names; one is the generic name as listed by the Food and Drug Administration (FDA); the other is the trade name given by the producer. These are:

Generic name	*Trade name*
Tolbutamide	Orinase (Upjohn Co.)
Acetohexamide	Dymelor (Eli Lilly Co.)
Tolazamide	Tolinase (Upjohn Co.)
Chlorpropamide	Diabinese (Pfizer, Inc.)
Glyburide	Diabeta (Hoechst-Roussel) Micronase (Upjohn Co.)
Glipizide	Glucotrol (Roerig)

Pancreas—An organ that is about the size of a hand and is located behind the lower part of the stomach. It makes insulin. It also makes enzymes that help the body digest food. Spread all through the pancreas are areas called the islets of Langerhans. The cells in these areas each have a special purpose. The alpha cells make glucagon, which raises the level of glucose in the blood; the beta cells make insulin; the delta cells make somatostatin. There are also the PP cells and the D_1 cells, about which little is known.

Pancreatic transplantation—An experimental procedure which involves replacing the pancreas of a person who has diabetes with a healthy pancreas that can make insulin. The healthy pancreas comes from a donor who has just died or from a living relative who can donate half a pancreas and still have enough to take care of his or her own needs.

Peripheral vascular disease (PVD)—Disease in the blood vessels of the arms, legs, and feet. People who have had diabetes for a long time may get this because their arms, legs, and feet do not receive enough blood. The signs of PVD are aching in the arms, legs, and feet (especially when walking) and foot sores that heal slowly. Although people with diabetes cannot always avoid PVD, doctors say they have a better chance of avoiding it if they take good care of their feet, do not smoke, and keep their blood pressure and diabetes under good control.

Polydipsia—A great thirst that lasts for long periods of time; a sign of diabetes.

Polyphagia—Very great hunger; a sign of diabetes. People with this great hunger often lose weight.

Polyuria—Having to urinate often; a common sign of diabetes.

Postprandial blood glucose—The amount of glucose (sugar) in the blood one to two hours after eating.

Protein—One of the three main classes of food. Proteins are made of amino acids which are called the building blocks of the cells. The cells need proteins to grow and to mend themselves. Protein is found in many foods, such as meat, fish, poultry, and eggs. *See also* Carbohydrate; Fat.

Proteinuria—Too much protein in the urine. This may be a sign of kidney damage.

Risk factor—Anything that raises the chance that a person will get a disease. For example, people have a greater risk of having non-insulin-dependent diabetes if their weight is above normal by 20 percent or more.

Saccharin—A man-made sweetener that is used in place of sugar because it has no calories.

Sorbitol—A sugar alcohol the body uses slowly. It is a sweetener used in diet foods. It is called a nutritive sweetener because it provides 4 calories per gram, just like table sugar and starch.

Sugar—A class of carbohydrates that tastes sweet. Sugar is a quick and easy fuel for the body to use. Types of sugar are lactose, glucose, fructose, and sucrose.

Sulfonylureas—Drugs that lower the level of glucose (sugar) in the blood. *See also* Oral hypoglycemic agents.

Symptom—A sign of disease. Having to urinate often is a symptom of diabetes.

Triglyceride—A type of blood fat. The body needs insulin to remove this type of fat from the blood. When diabetes is under control and a person's weight is what it should be, the level of triglycerides in the blood is usually about what it should be.

Urine testing—Checking the urine to see if it contains glucose (sugar) or ketones. Special strips of paper or tablets (called reagents) are put into a small amount of urine or urine plus water. Changes in the color of the strip show the amount of glucose or ketones in the urine.

FOR ADDITIONAL HELP AND INFORMATION

National Diabetes Information Clearing House
Box NDIC
Bethesda, MD 20205
301-496-7433
301-468-2162

Send for a list of excellent publications on all aspects of diabetes; available without charge to diabetics, their families, and those working with diabetics.

Diabetes Care and Education Practice Group
c/o American Dietetic Association
430 North Michigan Avenue
Chicago, IL 60611

A group of dietitians and nutritionists with a special interest in diabetes care. Send for the names of those in your area who are available for individual counseling if you need help with your diet.

Juvenile Diabetes Foundation International
60 Madison Avenue
New York, NY 10010
212-889-7575
and
4632 Yonge Street
Willowdale, Ontario
Canada M2N 5M1

An organization founded in 1970 to further research and education on diabetes, particularly in the young. There are over 160 local chapters worldwide providing education and counseling services to diabetics, their families, hospitals, schools, and community organizations. Membership fee is $10 a year and includes a subscription to *Countdown*, a quarterly publication.

American Diabetes Association
National Service Center
1660 Duke St.
Alexandria, VA 22314
800-232-3472

With affiliates in every state, this organization is an important on-going source of information and help to the diabetic. Membership fee includes membership in your local affiliate and a subscription to *Diabetes Forecast,* a magazine for diabetics. The Association publishes numerous educational materials.

International Diabetes Federation
c/o James G. L. Jackson, Secretary General
10 Queen Anne Street
London W1M OBD
England

This organization can provide a list of the names and addresses of member associations around the world.

Canadian Diabetes Association
Suite 601
123 Edward Street
Toronto, Ontario
M5G 1E2
Tel. 416-593-4311

AFFILIATES OF THE AMERICAN DIABETES ASSOCIATION

American Diabetes Association
ALABAMA AFFILIATE, INC.
904 Bob Wallace Avenue, S.W.
Suite 222
Huntsville, AL 35801
(205) 533-5775, (205) 533-5776

American Diabetes Association
ALASKA AFFILIATE, INC.
201 East 3rd Avenue
Suite 301
Anchorage, AK 99501
(907) 276-3607

American Diabetes Association
ARIZONA AFFILIATE, INC.
7337 North 19th Avenue
Room 404
Phoenix, AZ 85021
(602) 995-1515

American Diabetes Association
ARKANSAS AFFILIATE, INC.
Suite 229
Tanglewood Shopping Center
7509 Cantrell Road
Suite 227
Little Rock, AR 72207
(501) 666-6345

American Diabetes Association
NORTHERN CALIFORNIA AFFILIATE, INC.
2550 9th Street
Suite 114
Berkeley, CA 94710
(415) 644-0920

American Diabetes Association
SOUTHERN CALIFORNIA AFFILIATE, INC.
3460 Wilshire Blvd.
Suite #900
Los Angeles, CA 90010
(213) 381-3639

American Diabetes Association
COLORADO AFFILIATE, INC.
2450 South Downing Street
Denver, CO 80210
(303) 778-7556

American Diabetes Association
CONNECTICUT AFFILIATE, INC.
P.O. Box 10160 (mailing address)
40 South Street
West Hartford, CT 06110
(203) 249-4232 or 1 (800) 842-6323

American Diabetes Association
DELAWARE AFFILIATE, INC.
2713 Lancaster Avenue
Wilmington, DE 19805
(302) 656-0030

American Diabetes Association
WASHINGTON, D.C. AREA AFFILIATE, INC.
1819 H Street, N.W.
Suite 1200
Washington, D.C. 20006
(202) 331-8303

American Diabetes Association
FLORIDA AFFILIATE, INC.
P.O. Box 19745 (mailing address)
Orlando, FL 32814
3101 Maguire Blvd., Suite 288
Orlando, FL 32803
(305) 894-6664

American Diabetes Association
GEORGIA AFFILIATE, INC.
3783 Presidential Parkway
Suite 102
Atlanta, GA 30340
(404) 454-8401

American Diabetes Association
HAWAII AFFILIATE, INC.
510 South Beretania Street
Honolulu, HI 96813
(808) 521-5677

American Diabetes Association
IDAHO AFFILIATE, INC.
1528 Vista
Boise, ID 83705
(208) 342-2774

American Diabetes Association
DOWNSTATE ILLINOIS
AFFILIATE, INC.
965 North Water Street
Decatur, IL 62523
(217) 422-8228

American Diabetes Association
NORTHERN ILLINOIS
AFFILIATE, INC.
6 North Michigan Avenue
Suite 1202
Chicago, IL 60602
(312) 346-1805

American Diabetes Association
INDIANA AFFILIATE, INC.
222 S. Downey Avenue, Suite 320
Indianapolis, IN 46219
(317) 352-9226

American Diabetes Association
IOWA AFFILIATE, INC.
888 Tenth Street
Marion, IA 52302
(319) 373-0530

American Diabetes Association
KANSAS AFFILIATE, INC.
3210 East Douglas
Wichita, KS 67208
(316) 684-6091

American Diabetes Association
KENTUCKY AFFILIATE, INC.
McClure Building #513
P.O. Box 345 (mailing address)
306 West Main #513
Frankfort, KY 40602
(502) 223-2971

American Diabetes Association
LOUISIANA AFFILIATE, INC.
9420 Lindale Avenue, Suite B
Baton Rouge, LA 70815
(504) 927-7732

American Diabetes Association
MAINE AFFILIATE, INC.
59 Northport Avenue
Belfast, ME 04915
(207) 338-5132

American Diabetes Association
MARYLAND AFFILIATE, INC.
3701 Old Court Road, Suite 19
Baltimore, MD 21208
(301) 486-5516

American Diabetes Association
MASSACHUSETTS AFFILIATE,
INC.
190 North Main Street
Natick, MA 01760
(617) 655-6900

American Diabetes Association
MICHIGAN AFFILIATE, INC.
The Clausen Bldg. No. Unit
23100 Providence Dr., Suite 475
Southfield, MI 48075
(313) 552-0480

American Diabetes Association
MINNESOTA AFFILIATE, INC.
3005 Ottawa Ave., South
Minneapolis, MN 55416
(612) 920-6796

American Diabetes Association
MISSISSIPPI AFFILIATE, INC.
10 Lakeland Circle
Jackson, MS 39216
(601) 981-9511

American Diabetes Association
MISSOURI AFFILIATE, INC.
P.O. Box 11 (mailing address)
811 Cherry, Suite 304
Columbia, MO 65201
(314) 443-8611

American Diabetes Association
MONTANA AFFILIATE, INC.
Box 2411 (mailing address)
Great Falls, MT 59403
600 Central Plaza, Suite 304
Great Falls, MT 59401
(406) 761-0908

American Diabetes Association
NEBRASKA AFFILIATE, INC.
2730 South 114th Street
Omaha, NE 68144
(402) 333-5556

American Diabetes Association
NEVADA AFFILIATE, INC.
4000 E. Charleston Blvd.
Las Vegas, NV 89104
(702) 459-7099

American Diabetes Association
NEW HAMPSHIRE AFFILIATE, INC.
P.O. Box 595 (mailing address)
Manchester, NH 03105
104 Middle Street
Manchester, NH 03101
(603) 627-9579

American Diabetes Association
NEW JERSEY AFFILIATE, INC.
312 North Adamsville Road
P.O. Box 6423
Bridgewater, NJ 08807
(201) 725-7878

American Diabetes Association
NEW MEXICO AFFILIATE, INC.
525 San Pedro, N.E., Suite 101
Albuquerque, NM 87108
(505) 266-5716

American Diabetes Association
NEW YORK DIABETES AFFILIATE, INC.
505 8th Avenue
New York, NY 10018
(212) 947-9707

American Diabetes Association
NEW YORK STATE AFFILIATE, INC.
P.O. Box 1037 (mailing address)
Syracuse, NY 13201
113 East Willow Street
Syracuse, NY 13202
(315) 472-9111

American Diabetes Association
NORTH CAROLINA AFFILIATE, INC.
2315-A Sunset Avenue
Rocky Mount, NC 27801
(919) 937-4121

American Diabetes Association
NORTH DAKOTA AFFILIATE, INC.
101 North 3rd Street
(Mailing Address)
Suite 502
P.O. Box 234
Grand Forks, ND 58201
(701) 746-4427

American Diabetes Association
OHIO AFFILIATE, INC.
1855 Fountain Square Court
Suite 310
Columbus, OH 43224-1360
(614) 263-2330

American Diabetes Association
OKLAHOMA AFFILIATE, INC.
Warren Professional Building
6465 South Yale Avenue
Suite 423
Tulsa, OK 74136
(918) 492-3839 or 1 (800) 722-5448

American Diabetes Association
OREGON AFFILIATE, INC.
3607 S.W. Corbett Street
Portland, OR 97201
(503) 228-0849

American Diabetes Association
GREATER PHILADELPHIA AFFILIATE, INC.
Bourse Bldg. Suite 570
21 South Fifth Street
Philadelphia, PA 19106
(215) 627-7718

American Diabetes Association
WESTERN PENNSYLVANIA AFFILIATE, INC.
4617 Winthrop Street
Pittsburgh, PA 15213
(412) 682-3392

American Diabetes Association
MID-PENNSYLVANIA AFFILIATE, INC.
2045 Westgate Drive
Suite B-1
Bethlehem, PA 18017
(215) 867-6660

American Diabetes Association
RHODE ISLAND AFFILIATE, INC.
4 Fallon Avenue
Providence, RI 02908
(401) 331-0099

American Diabetes Association
SOUTH CAROLINA AFFILIATE, INC.
P.O. Box 50782 (mailing address)
Columbia, SC 29250
2838 Devine Street
Columbia, SC 29205
(803) 799-4246

American Diabetes Association
SOUTH DAKOTA AFFILIATE, INC.
P.O. Box 659 (mailing address)
Sioux Falls, SD 57101
1524 West 20th Street
Sioux Falls, SD 57105
(605) 335-7670

American Diabetes Association
TENNESSEE AFFILIATE, INC.
1701 21st Avenue, South
Room 403
Nashville, TN 37212

American Diabetes Association
TEXAS AFFILIATE, INC.
8140 North Mopac
Building 1, Suite 130
Austin, TX 78759
(512) 343-6981

American Diabetes Association
UTAH AFFILIATE, INC.
564 East 300 South
Salt Lake City, UT 84102
(801) 363-3024

American Diabetes Association
VERMONT AFFILIATE, INC.
217 Church Street
Burlington, VT 05401
(802) 862-3882

American Diabetes Association
VIRGINIA AFFILIATE, INC.
404 8th Street, N.E.
Suite C
Charlottesville, VA 22901
(804) 293-4953

American Diabetes Association
WASHINGTON AFFILIATE, INC.
3201 Fremont Avenue North
Seattle, WA 98103
(206) 632-4576

American Diabetes Association
WEST VIRGINIA AFFILIATE, INC.
Professional Building
1036 Quarrier Street, Room 404
Charleston, WV 25301
(304) 346-6418, (800) 642-3055

American Diabetes Association
WISCONSIN AFFILIATE, INC.
10721 West Capitol Drive
Milwaukee, WI 53222
(414) 464-9395

American Diabetes Association
WYOMING AFFILIATE, INC.
2908 Kelly Drive
Cheyenne, WY 82001
(307) 638-3578

GENERAL INDEX

RECIPE INDEX